D0918692

CAREERS in CLINICAL RESEARCH

Obstacles and Opportunities

Committee on Addressing Career Paths
for Clinical Research

Division of Health Sciences Policy
INSTITUTE OF MEDICINE

William N. Kelley and Mark A. Randolph, Editors

NATIONAL ACADEMY PRESS
Washington, D.C. 1994

610.72
C271

National Academy Press   •   **2101 Constitution Avenue, NW**   •   **Washington, DC 20418**

NOTICE: The project that is the subject of this report was approved by the Governing Board of the National Research Council, whose members are drawn from the councils of the National Academy of Sciences, the National Academy of Engineering, and the Institute of Medicine. The members of the committee responsible for the report were chosen for their special competencies and with regard for appropriate balance.

This report has been reviewed by a group other than the authors according to procedures approved by a Report Review Committee consisting of members of the National Academy of Sciences, the National Academy of Engineering, and the Institute of Medicine.

The Institute of Medicine was chartered in 1970 by the National Academy of Sciences to enlist distinguished members of the appropriate professions in the examination of policy matters pertaining to the health of the public. In this, the Institute acts under both the Academy's 1863 congressional charter responsibility to be an adviser to the federal government and its own initiative in identifying issues of medical care, research, and education. Dr. Kenneth I. Shine is president of the Institute of Medicine.

This study was supported by the National Institutes of Health, the former Alcohol, Drug Abuse and Mental Health Administration, the Agency for Health Care Policy and Research, the Department of Veterans Affairs, the American Cancer Society, the American Heart Association, Pfizer, Inc., and the Drug Information Association. Additional support for this project was provided by independent Institute of Medicine funds and the National Research Council Fund, a pool of private, discretionary, nonfederal funds that is used to support a program of Academy-initiated studies of national issues in which science and technology figure significantly.

Library of Congress Cataloging-in-Publication Data
Careers in clinical research : obstacles and opportunities / Committee on Addressing Career Paths
    for Clinical Research, Division of Health Sciences Policy, Institute of Medicine : William N.
    Kelley and Mark A. Randolph, editors
        p.   cm.
    Includes bibliographical references and index.
    ISBN 0-309-04890-7
    1. Medicine—Research—Government policy—United States. 2. Medicine—Research—
    Study and teaching—Goverment policy—United States. I. Kelley, William N., 1939–
    II. Randolph, Mark A. III. Institute of Medicine (U.S.). Committee on Addressing Career Paths
    for Clinical Research.
    [DNLM: 1. Career Choice. 2. Research. W 21 C271 1994]
    R854.U5C34 1994
    610′.72073—dc20
    DNLM/DLC
    for Library of Congress   94-13014
                                                    CIP

Additional copies of this book are available from the National Academy Press, 2101 Constitution Avenue, N.W., Box 285, Washington, D.C., 20055. Call 800-624-6242 or 202-334-3313 (in the Washington metropolitan area).

Copyright 1994 by the National Academy of Sciences. All rights reserved.

Printed in the United States of America.

The serpent has been a symbol of long life, healing, and knowledge among almost all cultures and religions since the beginning of recorded history. The image adopted as a logotype by the Institute of Medicine is based on a relief carving from ancient Greece, now held by the Staatlichemuseen in Berlin.

COMMITTEE ON ADDRESSING CAREER PATHS
FOR CLINICAL RESEARCH

WILLIAM N. KELLEY, *Chair*, Dean, School of Medicine, and Chief Executive Officer, Pennsylvania Medical Center, University of Pennsylvania, Philadelphia, Pennsylvania

KAREN H. ANTMAN, Professor of Medicine and Chief, Division of Medical Oncology, College of Physicians and Surgeons of Columbia University, Columbia Presbyterian Medical Center, New York, New York

DOROTHY BROOTEN, Professor and Chair, Health Care of Women and Childbearing, Director, Low Birthweight Research Center, School of Nursing, University of Pennsylvania, Philadelphia, Pennsylvania

MARY E. CHARLSON, Associate Professor of Medicine, Cornell University School of Medicine, New York Hospital, New York, New York

ROBERT C. COLLINS, Professor and Chairman, Department of Neurology, School of Medicine, University of California at Los Angeles, Los Angeles, California

HAILE T. DEBAS, Professor and Chairman, Department of Surgery, University of California at San Francisco, School of Medicine, San Francisco, California

WILLIAM LEO DEWEY, Professor of Pharmacology, Associate Provost for Research and Graduate Affairs, Dean of the Graduate School, Virginia Commonwealth University, Richmond, Virginia

JANICE G. DOUGLAS, Professor of Medicine, School of Medicine, Case Western Reserve University, Cleveland, Ohio

IRVING H. FOX, Vice President for Medical Affairs, Biogen, Inc., Cambridge, Massachusetts

ROBERT J. GENCO, Associate Dean for Graduate Studies, Distinguished Professor and Chairman, Department of Oral Biology, School of Dental Medicine, State University of New York at Buffalo, Buffalo, New York

DAVID J. KUPFER, Professor and Chairman of Psychiatry, School of Medicine, University of Pittsburgh, Director of Research, Western Psychiatric Institute and Clinic, Pittsburgh, Pennsylvania

NICHOLAS F. LARUSSO, Professor and Chairman, Division of Gastroenterology, Director, Center for Basic Research in Digestive Diseases, Mayo Clinic and Research Foundation, Rochester, Minnesota

ALBERT G. MULLEY, JR., Harvard Medical School, General Internal Medicine Unit, Massachusetts General Hospital, Boston, Massachusetts

University Libraries
Carnegie Mellon University
Pittsburgh PA 15213-3890

JOHN D. STOBO, William Osler Professor of Medicine, Director and
Physician-in-Chief, Department of Medicine, The Johns Hopkins
University School of Medicine, Baltimore, Maryland

MYRON L.WEISFELDT, Samuel Bard Professor of Medicine, Chair,
Department of Medicine, College of Physicians and Surgeons of
Columbia University, Columbia Presbyterian Medical Center, New
York, New York

CATHERINE M. WILFERT, Professor of Pediatrics and Microbiology, Duke
University Medical Center, Durham, North Carolina

Study Staff

Mark A. Randolph, Study Director
Joseph Cassells, Special Assistant
Ruth Ellen Bulger, Director, Division of Health Sciences Policy
(until August 1993)
Valerie P. Setlow, Director, Division of Health Sciences Policy
(from August 1993)
Sarah Zielinski Quinn, Project Assistant
Mary Jane Ball, Project Assistant
Philomina Mammen, Division Assistant

Preface

Concerns about the numbers of individuals pursuing careers in clinical investigation led the Board of Health Sciences Policy of the Institute of Medicine (IOM) to propose a study to review issues surrounding the career pathways of clinical investigators. For this review the President of the National Academy of Sciences and the Chair of the National Research Council appointed a 16-member committee, the Committee on Addressing Career Paths for Clinical Research, in 1991. The committee was composed of academic and industrial clinical investigators and administrators with expertise in nursing, dentistry, evaluative clinical sciences, surgery, epidemiology, and various medical subspecialties.

The committee was charged with identifying and evaluating issues in the education and training pathways for individuals pursuing careers in clinical investigation. In particular, the committee was asked to investigate ways to improve the quality of training for clinical investigators and to delineate pathways for individuals pursuing careers in clinical investigation in nursing, dentistry, medicine, and other related health professions engaging in human research. The committee was charged with addressing the following:

- define clinical research,
- how to stimulate individuals to pursue careers in clinical investigation,
- how to define appropriate curricula for training,
- how to identify mechanisms to bridge the gap between the basic and clinical sciences,

- how to address funding mechanisms for clinical investigation,
- how to establish measures of success in clinical research in addition to obtaining R01 grant support,
- how to encourage academic and industrial institutions to protect and reward these valuable investigators, and
- how to ensure adequate support mechanisms for retaining clinical researchers.

The study focused on how existing structures and mechanisms in government, academia, and industry might be used in new and innovative ways to foster careers for these groups of researchers. To the extent possible the committee searched for data to inform the committee in making its recommendations. Eleven background papers were commissioned; task forces were established to examine clinical research in nursing and clinical psychology, dentistry and surgery; a workshop was held to analyze training and research funding data and to reveal innovative approaches to training and support of clinical investigators; and a special effort was mounted to screen individual grant awards at NIH in an effort to quantitate the amount of patient-oriented clinical research supported.

Unfortunately, the data the committee was able to find on patient-oriented clinical investigation were not extensive, and those data that were available were not very reliable. Although the committee was unable to find incontrovertible evidence to support some of the committee's claims, the committee is convinced they are valid. Thus, many of the recommendations found in this report represent only the best judgments of this committee. Furthermore, when the committee began its deliberations more than two years ago, serious discussions about health care reform were only beginning to surface. After the inauguration of President Clinton and the initiation of his administration's analysis of the problem and presentation of a plan to reform health care, the committee found itself grappling with the issues regarding the impact that any new (yet, undefined) program might have on the clinical research and training environment. Because of the many intersections of patient care with clinical research, the committee feels that discussions about health care reform must not neglect the crucial role that clinical investigation has played in improving patient care in the past and the opportunities that clinical investigation has to continue to improve human health.

For example, from the health care reform discussions have come the proposal that 55 percent of all trainees in postgraduate medicine be committed to careers in primary care, whereas 45 percent be committed to careers in medical subspecialties. This proposal does not take into account the subset of individuals who are training for careers in academic medicine, where they will contribute to the development and transfer of new technology rather than to the continued expansion of individuals fully committed to the practice of a subspecialty. One possible solution would be to develop a separate track, the "academic track," as contrasted to the "clinical track." This academic track would be separate from the 55/45 percent split and would not have limits on it with regard to the distribution between primary care and medical specialty disciplines. It would, however, be a small portion (e.g. perhaps 10 percent) of all training positions. If the committee's recommendations are implemented, the committee believes that many barriers will be lowered or removed to recruit, retain, and support clinical investigators who the committee feels are necessary for realizing the promise of science for improved patient care.

William N. Kelley, M.D.
Chair
Committee on Addressing Career
Paths for Clinical Research

Contents

EXECUTIVE SUMMARY   1

1   INTRODUCTION   23
    Scope of Clinical Research, 24
    Origins of the Study, 29
    Charge to the Committee, 31
    Defining Clinical Research, 32
    Limits on the Scope of the Study, 36
    Conduct of the Study, 36
    Structure of the Report, 40

2   NURTURING CLINICAL RESEARCHERS   41
    Environment for Clinical Research, 43
    Clinical Research Workforce, 44
    Research Involvement of Faculty, 50
    Academic Recognition, 50
    Faculty Tracks, 55
    Competing Time Demands, 57
    Clinical Research Training, 57
    Mentoring, 58
    Lifestyle Issues, 60
    Conclusions, 60

3   CLINICAL RESEARCH FUNDING AND INFRASTRUCTURE   63
    The Big Picture, 64
    Federal Support for Health Sciences R&D, 67
    Nonprofit Organizations, 106
    Industry, 109
    Clinical Research and Third-Party Payers, 112
    Models of Cooperation, 119
    Conclusions, 121

4   TRAINING PATHWAYS   123
     Demographics, 127
     Kindergarten to College, 127
     Research Experiences for Undergraduate Students, 133
     Health Professional Schools, 142
     Undergraduate Medical Education, 145
     Graduate Medical Education, 161
     Barriers to Clinical Research Training, 168
     Avenues for Postdoctoral Research Training, 171
     Assessing the Outcomes of Training Programs, 178
     Model Programs for Research Training, 190
     Conclusions, 194

5   ACADEMIC-INDUSTRY RELATIONSHIPS   197
     Objectives of Academic-Industry Relationships, 200
     Two Cultures, 201
     Types of Academic-Industry Linkages, 202
     Programs to Help Commercialize Faculty Research, 205
     Prevalence of Academic-Industry Relationships, 206
     Benefits for Industry, 207
     Benefits for Academic Institutions, Faculty, and Students, 209
     Risks, Concerns and Conflicts, 210
     Managing Academic-Industry Relationships, 215
     Summary and Conclusions, 216

REFERENCES   219

APPENDIXES

A   Report of the Task Force on Clinical Research in Dentistry   237
B   Report of the Task Force on Clinical Research in Nursing and
     Clinical Psychology   251
C   Report of the Task Force on Clinical Research in Surgery   279
D   Agenda for the Workshop on Clinical Research and Training:
     Spotlight on Funding   301
E   Contributors   305
F   Biographies of Committee Members   309

GLOSSARY   319

INDEX   323

CAREERS in
CLINICAL
RESEARCH

Obstacles and Opportunities

Executive Summary

Health care in the United States has improved markedly over the past five decades, in large measure because of the advances made in health research by investigators who were supported by a myriad of federal agencies, industry, the private nonprofit sector, and research institutions. Diverse teams of scientists composed of basic scientists, physicians, nurses, dentists, pharmacists, and other health professionals have been involved in research ranging from fundamental biological discoveries about life processes, to behavioral and social research, to clinical and population-based studies, and to research on the delivery of health care services.

Progress in many areas of fundamental biomedical research has led to a new threshold of opportunity. The techniques of genetic engineering and molecular biology have made available hundreds of new proteins with powerful effects on cell growth and behavior. Many of these will have important clinical applications for the treatment of human diseases. As another example, the ability to identify genes linked with disease through a new technology termed *positional cloning*, in concert with the strategic efforts to fully map the human genome, is rapidly bringing medical science to a stage where it will be possible to define the exact genetic basis for many human diseases. This explosion of new information will introduce novel diagnostic and therapeutic modalities requiring highly skilled clinical investigators trained to design and conduct human studies. For each new gene identified to be linked with a human disease, one has the potential to develop not only chemical approaches that use classical pharmacologic techniques but also new biological approaches that utilize the availability of appropriate biological products and, most recently, genetic

1

approaches that use the new science of gene therapy. The opportunities for translation of information gained from molecular biology to health care delivery have never been greater, and they can be expected to increase at a dramatic rate, creating unique societal pressures on the ability of science, medicine, and other health professional groups to respond.

Tremendous advances in biology are opening doors to new therapies, creating numerous clinical research opportunities for evaluating the effectiveness of current or standard therapies. When numerous treatment regimens are possible for some conditions, the outcomes of treatment are often variable and dependent on the diverse social and behavioral attributes of patients. As more and more therapies are added to the medical armamentarium, prospective and retrospective studies of standard therapies also need to be performed. These types of questions have spawned an emerging area of clinical investigation often referred to as *outcomes research*. Such health services research will be needed to guide the nation's struggles to reorganize health care to expand coverage and improve quality while simultaneously holding down costs.

There continues to be debate on whether the current supply of individuals appropriately trained as clinical investigators is seriously deficient. Nevertheless, the explosion of the new knowledge in molecular biology, medicine, and health care, as well as in medical informatics will create the need for substantially more expertise—particularly for more fully trained physicians and other health professionals in academia, government service, and industry—to transform these discoveries into cost-effective diagnoses and treatments for human disease. Since most of these clinical investigators are trained in academia, it is important to recognize the crucial roles that academic health centers (AHCs) have in the career paths of clinical investigators and that there are many external factors that have an impact on the AHC environment.

The escalating costs of health care and the large number of uninsured and underinsured people in the United States have thrown health issues into the policy arena at all levels of government. In medicine, highly subspecialized medical training, a declining interest by U.S. medical students in primary care training, and shortages of physicians willing to practice in rural or inner-city areas are all cited as symptoms of a worsening problem. The spontaneous rise of human immunodeficiency virus infection and the rapid transmission of HIV infection to all segments of society has demonstrated that new diseases can arise at any time, and that a multifaceted approach spanning a variety of fields of research and a range of professional research scientists is needed to develop fundamental knowledge about a disease process, develop and test new diagnostic and therapeutic approaches, design prevention strategies, and assess the subsequent outcomes of health care practices. This can only be accomplished with a sufficient supply of highly talented and well-trained researchers in all areas of research.

FOCUS OF THIS REPORT

The Institute of Medicine Committee on Addressing Career Paths for Clinical Research sought to derive a definition of clinical research in terms of research activities or goals that would cut across artificial boundaries. Although it is difficult to arrive at an unambiguous definition agreeable to all parties, the committee believes that clinical research should be broadly defined as the elucidation of human biology and disease, and its control. Thus, there is a continuum of research spanning a wide range of activities that can be regarded as clinical research.

Using this definition (Chapter 1, page 35) as a departure point, **the special theme and focus of this study was patient-oriented clinical research, defined as that research which requires "hands-on" participation with a human subject. This subset of clinical research was defined as human research and was considered a subset of the entire spectrum of clinical research.**

Furthermore, the committee emphasizes that investigators in many professions are engaging in human research, including dentistry, nursing, pharmacy, and the behavioral sciences, among others. Each of these groups has developed its own clinical research capabilities to different degrees, depending on the research focus and resource base. For example, the diversity of the spectrum of research, from basic to clinical, in dentistry probably parallels that in medicine. However, dental training paths and the reduced level of third-party reimbursement for dentistry differ significantly from those in medicine, and have certain implications for training clinical investigators and performing clinical studies. Nursing, however, has historically been a discipline whose research has focused on patients rather than bench-type research. The formation of the National Center for Nursing Research at The National Institutes of Health (NIH) and its recent elevation to institute status have provided a solid foundation for peer-reviewed, patient-oriented clinical research in this discipline. The similarities and differences among the various disciplines added another dimension to this study, particularly with regard to making crosscutting recommendations. Nonetheless the committee felt that it was vitally important to include the perspectives of all groups engaged in human research.

The committee posed the following global questions about clinical research and the clinical research workforce:

- What can clinical research accomplish now and in the future to improve medical care?
- Is the current clinical research community poised and prepared to accomplish these goals?

• If the clinical research community is not prepared to accomplish these goals, what is the evidence that there is either inadequate clinical investigation or an inadequate number of well-trained clinical investigators to meet this need?

• What are the best approaches or best vehicles for change to improve clinical investigation and ensure a supply of highly competent clinical investigators to meet these needs and accomplish the research goals?

FINDINGS

Accurate data on the number of active clinical investigators or clinical research trainees are unobtainable from any current database. The complexities and heterogeneities of the medical and other health professional research workforces have confounded previous analyses, and this committee, too, was unable to apply existing models to estimate future workforce needs. Nonetheless, recognizing that vast opportunities are arising and the current state of the enterprise, the committee believes that the human resource pool will be seriously deficient for conducting investigations with human subjects in the near future—if it is not already. The committee drew several conclusions from their analyses:

• The current level of training and support for health professionals in clinical research is fragmented, frequently undervalued, and potentially underfunded. This is especially true for those concerned with human research, that is, research focused on the human subject.

• A number of variables make the pursuit of clinical investigation relatively unattractive for medical students and students of the other health professions. These include the prolonged period of clinical training required of current medical graduates; the effect of the accumulated debt burden on career choice; the relative lack of role models and mentors; the perceived instability of research funding from NIH and other federal agencies; the real funding instability as it pertains to the individual investigator; the perceived lack of support for research, particularly as it relates to human research; the lack of emphasis on clinical research training in the curriculum; and the multiple demands upon the trainees not only during their period of training, but also as they begin their careers on the faculty, in industry, or in government service.

• The voluntary and certifying accrediting bodies have a significant influence over individual career decisions, and in an effort to improve quality in one area, they may create significant hurdles in other areas. For example, meeting the new requirements for specialty or subspecialty board recertification which requires a broad overview of the entire discipline may conflict with the necessity of maintaining a narrow focus in a particular area of clinical research.

• Relatively few programs adequately prepare physicians and other health professionals to undertake research involving human subjects, and their successes are unproven.

• Managed competition represents the new paradigm for the funding of health care. The development of this model is likely to lead to the formation of large organizations of provider groups or health plans, which in turn will contract with consortia of employer groups or alliances to provide health coverage for employees and their families. This change will have a major impact on the ability of academic health centers to support their academic missions and thus will have a direct effect on the support of research and education. Unless new approaches to the support of clinical investigators and academic health centers involving the participation of third-party payers are forthcoming, it is likely that this paradigm shift in health care financing will seriously compromise the translation of results from fundamental research into improved health care.

• Funding for investigator-initiated human research is difficult to obtain. Whereas industry is obligated to conduct clinical trials during product development to meet regulatory conditions for market approval, there is no profit motive to support investigator-initiated studies on medical practice. The committee performed an analysis on a subset of R01 grants that were active in 1991. The purpose of that analysis was to determine the number of awards and amount of funding that were actually committed to patient-oriented research. Of the approximately 30 percent of all R01 grants indicating the use of humans or human materials, the committee determined that only one third (or about 10–12 percent of total R01s) of this grant pool actually involved human subjects. Although there are other mechanisms for funding human research, the R01 pool is the largest source of funds for investigator-initiated studies, both basic and clinical.

• Clinical investigators devote months or years to developing the appropriate design for a clinical study. Barriers include the need to submit numerous protocols for approval within their institutions, the need to have adequate infrastructure and personnel for conducting a clinical study, the competing demands on their time to provide patient care as well as teaching and research, and the amount of funding available for investigator-initiated human research. The measures of scholarly productivity for clinical investigators are not well defined, and to many university promotion committees, the research activities of clinical investigators may be considered nontraditional.

• Responsibility for oversight of the nation's clinical research capacity is fragmented at every level, whether academic or governmental. Thus, there appears to be little prospective planning involving all interested parties to identify clinical research needs or new opportunities. As a consequence, no organized segment of society, public or private, focuses attention on the clinical investigator to ensure and encourage a career path(s) at so critical a phase in the history of human health.

The committee concluded that new opportunities for clinical research are growing at a rapid pace. In addition, the committee believes that the present cohort of clinical investigators is not adequate and many are not suitably prepared to address many of the important questions that are arising, particularly in areas like gene therapy and outcomes research. Furthermore, numerous obstacles confront clinical researchers and clinical research trainees at various points in their career pathways, and these obstacles may dissuade them from pursuing clinical research careers. The committee is concerned that the health research community may be unable to address even a fraction of these opportunities, and this may delay substantially the development of new advances in medicine.

To foster improved clinical investigation, to facilitate and stimulate high-quality training for clinical investigators, and to ensure a supply of highly skilled clinical investigators, the committee calls for a multifaceted and concerted effort. The U.S. congress, industry, professional organizations, organized medicine, NIH and other federal agencies, as well as the nation's universities and academic health centers will need to work in partnership to meet these research and training needs.   Voluntary health organizations, accrediting and certifying agencies, and medical professional societies all have a role to play in the careers of clinical investigators.   Most of the committee's recommendations do not necessarily require increased funding to effect change. The committee emphasizes that effective and strong leadership in academic health centers, in government, and in industry is a critical ingredient in the process for improving clinical research and developing rewarding clinical research career pathways. Whereas each individual recommendation is directed to a specific group or organization, collectively the recommendations represent a package of reforms needed for redefining careers in clinical investigation.

RECOMMENDATIONS

NIH and Other Federal Agencies Supporting Research

Among the federal agencies, NIH continues to be the trendsetter in the support of biomedical research, both basic and clinical, and in the training of clinical investigators. Accordingly, efforts carried out by NIH will have a major impact on progress in the development of the clinical investigator. A number of approaches are recommended to enhance the effectiveness of NIH as a leader in patient-oriented clinical research.

Data Analysis

NIH and the other federal agencies that sponsor human research must develop and implement a process to prospectively collect data that accurately identify the subsets of human research.

The present system of classifying clinical versus nonclinical research is woefully inadequate and that for identifying human research is nonexistent. A large amount of research is recorded as clinical only because it is necessary to identify those grants that use human materials as well as human subjects. The absence of such categorization makes it impossible to accurately determine the level of investigator-initiated support for human research. Even the retrospective analysis performed by the committee (see Chapter 3) was not adequate for understanding either the levels or trends in support for human research. NIH and other federal science agencies should prospectively collect data that document the extent to which patient-oriented clinical investigations are being supported and the success rates of such grant applications in the peer review process. At a minimum, this should include the collection of information and separate documentation as to the use of human materials, the study of human subjects, and the conduct of human epidemiology.

Study Section Oversight

The committee recommends that the NIH director appoint a standing committee to regularly review the compositions, functions, and outcomes of study section activities, particularly as they relate to human research.

Rigorous application of scientific methods spanning the spectrum from fundamental to clinical research and within clinical research to human and population-based research requires specialized knowledge and skills. Therefore, it is important to ensure that the study sections at NIH are composed of individuals with the appropriate breadth and depth of knowledge to evaluate the research proposals assigned to that study section. An oversight committee that would largely comprise extramural investigators with expertise ranging across the entire spectrum of research should be established. A similar recommendation to form a Peer Evaluation of Extramural Research (PEER) was put forward by a 1992 internal review panel convened to examine the peer review system at NIH.

Newly Independent Investigators

The committee recommends that new mechanisms for supporting newly independent clinical investigators be developed.

Funding must be available to support newly independent clinical investigators who are just initiating their investigative careers. This segment of one's career development often becomes the most critical and the time when so many of the disincentives converge to dissuade newly trained clinical investigators from continuing to pursue clinical research career paths. Many believe that First Investigator Research Support and Transition (FIRST) awards have been highly successful in nurturing the careers of newly independent investigators. Indeed, FIRST awards could also be an avenue for launching a career in clinical investigation, but the structure of the awards and the ceiling on costs are more suited for bench-type research rather than human subject research. Stabilization of funding could well represent the single most important factor to the individual clinical investigator. This support has come from many sources in the past, perhaps most importantly from the academic health center. As noted later, this type of support is in jeopardy because of the changing health care system.

Centers and Program Projects

The committee strongly supports the efforts by NIH to develop centers and program projects to support research and infrastructure in exciting new areas of multidisciplinary, crosscutting research.

Not only is the development of these programs critical to the support of clinical research but they also provide one of the few mechanisms available for the development and support of core facilities. Such core facilities are essential to individual clinical investigators attempting to overcome obstacles in the progress of their own research. Centers not only provide physical infrastructure but also serve as a locus of intellectual capital and collaboration necessary for conducting human research. The availability of small feasibility grants as part of larger center grants often stimulates investigators to extend their expertise to new areas beyond their current levels of interest.

General Clinical Research Centers

The committee recommends that Congress be made aware of the clinical research and training potential of the General Clinical Research Centers (GCRCs) and recommit its support for this vital resource.

GCRCs serve as an important infrastructural resource for those institutions fortunate enough to have one. In the federation of disease and organ institutes of NIH, it is frequently difficult to muster support from Congress or special interest groups for centers like the GCRCs that do not focus on any one disease or organ. Strong GCRCs are, and will continue to be, critical in meeting the future promise of the advances in biomedical research as they will be applied to improving the quality and cost-effectiveness of patient care. In the past, GCRCs have played a pivotal role as a resource for investigators attempting to elucidate physiological parameters of healthy and disease states in human subjects. In the future, GCRCs must also serve as a vital link in elucidating the applications of biological products and gene therapy in human populations. GCRCs also provide attractive sites for studies related to the clinical development of novel drugs and could serve as important resources or loci for establishing programs for outcomes assessment. There are presently 75 GCRCs in the United States. The budget for GCRCs has not grown in real terms for a number of years, and actually has declined when corrected for inflation. The GCRCs require strong federal, corporate, and institutional support.

Multiyear Stabilization

The committee recommends that Congress make multiyear appropriations to NIH and other federal agencies that sponsor research. Similar recommendations have been made by other groups examining research funding and the appropriations process.

Research in all areas, and particularly human research, requires a long-term commitment to develop appropriate hypotheses, gain the requisite protocol approvals, and recruit a patient population for study. The perceived instability of federal funding for research, as well as the actual instability for the individual clinical investigator, appears to be an important obstruction in the choice of clinical research as a career for the young health professional. A multiyear commitment from the executive and legislative branches of the federal government for the support of NIH and other research agency appropriations would represent a major benefit to this perceived instability—which often translates into real instability related to grant cycling—of grant funding for the scientific community. In addition to multiyear stabilization of research funding, the formalization of administrative mechanisms to provide interim support from NIH during gaps in funding would provide further stability.

Support of Training Programs

The committee recommends that NIH and other federal agencies develop tracking mechanisms to be able to determine the outcomes of their training programs as they relate to clinical research. Model programs should be studied, and those that have proven track records in preparing successful clinical investigators should be expanded and replicated. Those with poor track records should be closed or replaced with successful models.

The conduct of patient-oriented clinical research requires a broad knowledge base and multiple skills. For some areas of investigation, a working knowledge of fundamental science is essential; for others, uncommonly strong clinical skills are necessary. And for some studies, a sophisticated analytic capability is needed to make valid inferences from experimental and nonexperimental data. The committee believes, however, that there is a core of knowledge and skills common to clinical investigation that serves not only as the foundation for scientific discovery but also as the basis for clinical appraisal of evidence in decision making in health care for all health care professionals. Furthermore, if the problem with obtaining funding for human studies through peer review is the poor quality of grant proposals, action must be taken to improve the ability of newly independent investigators to draft sound proposals for clinical studies.

The current training grants (T series awards), fellowships (F series), research career development awards (RCDAs), physician or dentist scientist awards (K series), and other training avenues provided through NIH should be reviewed with regard to their efficacies and successes in training creative and productive investigators. One earlier analysis by NIH in 1989 demonstrated that clinical trainees who serve for less than 9 months on training grants (T32) in clinical departments do not receive adequate training to become competitive in the NIH grant system.   An effort should be made to identify and expand programs that are the most successful in supporting human research. The method of review should include prospective mechanisms for tracking the professional outcomes of trainees, the total financial support required to relieve the individual candidates of the need to obtain funding through other sources, and a component of the training that fosters the transition from trainee to principal investigator status.

Such programs should continue to include at least three years of research training in addition to standard residency training. Again, experience in applying research skills under the supervision of experienced investigators is essential. Combination of residency and such fellowship programs, with integration of clinical and research training over a 6- to 10-year period, should be encouraged for trainees who make early commitments to careers in clinical research. Such combined programs could be particularly advantageous for patient-based research, which necessarily requires long periods of patient observation and data collection.

The committee recommends that selected centers be encouraged to develop programs of interdisciplinary studies that lead to advanced degrees in evaluative sciences related to clinical research.

Here the goals would be to enhance the theoretical basis for clinical research as well as the development of more efficient and effective research methods. Funding for these model programs must not compromise current research funding, and therefore should be derived from incremental new financial resources, possibly through congressional appropriations or funds derived from private sources (pharmaceutical industry, insurance companies, or nonprofit organizations).

The committee recommends that NIH expand the medical scientist training program and the dentist scientist training program specifically for training investigators in the skills of performing patient-oriented clinical research. Data should be collected and analyzed to identify those programs that have proven track records in preparing successful clinical investigators. Successful programs should be expanded and replicated and those with poor track records should be closed or replaced with successful models.

Successful medical scientist training programs and the dentist scientist training programs leading to the combined M.D. or dental degree and Ph.D. degree appear to represent the most useful approaches to the production of highly qualified physician and dentist scientists and should be expanded. The number of applications for these programs far exceeds the capacity; an expanded number of funded positions would be filled by highly qualified applicants seeking careers in clinical research. Some of the positions should be designed to focus on training in human research. The committee also encourages the expansion of NIH-funded combined programs that lead to the M.D. degree (or other professional degrees) with other advanced degrees in disciplines such as economics, epidemiology, public health, biostatistics, and ethics.

The committee recommends that each General Clinical Research Center (GCRC) evaluate the outcomes of the Clinical Associate Physician (CAP) program and consider expanding it if it is found to be effective for training patient-oriented clinical researchers. GCRCs should also develop a program to involve medical students and residents in clinical research activities in the centers.

This recommendation, in concert with an earlier recommendation, would represent a recommitment to the GCRC program to make these centers the loci of pioneering clinical studies in numerous disciplines. The CAP program of GCRC, is an important source of support for the training of clinical investigators committed to the field of human research. GCRCs and the CAP program deserve a careful analysis, and expansion if deemed appropriate.

Other federal agencies should reexamine their roles in supporting clinical research. Indeed, the successes of these agencies in support of both basic and clinical research for the future will be extremely important to facilitating the flow of information between the laboratory bench and the patient's bedside, and each agency can play a very specific and relevant role. Included in this group of agencies are the Departments of Veterans Affairs, Defense, Energy, Agriculture, and Education, the Centers for Disease Control and Prevention and the Agency for Health Care Policy and Research within the Department of Health and Human Services, and the National Science Foundation. The committee encourages the U.S. Congress to expand the support of research and training by each of these federal agencies as they define their priorities at this critical time in the history of health care.

The committee recommends that NIH, the other federal agencies that sponsor clinical research, industry, and the private, nonprofit agencies develop or expand debt relief packages for individuals desiring to pursue clinical research career paths.

The accumulating debt burden that students engender in pursuing professional training, particularly in medicine, creates a serious concern for many as they consider career options during their period of training. The committee believes that the pursuit of careers in clinical investigation may be seriously affected today by the prolonged period of training required, the instability of clinical research as a career option, and the modest levels of compensation that can be expected compared with those for other available career pathways for similarly trained individuals. Existing programs that pay medical school tuition, such as the longstanding Medical Scientist Training (MST) program, or that pay back educational debt, such as NIH's AIDS Research Debt Relief Program, to promote research careers have demonstrated positive results, and the committee encourages their expansion if they are proven to be effective. Medical schools have demonstrated their support for such programs, as evidenced by investing their own resources to fund nearly 50 percent of the M.D.-Ph.D. slots in the country. The committee believes strongly that mechanisms should be found to develop a funding base to underwrite a debt relief program for individuals who are committed to a career in clinical investigation. Although resources for supporting such program areas most likely must come from some new funds, the committee feels that a growing investment should begin now to ensure the availability of talent in the next several years. The committee believes that NIH is best equipped to implement these programs for the federal government and recommends that NIH be empowered to develop the appropriate organization and infrastructure. The committee urges the sponsors of clinical research and clinical research training to act independently to initiate programs of debt relief for these individuals.

UNIVERSITIES AND ACADEMIC MEDICAL CENTERS

The key to the success of individual clinical investigators is the university academic health center where most are likely to have acquired their research skills and where many conduct clinical investigation studies during a significant portion of their careers. The academic medical center is defined as the medical school and its related university hospital(s). The attractiveness of careers in clinical research can be enhanced substantially by the leadership at many levels within these institutions. The institutions and their leadership are now under considerable stress as a result of health care reform. Nevertheless, the support of teaching and research must continue to be among the highest priorities.

Academic Recognition and Rewards

The committee recommends that academic institutions where clinical research is conducted review their promotion guidelines to prevent bias against clinical investigators and establish reward mechanisms to acknowledge the scholarly contributions of clinical investigators.

The scholarship of the successful clinical investigator should be appropriately recognized in the academic setting. This would include recognition that the nature of their research, the sources of their funding, and the journals in which they publish may differ substantially from those of the investigators in fundamental research. Some institutions have chosen multiple pathways for clinicians, whereas others have adhered to single promotion pathways for all investigators. Whatever the pathway, it is incumbent on institutions to create a fair and equitable means for recognizing and rewarding the scholarly contributions of clinical investigators.

Faculty Protection

The committee recommends that academic institutions establish reward mechanisms to acknowledge the importance of teaching, advising, and mentoring by clinical investigators.

The existence of faculty in clinical investigation who teach, advise and mentor trainees, and serve as role models is important in attracting students to careers in clinical investigation. These faculty activities, therefore, must be recognized and rewarded. Such recognition in the academic health center includes promotion, protected time, and financial support. Leaders at all levels within these institutions must define their expectations of junior faculty and support them so that these young men and women can meet or exceed those expectations. In many institutions support has been successfully facilitated by the formation of specific clinical faculty tracks; others have developed equally successful single-track systems that are capable of recognizing the diversity of academic productivity. The committee does not endorse one system over another; rather, it encourages institutions to establish suitable means for recognizing the contributions of clinical investigators and developing appropriate reward systems.

Infrastructure

The committee recommends that research institutions provide clinical investigators with the appropriate infrastructure in order to conduct high-quality clinical studies.

In addition to well-trained and adequately funded patient-based clinical investigators, the successful execution of clinical and especially human research requires a suitable institutional infrastructure. University-based and research-intensive medical centers should develop mechanisms to achieve the optimal infrastructure to support inpatient- and outpatient-based human research. The features of such an infrastructure may include a clinical practice that is structured to deliver health care in a scholarly and investigative fashion and the integration of students, residents, fellows, and other health care professionals into human research activities. In addition, multidisciplinary facilities are required at academic institutions to support core requirements for clinical research; these might include such elements as biostatistics, data management, and an opportunity to work with other health professionals. Creative start-up efforts through academic institutional mechanisms to establish core facilities that will seek continued funding through extramural sources represent an important activity that should be strongly encouraged within the academic setting.

Medical School Curriculum

The committee recommends that the curriculum of the medical school and those of other health professional schools should cut across departmental lines and be led by a team of educators committed to discovery in the basic laboratory, the clinic, and the community.

Exposure to the principals of clinical research should occur in the first year of the medical school curriculum. This would include, but not be limited to, practical application of disciplines such as epidemiology, statistics, and the design and ethics of clinical trials in a setting such as a general clinical research center. Thus, the committee strongly encourages increased opportunities for early participation of students in high-quality research, including human research, and exposure to role models.

The committee recognizes the health care needs of society and the pressure to increase the proportion of practicing generalists. These individuals will best meet the needs of society if they are educated by a process that emphasizes discovery. Indeed, many of these individuals can and should contribute to clinical investigations as their careers in primary care develop.

Furthermore, the committee believes that each health professional school should have a program in place that requires in-depth, meaningful participation in research, including patient-based clinical research. Such programs might include a required thesis for research performed over an extended period of time (for example, one year involved in research) or an article submitted for publication in a peer-reviewed journal. Although this approach may not be possible in all settings, the committee recommends, as a minimum, a program that seeks out medical students and other health professionals with an ability and interest in research and that provides a concrete opportunity, it is hoped with funding, for a program of research training. The committee encourages other health professions to examine their training programs and curricula to ensure that they attract and support individuals capable of performing human research related to their professions. Such funding could be provided by academic institutions, foundations, industry, government, or an alliance thereof.

Postgraduate Training

The committee recommends that postgraduate training programs implement programmatic changes to ensure that residency and fellowship training programs include ongoing exposure to basic elements of experimental design, biostatistics, epidemiology, and decision theory in relation to measures of therapeutic effectiveness, diagnostic accuracy, prognosis, and screening and disease prevention.

The importance of expanding current model postgraduate training programs, which have proven to be successful in the training of clinical investigators, has been noted earlier and deserves reemphasis here. Ideally, these programs will be integrated with clinical teaching as well as relevant areas of investigation that emphasize the translation of research to clinical decision making and the role of the clinical appraisal of evidence in that process. Teaching and research institutions cannot rely on other sectors to effect change in clinical research and clinical research training and must begin to make the necessary changes in their own programs. The committee feels that these changes will not only produce clinical researchers with better skills but physicians who can provide better care as well.

ACCREDITATION AND CERTIFICATION ORGANIZATIONS

The voluntary accrediting agencies responsible for overseeing the education and training programs for health professionals in the United States are highly developed and successful. This includes the Liaison Committee for Medical Education, the Accreditation Committee for Graduate Medical Education, the Accreditation Committee for Continuing Medical Education, the Joint Commission for Accreditation of Health Care Organizations, and the accreditation bodies for other health professions. In addition, there is a voluntary certification process to recognize individual qualifications in pursuit of specialty careers in organized medicine and dentistry. Some of these certifying bodies, such as the American Boards, are organized under the umbrella organization the American Board of Medical Specialties. Each of these organizations plays a major role in establishing standards and ensuring continuous quality improvement in the education and training process, both for the program and for the individual. Hence, evolving changes in the nature of the education and training programs that affect clinical research will, of necessity, require cooperation and participation of the accrediting and certifying bodies. Their strong support and cooperation would be extremely helpful in facilitating the entire process.

Liaison Committee on Medical Education

The committee recommends that the Liaison Committee on Medical Education (LCME) recognize the importance of scientific inquiry by effecting changes in the medical school curriculum that encourage an appreciation of clinical investigation and participation in clinical research.

LCME is the national authority for the accreditation of medical education programs leading to the M.D. degree. The committee believes that LCME must play a key role in effecting changes in medical school curricula that will encourage lifelong learning and intellectual curiosity. Such curriculum changes in medical schools, as well as changes in other health professional schools, must recognize the crucial role of scientific inquiry and incorporate necessary changes that are supportive of individuals pursuing research career pathways, particularly clinical research pathways.

Accreditation Committee for Graduate Medical Education

The committee recommends that the Accreditation Committee for Graduate Medical Education (ACGME), through its Residency Review Committees (RRCs), ensure that the environment of graduate medical education and training programs is conducive to and supportive of an atmosphere of intellectual growth and scientific inquiry, particularly as it relates to clinical investigation.

ACGME is made up of the 24 RRCs, which accredit the individual residency training programs. The committee fully recognizes the need for a long period of training and for the rigid clinical requirements that exist. Nevertheless, the explosion of knowledge in basic and clinical research requires that the health professionals of the future develop the ability to critique study designs and published results. In addition, physicians, dentists, and other health professionals trained and expert in clinical research are needed to transfer the advances of basic science to the clinic and to ensure that epidemiologic and outcomes studies are conducted appropriately.

Such an atmosphere could be achieved by the organization of specific clinical investigator pathways and the development of a curriculum that provides exposure to elements important in translating basic advances to the resolution of clinical problems. For those programs designed to train clinical investigators, a mechanism to measure the quality and success of research training must be developed.

American Board of Medical Specialties

The committee recommends that the member boards of the American Board of Medical Specialties (ABMS) establish appropriate criteria to recognize and encourage the development of clinical investigators in their respective specialties, including a careful analysis of the recertification process on clinical investigator careers.

The certifying boards of ABMS, which establish the basic requirements for individuals to receive certification in specialty disciplines, should be strongly encouraged to develop specific clinical investigator pathways to allow individuals who pursue their disciplines to substitute experience and training in clinical investigation for other requirements. Familiarity with clinical research methodologies and interpretation should be tested during the certification process.

Most boards that provide certification in organized medicine within the United States have developed time-limited certifications. Individuals in their disciplines must participate in a recertification process within a specific time frame (generally every 10 years) to continue to be recognized as a specialist in the field. The committee is concerned that this process, although appropriate from the perspective of ensuring the clinical excellence of the certified physician, could provide a major disincentive for the pursuit of a career in clinical research. This issue deserves special review and analysis by the certifying boards in medicine and other bodies governing specialists in other health professions.

EXECUTIVE BRANCH, CONGRESS, INDUSTRY, FOUNDATIONS, AND PROFESSIONAL SOCIETIES

Health care reform is a national goal that is focused on bringing cost-effective quality care to all Americans. The issues involved currently occupy much of the national agenda. Clinical research must be a critical element in health care reform because it produces efficient and effective therapies and strategies for patient care in the future. The prevention and cure of disease are the ultimate benefits of clinical research. Indeed, the return on investment will be enhanced substantially by the removal of the obstacles and constraints in the smooth translation of advances in science to health care.

Federal science agencies, the pharmaceutical and biotechnology industry, private nonprofit organizations, research institutions, the insurance industry, society at large, and medical professional societies all have a vested interest in clinical research. However, the committee is concerned that the fragmented interest in clinical investigation among many institutions and organizations and the lack of cooperation or coordination among the various groups is an impediment to a systematic approach to the training of highly skilled clinical investigators. The committee believes that some means to bring together all the interested parties with the appropriate resources and authority to effect change could provide the critical catalytic process necessary to redefine clinical investigator career pathways in this new era of health care. Although this report analyzes the current status of clinical research, the changing dynamics of clinical research within the rapidly changing realm of biomedical research and health care reform require that consistent attention be paid to this vital segment of the research enterprise. Thus, the committee felt that such a forum needs to be an ongoing effort to provide data analysis and continuing attention to the problems of the clinical investigator. The committee considered several proposals for action including the following:

• **Create a panel with broad representation by all interested parties that is funded through membership fees and that has the authority to distribute funds for training and research. Such an organization might be a private- or public-sector organization with combined funding from the federal government and the private sector. For clinical research, which the committee views as critical to national security and economic competitiveness, such an organization could include funding and representation from the federal science agencies, the pharmaceutical and biotechnology industry, third-party payers, the health and life insurance industries, and other interested groups.**
• **Another option could be the establishment of a permanent federal commission or council to monitor the nation's clinical research activities and advise the Congress and other sponsors on the needs of clinical investigation and the clinical investigator. Such a commission or council may or may not have authority over funds. For example, the President's Commission on AIDS is a senior-level advisory body to the administration and federal science agencies.**
• **The private sector could act alone by forming a coalition of special interest groups (industry, third-party payers, academia, and nonprofit organizations) that could act on behalf of the groups' collective interests to identify critical areas for investment in clinical research. For example, the Alliance for Aging Research promotes research in this particular field as well as collects funds from many sectors to establish national centers of excellence in aging research.**

The committee does not endorse any one proposal, but presents them for consideration and to raise the consciousness of all concerned about the difficulties related to clinical research and clinical research training in hopes of ensuring that they are not overlooked as the nation grapples with health care reform.

Conflicts of Interest

The committee recommends that the government, universities, research institutes, and industry develop appropriate guidelines and means to resolve conflicts of interest to encourage strong cooperation in clinical studies.

The committee believes strongly that the translation and application of advances in research to patient care require a strong partnership between research universities and medical centers and industry. Effective interdependent relationships between clinical investigators, their institutions, and industry are necessary for the United States to continue to lead the world in developing innovative therapies. Facilitating technology transfer by both parties with the support of the federal government is vitally important and deserves special attention. This will require new standards in the definition and resolution of conflicts of interest at all levels. Healthy relationships that encourage full cooperation can build on this interdependence and can be synergistic.

Preserving Academic Health Centers

The committee emphasizes that the federal government and third-party payers recognize the vital contributions that academic health centers (AHCs) make in medical education and clinical research to improve health care and recommends that they take appropriate action to reimburse AHCs according to their broad mission.

The committee acknowledges that the costs of health care in the nation's AHCs appear to exceed those of health care providers without a broader mission for teaching and research. Because of AHCs' commitment to research and teaching, these institutions frequently cannot compete on a pure cost basis with other providers, and payers must be made aware of their broad mission. The committee believes that there is a need to identify, isolate, and detach those costs unique to the AHCs that provide benefit to all stakeholders and to provide payment through a separate income stream funded by all payers. This in effect would provide parity so that AHCs could compete fairly in the provision of patient care on the basis of quality and price. Providing state-of-the-art care and continued innovation requires a sound underpinning of basic and clinical research. It is important that the level of payments for graduate medical education recognize all the costs involved in graduate training, including residents' stipends and benefits, salaries and benefits related to faculty teaching, and overhead costs related to the graduate education process to preserve the most creative and innovative health care and health research systems in the world.

Graduate medical education is not the only factor that accounts for the higher costs at AHCs. Health care professionals at AHCs often treat patients who are more seriously ill, provide infrastructure for biomedical and health services research, and offer clinical training experiences for undergraduate medical and other health professional students—costs that add to an institution's cost base. In recognition of these additional costs, the Medicare program has historically paid teaching hospitals an indirect medical education adjustment. Likewise, some modified version of an adjustment to account for those costs unique to AHCs, above and beyond the direct costs of graduate medical education, will be necessary in a managed competition environment. The adjustment should be formula driven rather than based on year-to-year appropriations and, again, should be funded by all payers.

Finally, all accountable health plans, when feasible, should include an academic health center as a centerpiece of their networks. Such a requirement would guarantee all citizens access to the latest in state-of-the-art care when medically necessary. At the same time, it would help to ensure an adequate flow to academic health centers of the patients on whom their educational and human research programs are completely dependent. Without access to suitable patient populations for clinical studies, the United States will lose its leadership in opening the frontiers of innovative and effective health care. This approach might be further complemented if regional "centers of excellence" were established in AHCs for the evaluation of emerging technologies and specialized methods of treatment. AHCs would be the natural place for locating such centers, given their strong emphasis on research, particularly if they have a health services research component. The regionalization of certain emerging technologies would also help to control the widespread diffusion of new technologies absent sufficient outcomes research that could be used to judge their cost-effectiveness.

1

Introduction

Health care in the United States has improved markedly over the past five decades, in large measure because of the advances in health research that have been supported by a myriad of federal agencies, industry, the private nonprofit sector, and research institutions. Diverse teams of scientists composed of basic scientists, physicians, nurses, dentists, pharmacists, and other health professionals have been involved in research spanning a spectrum from fundamental biological discoveries about life processes, to behavioral and social research, to clinical and population-based studies, and to research on the organization, financing, and delivery of health care services. For example, imaging technology that allows investigators to peer into the human brain and observe the circuitry and biochemical reactions as humans construct thoughts and words is now available. Progress in genome mapping promises to provide monumental advances in understanding of genetic diseases and to aid investigators in finding biological therapies. Rational drug design is allowing researchers to custom design pharmacologic agents that can act on specific tissues, organs, or cell receptors and treat a broad spectrum of human maladies. Entirely new approaches to the treatment, cure, and prevention of human diseases are evolving with the availability of biological products and gene therapies. Research methods are being developed to permit investigators to evaluate the outcomes and effectiveness of health care practices. Research in these and other areas has formed a dynamic synergy that has positioned the United States at the forefront of innovation in medicine.

Despite all the advances, however, signs of stress are surfacing throughout the health care and health research systems. The soaring costs of health care and the escalating number of uninsured and underinsured people in the United States have thrown health issues into the policy arena at all levels of government. In medicine, highly subspecialized medical training, a declining interest by U.S. medical students in primary care training, and shortages of physicians willing to practice in rural or inner-city areas are all cited as symptoms of a worsening problem. The emergence of human immunodeficiency virus infection has demonstrated that new diseases can arise unexpectedly, and that a multifaceted approach spanning a variety of fields of research and a range of professional research scientists is needed to develop fundamental knowledge about a disease process, diagnosis, effective therapies, and prevention strategies and to assess the subsequent outcomes of health care practices. This can only be accomplished with highly talented and well-trained researchers in all areas of research, from basic to clinical research to outcomes and health services research.

Research is a highly social and political process of communication, interpersonal relationships, and scientific exchange that seeks to describe, explain, and modify biological and pathological processes. Researchers develop hypotheses and test them by collecting and analyzing data. The results add to existing knowledge. The unique feature of clinical research that distinguishes it from laboratory research is the direct involvement of human subjects. Although both laboratory and clinical research employ the same scientific principles for experimental procedures, the use of human subjects increases the complexities of scientific investigations. Whereas laboratory studies can more easily control for as many variables as possible to yield reproducible results, clinical research involves more heterogeneous populations, often is more expensive, takes longer to develop, requires long periods of time for data collection, and may be difficult to reproduce (Kimes et al., 1991). To advance medical care in patients, however, research must be performed in populations of patients with diseases.

Many research activities performed by a broad spectrum of professionals fall under the rubric of clinical research. Whereas many kinds of clinical research require similar skills and abilities, others may require different tools to achieve research objectives. Examples of how earlier investigations have influenced today's medical care are well known. Present research studies will improve tomorrow's medical practice, while future clinical research opportunities will affect care in the twenty-first century. What is the scope of clinical research, and what are the settings for conducting clinical research and the opportunities for future research?

SCOPE OF CLINICAL RESEARCH

Clinical research is a relatively new discipline. Although the American Society for Clinical Investigation was formed in 1908, clinical advances prior to the 1950s were often based on imprecise observations by practicing clinicians

(Cadman, 1994; Fox et al., 1992). In 1948 the British published the first randomized clinical trial, evaluating streptomycin in the treatment of malaria (Medical Research Council, 1948); the first clinical trial published in the United States was a study evaluating the effectiveness of penicillin for treating pneumoccocal pneumonia (Austrian et al., 1951). As methods for large-scale clinical studies became more refined, investigators gained an appreciation for new study designs, methodological advances, and the power of statistical analysis that permitted the validation of small differences between treatment regimens. Clinical research quickly became accepted as scholarly work and as an academic discipline (Fye, 1991; Ledley, 1991).

A major paradigm shift in clinical research was initiated in the 1970s when human cells were grown in vitro. As a result, some forms of clinical research could be performed on human cell lines grown in culture. This initiated a period some refer to as *reductionism* in which patients were no longer used as the primary focus of clinical research. This idea was extended by using the techniques of molecular biology, which permitted the study of human nucleic acid alterations in disease instead of requiring the study of the entire patient. Yet, in the final analysis, the application of these discoveries to improve medical care requires that these findings be used on the whole patient.

In parallel, during the last decade the discipline of clinical research has undergone a remarkable evolution in the scope, sophistication, and power of its methodologies. Changes have occurred in the approach to data collection, experimental design, and data analysis, and these changes provide a stronger basis for clinical research. In addition, understanding of the pathogenesis of diseases has provided more precise concepts of preclinical and subclinical disease states. The application of molecular epidemiology is a prime example of these changes in clinical research. Now the results of new biology are ripe for application to improve medical care, but many fear that a talented cohort of clinical investigators has not been prepared to translate these fundamental advances into improved medical care.

The revolution of fundamental research discovery is expected to accelerate in the future, driven by the explosion of science in biotechnology, molecular biology, computer technology, diagnostic systems, decision modeling, and clinical measurements technology. The sophisticated methods for clinical research require investigators with the requisite talents to design excellent clinical studies, recruit adequate numbers of research subjects, and analyze the large amounts of data collected. The need for cross-disciplinary teams to accomplish the objectives of multicenter, complex clinical trials is readily apparent. It is clear that training for a career in clinical research must be as rigorous as training for a career in the traditional basic sciences. Understanding of both the basic sciences and the evaluative sciences is essential to the success of clinical researchers. Moreover, novice clinical investigators require the same mentoring and nurturing in a supportive environment as those engaged in fundamental research disciplines if they are to develop into mature, independent scientists who remain competitive and productive over an extended period of time.

Numerous advances can be cited to describe opportunities in clinical research; the following allow one to comprehend their broad scope. One dramatic example of progress in fundamental research that has opened up immeasurable clinical research opportunities is the discovery in 1989 of the gene that is mutated in patients with cystic fibrosis. The gene was identified by using the advanced methodologies of positional gene mapping. Investigators delineated the nature of the mutation that leads to the production of a defective protein in the membranes of cells from patients with cystic fibrosis patients. Subsequent research demonstrated that this protein is associated with a membrane channel involved in the transport of chloride ions. This understanding has led to a number of chemical approaches to treat the disease. In addition, new efforts are under way to treat or cure the pulmonary manifestations of the disease by employing methods that are being developed in DNA transfer therapy. Research that is now being conducted in the laboratory will soon be carried over to use in patients with cystic fibrosis. Clinical investigators are crucial to the performance of this work and in bringing these novel therapies into common practice. Their participation will also be necessary to help determine how to deliver the technology efficiently, under what conditions and to which patients, and to assess the outcomes of these new therapies.

Hundreds, if not thousands, of other genetic disease are now being studied in the same fashion. As knowledge about the underlying genetic mechanisms for these diseases grows, new treatment approaches developed from basic laboratory techniques will be carried forward into clinical trials. In addition, genetic factors are being defined in diseases that have been regarded as multifactorial. For example, breast cancer scientists are on the threshold of discovering the genes that regulate its occurrence. Thus, approaches to modify the expression of these genes may be useful in the treatment of breast cancer. Genes that regulate the formation of atherogenic lesions in arteries, abnormalities that lead to coronary artery disease and heart disease have recently been identified. Blocking the activities of these genes using antisense gene therapy has been shown to block the progression of atherogenic lesions in arteries in animal models. On the basis of results of these promising studies, antisense gene therapies are being developed for use in humans. Novel therapies directed at blocking the genetic expression of the factors that determine atherogenesis as well as genetically directed products that can prevent or reverse these effects may be developed in the future and may lead to treatments or cures for ischemic heart disease and some forms of stroke. Clearly, clinical investigators will be critical for developing and testing these new therapies to determine their safety, efficacy, effectiveness, and cost-effectiveness in humans. Clinical investigators will also play a role in discussions regarding ethical considerations such as genetic testing and elucidating the behavioral or environmental factors influencing genetic diseases.

Although new therapies are being developed rapidly and require extensive clinical testing, old or current therapies should be rigorously evaluated as well. During the past few years several groups have initiated studies to examine the outcomes of current therapies for particular diseases or conditions (Eddy, 1984; Roper et al., 1984). For example, a broad-based research team has been investigating the treatment for benign prostate hypertrophy in a patient population in Maine (Wennberg et al., 1988). By taking into consideration the behavioral and social attributes of patients, the outcomes of the various treatments have been assessed. Not all treatment regimens are viewed favorably by patients, who have various needs and desired outcomes. Thus, the outcomes of particular therapies require sophisticated scientific methods to determine the effectiveness of therapy in patients with different expectations and needs. Other examples of opportunities for outcomes research can be cited by examining the topics under investigation by the Patient Outcomes Research Teams funded by the Agency for Health Care Policy and Research, such as low back pain, joint replacement, incontinence, and others. The research methods and tools used by those investigators are every bit as sophisticated as those needed to clone genes or isolate and characterize proteins. Similar studies in other fields of medical practice using these novel methodologies will be critical in the future.

The diversity of the preceding examples is a small sampling from a field rich in opportunity for improving medical care for millions of people in this country and around the world. An important interface in bringing these technologies to patients is the clinical investigator—the bridging scientist. The remarkable progress that has been evidenced in fundamental biology brings with it parallel opportunities for investigations in human populations. The realm of biomedical research can be viewed as a spectrum, with fundamental research occurring throughout the spectrum, some of which uses humans to answer crucial questions about human health and behavior. Thus, there is no discontinuity between fundamental biological science and clinical investigation. Indeed, it is progress throughout this research spectrum that frames the opportunities for progress in clinical research.

Increasing levels of sophistication and the assurance of an ample supply of excellent clinical investigators to carry technological advances to medical practice remain critical issues if the country is to continue to improve its health care system. There is growing evidence, however, of a discontinuity in the process of translating new research discoveries into improved health care; the process is further threatened by a potential lack of well-trained clinical investigators to provide the bridge to bring these discoveries into improved medical care (Kelley, 1988).

In the 20 years following World War II, bountiful resources were provided by the federal government to support research, primarily at the nation's research universities and medical schools (U.S. Department of Health, Education, and Welfare, Public Health Service, 1976). This paradigm of peer-reviewed, university-based research has been attributed to the wisdom and foresight of Vannevar Bush (Bush, 1945). Resources were not only plentiful for supporting research but numerous programs were also initiated to build the physical research infrastructure and train more highly talented scientists (Institute of Medicine, 1990). The biomedical research community responded, and the nation's health research capacity expanded significantly. During this period research that involved interactions with human subjects, possibly with the exception of psychological studies, was primarily the domain of physician-scientists. Many of these physician-scientists were motivated to pursue research careers because of the rapid advances in biomedicine and the potential to become critical players in medical discovery. Others may have pursued research to avoid military service in an unpopular war in Southeast Asia. Nonetheless, after completing their clinical training residencies, many physicians sought fellowships at the National Institutes of Health (NIH) and subsequently moved into academic and research positions around the country. Whatever their motivation, most of these scientists have contributed to the fount of knowledge that serves as the basis of modern health care.

In the late 1970s and early 1980s, many leaders in the medical research community expressed concern about a perceived decline in the participation rates of physicians engaged in all aspects of biomedical research (DiBona, 1979; Gill, 1984; Kelley, 1980 and 1985; Thier et al., 1980; Wyngaarden, 1979). This perception was supported by data demonstrating that the ratio of M.D.s to Ph.D.s successfully obtaining research grant awards from NIH was declining. More alarming was the notion that individuals who were highly trained in patient care and who were considered the technology transfer agents were not seeking rigorous scientific training, which widened the gap between basic research discoveries and application of these advances to improved health care (Glickman 1985; Healy, 1988). Furthermore, although some physicians were seeking training in the basic biological sciences, there was a perception that few were being trained to develop and test hypotheses in human subjects or populations (Forrest, 1980). Ironically, data show that the number of full-time faculty in medical schools has grown by more than 20,000 over the past decade, to nearly 65,000. (Data from the Association of American Medical Schools report that medical school faculty totaled 65,000 in 1990, whereas data collected for the Liaison Committee for Medical Education reports that faculty totals were nearly 80,000.) It has been hypothesized that this growth reflects a growing dependence on medical center profits to offset increasing constraints on research funds and shrinking subsidies for graduate medical education (Chin, 1985; Hughes et al., 1991). Although faculty members are required to perform scholarly activity, there appears to be an increasing demand on the clinical faculty to derive revenue through patient care. Furthermore, the growth in clinical faculty may have increased tensions between the faculty in basic science departments and those in the clinical departments. These tensions may arise because basic science faculty fear that their research funding base is being eroded by growing research activities in the clinical departments, and the growing number of clinical faculty bringing in patient care dollars positions the latter on a firmer financial footing. There is also a perception that some academic clinicians pursue research as a secondary interest and are not serious investigators. Many of these clinicians also feel that they cannot obtain tenure by performing human subject research, where the results may not be realized for many years and funding is believed to be extremely difficult to obtain. Moreover, those clinicians who focus on human research fear that they are perceived as second-rate scientists by their colleagues who perform fundamental research in both clinical and basic science departments.

A cause and effect has been difficult, if not impossible, to prove. Determining the size of the cohort of clinical investigators is fraught with error, because no database currently exists to track these investigators. Moreover, there has been no systematic way to collect and analyze data on the number of individuals who choose to perform clinical investigations, the availability of training pathways, or the outcomes of those few programs that do exist. Although many believe that quantitative factors such as debt and economic status directly influence decisions to pursue academic and research careers, there appear to be no measures for factoring in personal considerations such as the effects of mentors and role models, the desire to spend time with one's family, or having leisure time to pursue other personal interests. The growing base of fundamental science, the increasing complexity of medical care and understanding outcomes or effectiveness research, the difficulty (real or perceived) in obtaining research funding, and countless demands on an investigator's time all seem to weigh heavily against pursuing a career in research, particularly research that involves interactions with human subjects. The many employment sectors that require this expertise, such as federal agencies and industry, are also obstacles to conducting a thorough analysis.

Although most attention has been focused on the plight of physician-scientists, many other professional groups are experiencing similar difficulties in the area of human research. As in medicine, training for research careers in other professions is often fragmented, and the career pathways that young trainees should pursue are not clearly delineated. Although many of these other professions also provide outstanding training for delivering care, their programs may not be specifically structured for developing research capabilities. Thus, the Institute of Medicine (IOM) sought to undertake an analysis of the problems affecting the career paths leading to clinical research.

ORIGINS OF THE STUDY

IOM has had an ongoing concern about the problems in the biomedical research arena, and particularly those problems confronting researchers who perform studies that require human subject participation. In 1988, IOM was commissioned by NIH to conduct a study to assess the availability of resources for performing research using patients. The committee was asked to consider a series of issues, including the effects of changes in the health care system on the environment for clinical research; how to improve the recruitment of medical students and residents into clinical research careers; identification of barriers to translating basic research advances into clinical practice; how to improve the relationships among clinical researchers, federal sponsors, and industry; the organization of clinical research; and how to stimulate interest in evaluative clinical sciences. Whereas that committee was asked to examine clinical research in the narrow sense of human subject research, the data from NIH that were available to the committee included all research on humans or human materials approved by institutional review boards, as indicated on Public Health Service grant application form number 398. This included research on all human material such as DNA, RNA, proteins, cells, or body fluids for in use in vitro studies, not necessarily material related to a patient's disease or involving the patient. Moreover, the committee was not able to glean any information from the private sector, either for-profit or nonprofit, to construct a complete picture of the resource base for patient-oriented clinical research.

Following the release of its report, *Resources for Clinical Investigation* (Institute of Medicine, 1988), the IOM Board on Health Sciences Policy convened a working group to reexamine issues related to clinical research. The working group recognized that the heterogeneous nature of the research training pathways for physician-scientists and the broad spectrum of research questions pursued by those investigators had complicated earlier analyses. The working group met twice to develop a strategy for exploring problems associated with the clinical research training pathways, particularly for physician-scientists. The working group sought to refine an approach that would isolate only the small portion of physician-scientist training that it felt was in a particularly vulnerable stage— patient-oriented clinical research—and did not attempt to address all the problems associated with physicians engaging in basic or health services research.

In December 1989, the National Research Council released the quadrennial report *Biomedical and Behavioral Research Scientists: Their Training and Supply* (National Research Council, 1989), which examined research training supported by the Public Health Service through National Research Service Awards (NRSAs). Although that report presented a detailed analysis of the doctoral biomedical and behavioral research workforce and recommended the numbers of NRSA trainees that should be supported, it paid scant attention to physician-scientists and largely ignored dentist- and nurse-scientists. The reasons for these ommissions remain unclear, but they probably are the result of the inability to develop clearly defined populations of scientists in these professions. Whereas physicians, dentists, and nurses engage in a broad spectrum of fundamental research activities, they are critical players in clinical research. Although this group of scientists has often been referred to as clinical researchers because of their clinical degrees, they might be more appropriately referred to as clinician-researchers. Furthermore, the population of doctoral scientists engaged in human research also has remained undefined.

Following the release of the 1989 NRSA study, IOM's Committee on Policies for Allocating Health Sciences Research Funds released a report in 1990, *Funding Health Sciences Research: A Strategy to Restore Balance* (Institute of Medicine, 1990). That committee also acknowledged that the limited understanding of the physician-scientist population and barriers to effective training of that population hampered the committee's attempts to recommend ways to overcome the barriers confronting those investigators. Thus, they recommended that a thorough analysis be performed on physician-scientists to clarify many of these issues.

CHARGE TO THE COMMITTEE

The Committee on Addressing Career Paths for Clinical Research was formed in 1991 and was charged with identifying and evaluating issues in the education and training pathways for individuals pursuing careers in clinical investigation. In particular, the committee was asked to investigate ways to improve the quality of training for clinical investigators and to delineate pathways for individuals pursuing careers in clinical investigation in nursing, dentistry, medicine, and other related health professions engaged in human research. The committee was charged with the following: defining clinical research, how to stimulate individuals to pursue careers in clinical investigation, how to define appropriate curricula for training, how to identify mechanisms to bridge the gap between the basic and clinical sciences, how to address funding mechanisms for clinical investigation, how to establish measures of success in clinical research other than obtaining R01 grant support, how to encourage academic and industrial institutions to protect and reward these valuable investigators, and how to ensure adequate support mechanisms for retaining clinical researchers. For comparison, the committee also examined the pathways that lead physicians toward careers in basic research. The study focused on how existing structures and mechanisms in the federal government, universities, and industry might be used in new and innovative ways to foster careers for these groups of researchers.

The chair of the National Research Council appointed a 16-member committee to address the questions posed in the committee's charge. The committee was composed of active researchers and research administrators with expertise in nursing, dentistry, evaluative clinical sciences, surgery, epidemiology, and various medical subspecialties. The committee viewed several areas as deserving special attention, and these were addressed by task forces, including task forces in surgery, dentistry, nursing, and clinical psychology. The complete task force reports are included as appendexes to this report.

DEFINING CLINICAL RESEARCH

The first item on the committee's agenda was to derive a working definition of clinical research. Various definitions have been used to describe or inventory research and development activities. Many lexicons classify research and development expenditures into the following three general categories: (1) basic research, (2) applied research, and (3) development. Although this classification scheme is useful for describing various research activities for budgetary purposes, it becomes less appropriate for describing cross-disciplinary clinical research, which may encompass portions of each of these categories.

Classification schemes often portray a linear progression of scientific knowledge from basic biological research, to applied research and development, and to improved diagnosis, treatment, and prevention of human disease. Many would argue, however, that a broad spectrum of research activities, from the most basic discoveries of nature to the application of knowledge in humans to understand and treat disease, would more accurately portray biomedical research (Figure 1-1). Furthermore, research activity throughout the spectrum could be bidirectional or demonstrate circular feedback loops for generating new hypotheses. For example, many basic biomedical research questions arise from disease processes first observed in patients. Moreover, the boundaries between many of these subcategories are indistinct, with varying degrees of overlap and movement over time.

Several clinical research classification methodologies have been attempted, each with its own limitations. Clinical research encompasses a vast range of research activities that are conducted by investigators in numerous disciplines. Ahrens has categorized the disparate activities encompassed under the rubric of clinical research into the following seven areas (Ahrens, 1992, pp. 40–48):

1. Studies on the mechanisms of human disease
   - refinements in characterizations of disease processes
   - explorations of unresolved questions in human biology
2. Studies on management of disease
   - evaluations of new diagnostic and therapeutic techniques and devices
   - drug trials (phases II, III, IV)
   - studies of patient compliance and prevention measures
   - searches for accurate prognostic markers
3. In vitro studies on materials of human origin
4. Animal models of human health or disease
5. Field surveys

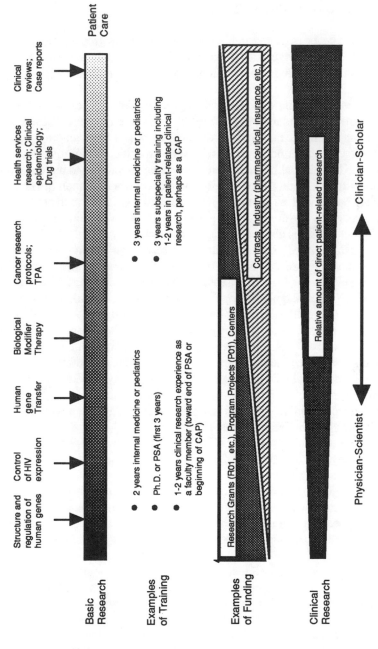

FIGURE 1-1 Diagram depicting the broad spectrum of clinical research, examples of training pathways, and possible sources of research funding. (Adapted from Kelley, 1988.)

6. Development of new technologies
7. Assessment of health care delivery.

All seven categories of research are essential to the progress of medical care and, ultimately, to the prevention of disease. Because the boundaries between these areas are indistinct, individuals can be working in more than one category at any given time.

The committee sought to derive a definition of clinical research that would cut across artificial boundaries to describe the universe of clinical research in terms of research activities or goals. Although there is a large amount of basic biological research that is not directly relevant to specific human diseases, such laboratory-based preclinical bench research may have direct links to understanding normal human function and disease. For example, control of human or retroviral gene expression as well as animal or cellular models of normal or diseased biological processes in humans is often clinically relevant, and under some classification schemes it is defined as clinical research.

At the other end of the spectrum is research on human subjects and populations that have direct application for understanding the prevention, diagnosis, and treatment of human disease by exploiting disciplines such as health services research, clinical epidemiology, and outcomes assessment. Undoubtedly, clinical research includes phase I–III human clinical trials to assess the effectiveness of new methods of intervention or patient management in defined populations. A body of research is also directed at understanding motivational factors for disease prevention and screening and the social and emotional impacts of disease and treatment by employing the disciplines of psychosocial, behavioral, and educational research, which can be considered clinical research. Thus, the committee agreed that there is a continuum of research spanning a wide range of activities that can be regarded as clinical research.

The committee emphasizes that clinical research is not simply that research performed by physicians or other professionals holding clinical degrees. Clearly, many scientists holding doctorates in the basic sciences are performing research that is very clinical in nature; many physicians are also outstanding basic scientists. Although it is very difficult to arrive at an unambiguous definition that will be agreeable to all parties, the committee believes that clinical research should be directed toward the elucidation of human biology and disease, and the control thereof.

The committee emphasized that a common definition should be as broad and inclusive as possible to accurately reflect the population of biomedical scientists generating knowledge about human "dis-ease." Furthermore, the committee acknowledges that clinical researchers may be performing research in more than one category; they may move back and forth along the spectrum as their line(s) of investigation matures or new research questions evolve. Thus, the committee proposes the following definition:

Clinical investigation, broadly defined, includes all studies intended to produce knowledge valuable to understanding the prevention, diagnosis, prognosis, treatment, or cure of human disease. This includes biomedical and health services research carried out in humans, usually by health care professionals, as well as research in organs, tissues, cells, subcellular elements, proteins, and genes derived from humans. It may also include the study of microorganisms as well as studies of other members of the animal kingdom when this research is directed toward human disease.

Whereas this definition is suitably inclusive for all the researchers engaged in clinical research in the broadest sense, the committee identified specific areas that it believes need particular attention. The evolution of the new biology has begun to erode the perceived boundaries among the various medical disciplines as well as the boundaries between basic and clinical research. Moreover, the importance of basic research or other training experiences for teaching research methodology and study design to young clinical investigators cannot be overstated. Thus, the committee felt compelled to develop a broad definition for clinical research and then to focus on areas that it believes need immediate remediation to foster continued progress in clinical research. **The special theme and focus of this study was patient-oriented clinical research, defined as that which requires "hands-on" participation with a human subject as opposed to the entire spectrum of clinical research.** Interpreting its charge, the committee recognized that many professions are engaged in clinical research, including dentistry, nursing, pharmacy, osteopathic medicine, and the behavioral sciences, among others, and sought to include the perspectives of members of those professions as well. Nevertheless, the committee reinforced the common theme of the study and posed the following global questions about clinical research and the clinical research workforce:

- What can clinical research accomplish now and in the future to improve medical care?
- Is the current clinical research community poised and prepared to accomplish these goals?
- If the clinical research community is not prepared to accomplish these goals, what is the evidence that there is either inadequate clinical investigation or an inadequate number of well-trained clinical investigators to meet this need?
- What are the best approaches or best vehicles for change to improve clinical investigation and ensure a supply of highly competent clinical investigators to meet these needs and accomplish the research goals?

LIMITS ON THE SCOPE OF THE STUDY

Although the committee developed a broad definition of clinical research, the major focus of the study was clinical research in which patients serve as the research subjects, often referred to as *patient-oriented, patient-related*, or preferably, *human research*. This category of clinical research includes research activities such as the characterization of healthy and diseased human function; evaluation of new diagnostic, therapeutic, and prognostic techniques, approaches, and devices; medical decision making; patient compliance and disease prevention research; health education research; drug trials; and the assessment of health care practices on patient populations. Thus, the committee's deliberations focused on the issues surrounding the preparation and training of clinical researchers who are engaged in research that requires the direct participation of human subjects. Lastly, although the committee frequently mentions areas of potential clinical research opportunities, it was not charged with developing a research agenda in clinical research and uses the examples only for reference.

CONDUCT OF THE STUDY

During the course of the study, the committee held four meetings to develop strategies and to analyze data. The committee used a variety of approaches to expand its expertise by involving as many avenues of input as possible to achieve its objectives, including four subcommittees, three task forces, a workshop, 11 commissioned papers, and information gained through solicitations of written input and interviews.

Subcommittees

First, the committee divided its members into the following four subcommittees to identify problems along the career pathways of clinical researchers: (1) undergraduate and precollege science education and research training, (2) research training during health professional school, (3) postdoctoral clinical research training, and (4) nurturing clinical research faculty. These subcommittees were convened separately to identify issues confronting their respective portions of the pathways and to develop approaches to collecting and analyzing data that could be used to draw conclusions.

Task Forces

Three task forces were convened in the spring of 1992 to address clinical research issues specific to (1) nursing and clinical psychology, (2) dentistry, and (3) surgery. Each of these task forces was chaired by a member of the committee and the membership was selected from those in the profession. They were charged with the following:

• Describe the clinical research performed by researchers in their respective professions and emphasize how it is different from that in other professions.
• Determine how many researchers in their profession are engaging in clinical research and estimate how many are needed.
• Identify the barriers to careers in clinical research in their profession, including the following:
— Identify what needs to be enhanced or changed to encourage recruitment and the retention of clinical researchers in the profession.
— Identify the funding sources for clinical research in their profession.
• Assess research training for clinical research in their profession.
— Explore the training backgrounds of the current cohort of clinical researchers in the profession.
— Identify the education and training requirements for preparing clinical researchers in the profession.
— Recommend changes necessary to address new clinical research questions for the profession in the future.
— Describe how changes can be implemented or interwoven into existing organizational structures.
— Identify the research training resources for individuals pursuing careers in clinical research for the profession.
• Recommend possible solutions to improving the career pathways leading to clinical research.

The complete task force reports can be found in Appendixes A, B, and C at the end of this report.

Workshop

In June 1992 the committee sponsored a one-and-one-half-day workshop entitled "Clinical Research and Research Training: Spotlight on Funding." The overall goal of the workshop was to analyze training and research funding data and to explore innovative approaches to the training and support of clinical investigators. The first day of the workshop focused on the roles and responsibilities of research sponsors including the federal government, industry, the private nonprofit sector, third-party payers, and academic health centers and research institutions. The second day concentrated on the organizational barriers to clinical research training as well as the funding available for training. A transcript of the meeting was made for the use of the committee in preparing this report, but the committee chose not to publish a separate workshop proceedings.

Commissioned Papers

The committee commissioned 11 background papers to analyze topics of particular importance to the committee's deliberations. Although the findings of the papers are incorporated into this report, the committee felt that the papers were of such high quality and made such significant contributions toward a better understanding of clinical research careers that they encouraged the authors to publish them separately. The following is a list of the paper titles and authors:

1.   "Early Exposure to Research: Opportunities and Effects," by Marsha Lake Matyas of the American Association for the Advancement of Science.
2.   "Advisers, Mentors, and Role Models in Graduate and Professional Education: Implications for the Recruitment, Training, and Retention of Physician-Investigators," by Judith P. Swazey of the Acadia Institute.
3.   "The Effectiveness of Federally Supported Research Training in Preparing Clinical Investigators: Important Questions but Few Answers," by Georgine Pion of Vanderbilt University.
4.   "Considerations of Educational Debt and the Selection of Clinical Research Careers," by Robert L. Beran of the Association of American Medical Colleges.
5.   "Models of Postdoctoral Training for Clinical Research," by Thomas Lee and Lee Goldman of the Brigham and Women's Hospital.
6.   "Models of Postdoctoral Training for Clinical Research," by David Atkins, Richard A. Deyo, Richard K. Albert, Donald J. Sherrard, and Thomas S. Inui of the University of Washington.
7.   "Role of the GCRC in Establishing Career Paths in Clinical Research," by Charles Pak of the University of Texas Health Science Center.
8.   "The Image of the Clinical Investigator," by Edwin Cadman of Yale University.
9.   "University-Industry Relationships in Clinical Research: University Perspective," by David A. Blake of Johns Hopkins University.
10.   "Roles and Responsibilities of Resident Review Committees and Certification Boards in Promoting Research Careers," by Linda Blank of the American Board of Internal Medicine.
11.   "Clinical Research in Allied Health," by Leopold G. Selker of the University of Illinois.

Grants Analysis

The committee also undertook a detailed analysis of R01 grant awards that have been approved by institutional review boards to determine the fraction of awards that are truly patient-oriented, apart from those that use human materials or body fluids. Because the R01 pool represents about 55 percent of the total extramural funds awarded by NIH and because of the large time commitment required to read through grant files, the committee chose to limit the analysis to R01-type grant awards that were considered by initial review groups (study sections) in the Division of Research Grants (DRG). Of the more than 16,000 R01 grants active in fiscal year 1991, about 14,535 were reviewed by DRG study sections; of those, about 4,284 indicated the involvement of human subjects or materials. Of this 4,284, a random sample of 450 from 11 institutes was used for this analysis. The committee reviewed grants provided by the National Cancer Institute, National Heart, Lung, and Blood Institute, National Institute of Deafness and Communicative Disorders, National Institute of Arthritis, Musculoskeletal and Skin Diseases, National Institute of Child and Human Development, National Institute of Neurological Diseases and Stroke, National Institute of Allergy and Infectious Diseases, National Institute of Aging, National Institute of General Medical Sciences, National Institute of Diabetes, Digestive and Kidney Diseases, and National Eye Institute. Since the committee convened task forces on nursing and dentistry that evaluated grants in these disciplines, it did not include grants from the National Institute of Nursing Research (formerly the National Center for Nursing Research at the time the task force was convened) or the National Institute for Dental Research in the analysis. Furthermore, because National Institute of Mental Health, National Institute of Drug Abuse, and National Institute of Alcohol and Alcohol Abuse were not officially part of NIH at the start of this project and the transfer of these institutes was not assured in mid-June of 1992, grants from these institutes also were not included in the analysis. The results of this analysis are presented in Chapter 3.

To supplement the information gleaned from each of the aforementioned mechanisms and to add breadth to the material available to the committee, IOM staff undertook several interviews of staff in various federal agencies, including NIH, the Food and Drug Administration, the Agency for Health Care Policy and Research, and Alcohol Drug Abuse and Mental Health Administration. Many of the data for the study came from NIH staff, to whom the committee is truly indebted. Because of the broad nature of the study, many sectors, public as well as private, contributed valuable information. Appendix E recognizes the many individuals who made important contributions to the report and are not cited elsewhere.

STRUCTURE OF THE REPORT

This report presents the findings from all the aforementioned methods of data collection and analysis. The following chapters elaborate on the issues the committee explored, presents its findings and conclusions, and offers its recommendations for improving clinical research career pathways. Chapter 2 examines the employment sectors and issues and obstacles confronting established clinical investigators, with an emphasis on academic clinical investigators. Chapter 3 discusses the available resources for funding clinical research. The obstacles and barriers to training pathways are presented in Chapter 4. Chapter 5 explores the academic-industry relationships and the roles and responsibilities of investigators in these alliances.

2

Nurturing Clinical Researchers

Despite the tremendous advances made over the past 50 years in the ability to understand, diagnose, and treat human disease, there is a growing and legitimate concern that the pace of clinical research will be significantly hampered at a time when some of the most exciting research developments in the history of medical science are ready for human testing. As more and more is understood about fundamental cellular and molecular biology from the study of cells and animal systems, many questions about basic human biology arise, and these questions can only be answered in human subject studies, or what Ahrens refers to as basic patient-oriented research (Ahrens, 1992). Furthermore, over the past two decades the measures for assessing medical practice and determining medical outcomes have been refined progressively, and this field of research stands on the crest of rapid implementation to improve the practice and delivery of effective health care (Wennberg, 1990).

Clinical investigation in the United Sates is currently threatened by fundamental changes in the organization of health care, major efforts to contain health care expenditures, the high costs of performing clinical studies, such as those associated with drug development, that add to the growing health care budget, and a perceived reduction in the number of individuals pursuing careers in patient-based research. It should be noted that new knowledge gained through scientific investigation is a public good (Pool, 1991). Thus, there is an inherent penalty for those who fund research and a reward for those who let others support it. There is grave danger in a cost-conscious health care reform environment that people will have the notion that clinical research is something

41

that should be supported by someone else. However, society and the payers as society's representatives must recognize the value to all society of support for clinical research. The committee fears that a health care environment that focuses solely on costs or the effort to contain costs will increase the disincentive to invest in clinical research.

Current medical practice and health care rely on sound scientific principles. Clinical research into new therapies, diagnostics, prevention strategies, as well as outcomes assessment of current medical practice requires methods every bit as sophisticated as those required to isolate and clone genes. To develop a sound scientific basis for health practices, a thorough understanding of hypothesis testing and knowledge base in areas such as biochemistry, pharmacology, cellular and molecular biology, statistical methodology, economics, medical informatics, and the social and behavioral sciences is necessary. Design of clinical research without attention to preclinical studies is inappropriate.

Identifying and enrolling suitable patients into clinical research protocols is very time consuming. It is estimated that in many studies only 20 percent of the pool of apparently suitable patients are actually appropriate candidates (Friedman, 1987; Hunter et al., 1987; Martin et al., 1984). Thus, considerable effort is expended by the physician member of a research team who screens patients to enroll suitable subjects into research protocols. Many feel that this time commitment is underappreciated by other scientists and research administrators.

Although clinical investigators are commonly sought for academic departments, highly skilled and talented individuals who understand and can perform complex human studies are also needed by industry and government agencies (Shaw, 1992; Spilker, 1992). Career trajectories are vague, however, and clinical research funding appears tenuous when compared with the funding base for laboratory-based research (Wyngaarden, 1983). For many, the lengthy periods of training required to become skilled in providing high-quality health care conflict with the time demands of becoming outstanding researchers. High levels of educational debt, pressures to develop a unique academic practice and earn one's salary, obligations to family, responsibility to serve on numerous committees, and other commitments add to the pressures confronting junior faculty. On top of these pressures, faculty often find that the institutional paperwork required for different committees overseeing human research activities is virtually endless. Although these are just a few of the barriers and obstacles confronting individuals who choose to perform a human study in academic institutions, these and other problems affect investigators in both the federal government and the private sector.

The academic model in the past was the "triple-threat" faculty member who was expected to be an outstanding researcher, teacher, and clinician simultaneously. Because of the increasing complexity in all three realms, many now believe that the triple threat is no longer feasible and that a clinician can focus on being outstanding in only one, or possibly two, of these areas. This chapter explores the number of faculty available for performing clinical research, examines some of the barriers to careers in clinical research, and suggests some solutions for overcoming the impediments to these career paths.

ENVIRONMENT FOR CLINICAL RESEARCH

Clinical research can be conducted in numerous sites, but the primary locus of most clinical research has been the academic medical center. There are currently 126 accredited allopathic medical schools in the United States, 14 of which are free standing and 112 of which are affiliated with a university. In addition, some academic medical centers are closely affiliated with schools of nursing, pharmacy, or allied health. To trace the course of development to the modern academically based clinical research environment, it is useful to reflect on the history of academic medical centers.

Prior to this century, medical education was the province of voluntary private practitioners. Over the past 100 years, medical education in the United States has undergone vast changes. At the turn of the century there were approximately 155 medical schools in the United States and Canada, and there were three predominant models: the hospital-based clinical model, in which students were trained through programs similar to apprenticeships; the university-based model; and the proprietary or for-profit schools (Burke, 1992). In 1910 Abraham Flexner published a report, "Medical Education in the United States and Canada," based on personal visits and surveys of medical schools (Flexner, 1910). By the time Flexner issued his report, the university-based teaching model was beginning to gain broad acceptance in the United States. Flexner endorsed this model and recommended that the responsibility of medical education be delegated to full-time faculty members who would also be involved in advancing knowledge in medical science as well as training physicians. Moreover, Flexner's description of the for-profit medical schools and the low educational standards of these schools led to the closure of many schools and reforms in a large number of the schools that remained. Flexner's report may thus have served as the catalyst for the shift to staff clinical departments with full-time faculty. This change to full-time faculty in the university-based medical centers, combined with an academic organization similar to those in the other parts of universities, made the medical school more like the rest of the university, with a greater emphasis on scholarly achievement (Fye, 1991).

Largely as a result of the Flexner report, the number of medical schools in the United States dropped to 80 by 1925. Following World War II, the number of medical schools began to rise again as a result of a variety of forces. In 1940 there were about 2,800 full-time medical school faculty. By 1950, the number of faculty had grown by more than 50 percent, to nearly 4,200, and it more than doubled again during the next decade, to reach 11,300 by 1960 (Burke, 1992). This rapid rate of growth was fueled by several policy changes by the federal government, most notably the surge in federal research monies flowing to universities, the government's decision to push for training of more doctors, and the concomitant funding made available for building new medical school facilities throughout the 1960s (Ahrens, 1992; Institute of Medicine, 1990). The number of medical schools grew to 95 by 1969 and to 127 by 1982. There has been only one closure, leaving the present total of 126 medical schools of which 74 are publicly supported institutions and 53 are private (Ahrens, 1992).

CLINICAL RESEARCH WORKFORCE

Obtaining demographic data on the subset of academic faculty performing patient-oriented clinical research is hampered by the lack of a database for recording these data, the heterogeneity of the disciplines engaged in clinical research, and the inability to separate clinical investigator faculty from those with predominantly laboratory-based research or clinical care responsibilities. Furthermore, many faculty may be involved in more than one of these areas, possibly both laboratory and human research or human research and patient care. Unlike the Doctorate Record File database maintained by the National Research Council, which records the doctorates conferred on all graduates of U.S. institutions and gives some indication of the talent pool for biomedical research, comparable listings for medical or dental school graduates do not provide insight into the potential researcher pool in these professions (National Research Council, 1989a). Also, Vaitukaitis has shown that almost half of all grant awards to investigators indicating the use of humans or human materials are to Ph.D.s (Vaitukaitis, 1991). Because clinicians are trained primarily to provide health care, they have alternate career options available if research pathways appear unappealing because of difficulties in funding or other reasons. In addition, there is no way to quantify the reserve pool of clinical investigator talent—the number of adequately trained clinicians who might apply for research funding if the chances for garnering funds were somewhat better.

To gain a clearer understanding of the physician-investigator workforce, it is useful to look at the total pool of U.S. physicians and its subsets, particularly those on the faculties of medical schools, where the majority of academically based clinical investigators are believed to be employed. According to the American Medical Association (AMA) Physician Masterfile, there were more than 615,000 M.D.s in the United States in 1990, of whom about 90 percent were active in medical practice (American Medical Association, 1992). What is very striking is that the number of women physicians has quadrupled since 1970, from 25,401 (7.6 percent of the 334,038 physicians in 1970) to 104,194 (16.9

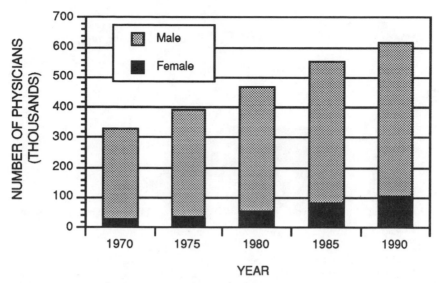

FIGURE 2-1 Total number of U.S. physicians by gender for selected years, 1970–1990. (Source: American Medical Association, 1991.)

percent) in 1990 (Figure 2-1) (American Medical Association, 1991). Moreover, women constitute more than 28 percent of the estimated 134,872 physicians under the age of 35. The growing number of women in the physician workforce implies that particular attention should be paid to clinical research career pathways for this subset as well.

Both the AMA and the Association of American Medical Colleges (AAMC) collect data on medical school faculty, and both sets of data are useful in describing the clinical research workforce. Data collected by the AMA for the Liaison Committee for Medical Education reveal that there were 80,086 medical school faculty in the 1991–1992 academic year (Jolin et al., 1992). The AAMC, however, reports that there were about 75,144 medical school faculty in 1993. Of the latter, 44,838 (59.7 percent) were M.D.s, another 5.4 percent (4,076) were M.D.-Ph.D.s or M.D.s with another health degree (for example, D.Sc., D.P.H., and the like), and the remainder had either a Ph.D. (19,589) or another degree (6,641) (Figure 2-2) (Association of American Medical Colleges, 1993).

Using Institute of Medicine, AMA, and National Institutes of Health (NIH) data, Ahrens has shown that distribution of faculty between clinical and preclinical departments is about 80 percent and 20 percent, respectively (Table 2-1) (Ahrens, 1992). Moreover, the proportion of Ph.D.s on medical school faculties has remained fairly stable, at about 29 percent, since 1970. Whereas

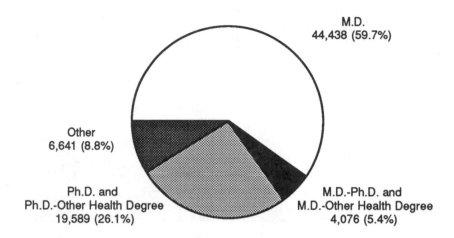

FIGURE 2-2 Distribution of U.S. medical school faculty (Total = 75,144) by degree in 1993. (Source: Reprinted, with permission, from Association of American Medical Colleges [1993], p. 4. Copyright 1993 by Association of American Medical Colleges.)

M.D.s have always been clustered in the clinical departments and more than 90 percent are so assigned, nearly half of the Ph.D.s now have their primary appointment in a clinical department (Ahrens, 1992; Herman, 1986). This represents about a 36 percent increase since 1970, but there is variability in the employment practices among medical schools as well as among departments. What is not known is how many faculty, M.D.s or Ph.D.s, have dual appointments in both the preclinical and clinical sciences, partially because of the inability to track investigators' appointments with any current database. Gaps also exist in quantifying the number of investigators, basic as well as clinical, who are employed by independent teaching hospitals and independent research institutions without medical school affiliations.

Also of interest is the gender, racial, and ethnic distributions of the faculty (Eisenberg, 1989; Grant, 1988). According to the AAMC data, women make up about 23.5 percent of medical school faculty (17,642 of the 75,144 total faculty) (Figure 2-3) (Association of American Medical Colleges, 1993). About 9,666 or slightly more than half (54.8 percent), of women medical school faculty are M.D.s (including M.D.s with Ph.D.s or other health degrees) compared with 68.7 percent (39,181 of 57,007) of male faculty who have an M.D. The proportion of women physicians on medical school faculty exceeds their representation in the overall population of physicians—about about 23 percent versus 17 percent, respectively (see Figures 2-1 and 2-3). Most of the women faculty, however, are clustered in the lower ranks of the faculty (Figure 2-4).

TABLE 2-1 Full-time Faculty in All U.S. Medical Schools, 1961–1989

Fiscal Year	Number of Schools	Number of Awards			Percent in Clinical Departments
		Total	Pre-clinical Departments	Clinical Departments	
1961	86	11,224	4,023	7,201	64.2
1962	86	12,040	4,342	7,698	63.9
1963	87	13,602	4,693	8,909	66.0
1964	88	15,015	5,541	9,474	63.1
1965	89	15,882	5,233	10,649	67.1
1966	89	17,118	5,671	11,447	66.9
1967	92	19,297	5,877	13,420	69.5
1968	99	22,293	6,639	15,654	70.2
1969	101	23,034	7,048	15,986	69.4
1970	103	24,093	7,287	16,806	69.8
1971	108	27,539	8,283	19,256	69.9
1972	112	30,170	8,714	21,456	71.1
1973	114	33,265	9,381	23,884	71.8
1974	114	34,878	9,928	24,950	71.5
1975	114	37,010	10,164	26,846	72.5
1976	116	39,346	10,743	28,603	72.7
1977	122	41,650	11,031	30,349	72.9
1978	125	44,358	11,736	32,622	73.5
1979	126	46,662	12,605	34,057	73.0
1980	126	49,446	12,831	36,665	74.2
1981	126	50,532	12,816	37,716	74.6
1982	127	53,371	13,223	40,148	75.2
1983	127	55,525	13,587	41,938	75.5
1984	127	57,003	13,560	43,443	76.2
1985	127	58,774	13,767	45,007	76.6
1986	127	61,397	14,204	47,193	76.9
1987	127	63,313	14,479	48,834	77.1
1988	127	66,798	14,580	52,218	78.2
1989	127	70,308	14,832	55,476	78.9
Average Annual Growth Rate 1961–1989	1.4%	6.7%	4.8%	7.6%	

Source: Reprinted, with permission, from Ahrens [1992], p. 21. Copyright 1992 by the Oxford University Press, Inc.

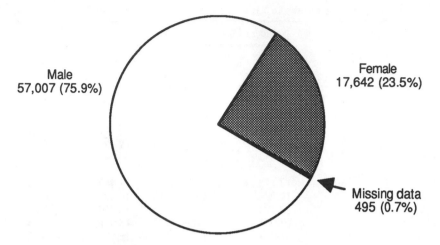

FIGURE 2-3 Distribution of U.S. medical school faculty (Total = 75,144) by gender in
1993. (Source: Association of American Medical Colleges, 1993.)

For example, only 9 percent are full professors, 19 percent are associate
professors, and 50 percent are assistant professors. The remainder are listed as
instructors (18 percent) or have other types of appointments. By comparison,
the male faculty are almost evenly stratified among professors (31 percent),
associate professors (25 percent), and assistant professors (35 percent).

The reasons for women being clustered in the lower professional ranks
remain unclear, but several suggestions have been postulated (Bickel, 1988;
Bickell and Whiting, 1991; Cotton, 1992a and 1992b; Dwyer et al., 1991;
Graves and Thomas, 1985; Levinson and Weiner, 1991). For example, women
did not begin to enter medical schools in significant numbers until the 1970s.
Thus, the age profile of faculty shows that women faculty are younger than their
male counterparts. For example, 36 percent of women faculty are under the age
of 39, compared with 23 percent of male faculty. Only 22 percent of the women
faculty are between the ages of 50 and 69, whereas 36 percent of the male
faculty are in the same age bracket (Association of American Medical Colleges,
1993). Women are only now beginning to enter the top ranks of medical school
faculties in large numbers. There has also been a perceived bias on the part of
promotion committees, which have been dominated by men in the past.

Another apparent barrier to clinical research careers for women is
balancing the responsibilities of family with the demands of a professional
career (Cole and Zuckerman, 1989; Levinson et al., 1989). It is estimated that
nearly 75 percent of women physicians are currently married (American Medical
Association, 1991). Of these, 93 percent of the spouses of married women

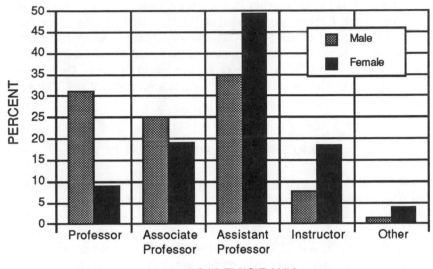

FIGURE 2-4 Distribution of U.S. medical school faculty by gender and academic rank for 1993. (Source: Reprinted, with permission, from Association of American Medical Colleges [1993], p. 8. Copyright 1993 by the Association of American Medical Colleges.)

physicians are employed outside the home, compared with 45 percent for married male physicians. Among married women physicians under the age of 40, about 45 percent are married to other physicians, while less than 10 percent of male married physicians in the same age bracket are married to physicians (American Medical Association, 1991). Another fraction is married to individuals in other professions who are as dedicated to their careers as physicians are. Moreover, about 85 percent of women physicians who are married have children. To maintain competence in their profession, it is believed that physicians must maintain continuity in their practices and that they do not exit and reenter the job market. For those pursuing research careers as well, it is nearly impossible to maintain active participation in research on a part-time or intermittent basis. Thus, the balancing of two-career families and the juggling of two-career families with children can often lead to career compromises by one or both of the parents. It is believed that women, even those in two-professional families, shoulder a disproportionately larger share of the responsibilities of child-rearing and household duties than their male spouses. No reliable data are available to substantiate whether these concerns affect women physicians more than male physicians, however.

Of the 17,642 women faculty, 2,835 (16.1 percent) are nonwhite (Figure 2-5). Most of this fraction are of Asian or Pacific Island descent (more than 9 percent of the total). Of the 57,007 male faculty, 7,105, or about 12.5 percent, are nonwhite (Figure 2-6). Here, too, most of the nonwhite male faculty (almost 8 percent of the total) is of Asian or Pacific Island descent. Only a small fraction of the men or women faculty are African American (1.9 and 3.7 percent, respectively).

RESEARCH INVOLVEMENT OF FACULTY

Data on the research involvement of medical school faculty are sparse. The only comprehensive study of faculty research activity was conducted in 1986 by the Association of Professors of Medicine in conjunction with the AAMC, *Research Activity of Full-Time Faculty in Departments of Medicine* (Beaty et al., 1986; Association of American Medical Colleges, 1987). The parameters of research involvement were effort, funding, laboratory space, and publications. The study concluded that the median research effort of M.D. faculty in departments of medicine was 25 percent, compared with the 95 percent effort of Ph.D.s in the same departments. About 45 percent of the M.D.s and 68 percent of the M.D.-Ph.D.s reported that more than 20 percent of their effort was devoted to research. While 68 percent of the M.D. faculty had some form of external funding to support their research, only 23 percent of the M.D. faculty were principal investigators on an NIH grant. Twenty-five percent reported no research funding. Moreover, 34 percent of the M.D.s and 22 percent of the M.D.-Ph.D.s reported that they had no laboratory space. More striking was the fact that nearly half of the M.D. faculty had not published an original, peer-reviewed article (Association of American Medical Colleges, 1987). Ahrens has also reported that half of the clinical faculty in three departments of his three-department analysis did not publish at least one research article (Ahrens, 1992).

A 1989 follow-up study of internal medicine faculty revealed that there was no difference among M.D., M.D.-Ph.D., and Ph.D. faculty who had been or were principal investigators on a peer-reviewed research grant application (60, 61, and 58 percent, respectively). Although 52 percent of those conducting research were doing laboratory research, only 7 percent were performing patient-related research; 29 percent were involved in both (Levey et al., 1988).

ACADEMIC RECOGNITION

Promotions committees, and particularly tenure committees at competitive medical schools, require proof of a candidate's scholarly contributions.

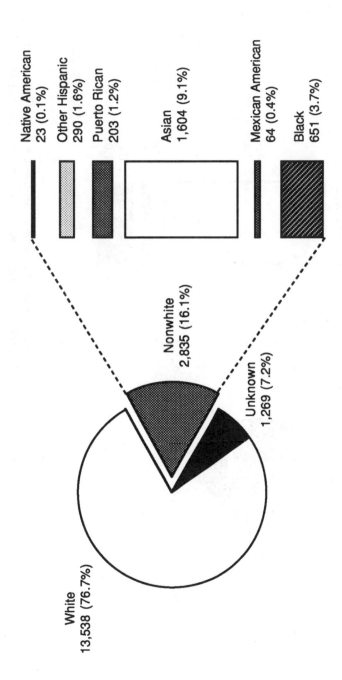

Native American
23 (0.1%)

Other Hispanic
290 (1.6%)

Puerto Rican
203 (1.2%)

Asian
1,604 (9.1%)

Mexican American
64 (0.4%)

Black
651 (3.7%)

Nonwhite
2,835 (16.1%)

Unknown
1,269 (7.2%)

White
13,538 (76.7%)

FIGURE 2-5 Distribution of female U.S. medical school faculty by race and ethnicity. (Source: Reprinted, with permission, from Association of American Medical Colleges [1993], p. 7. Copyright 1993 by the Association of American Medical Colleges.)

52

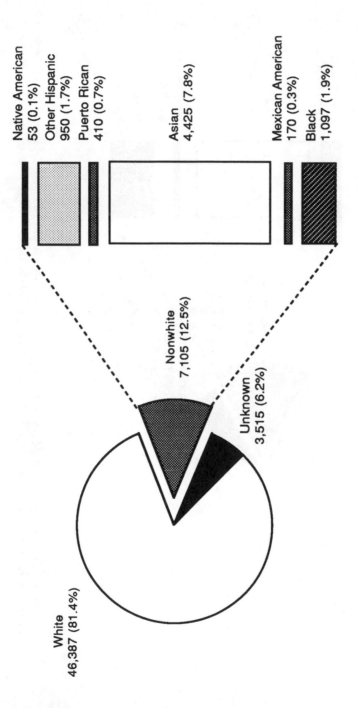

FIGURE 2-6 Distribution of female U.S. medical school faculty by race and ethnicity. (Source: Reprinted, with permission, from Association of American Medical Colleges [1993], p. 9. Copyright 1993 by the Association of American Medical Colleges.)

However, what constitutes scholarship is not clearly defined. Although Boyer has suggested a broadening of what constitutes scholarly activity, over the past few decades scholarship in biomedicine has become equated with research, particularly laboratory-based research that frequently allows rapid data collection and publication (Boyer, 1987). Scholarship is, in turn, measured by one's ability to obtain competitive grant funds and publish results in peer-reviewed journal articles (Abrahamson, 1991; Applegate, 1990). Laboratory investigators, who devote all their time to research, usually have protected time to pursue research that is secured by grant funds. Clinical investigators, however, less frequently have grants to support their salaries and protect a segment of time to perform research activity. Thus, defining reliable measures of scholarship based on research activities for clinical investigators is much more difficult than for bench scientists (Bickel, 1991; Bickel and Whiting, 1991).

Physician faculty in clinical departments have certain patient care responsibilities that are distinctly different from those of physicians in independent research institutes, private industry, or preclinical departments (Blackburn, 1979). Clinical research faculty are generally hired to care for patients and teach clinical medicine to students, house staff, and clinical fellows—demands that are not made on nonclinical faculty. The economic necessity of maintaining a clinical department in financial balance has placed a greater emphasis on the clinical care component of a department's activities (Chin, 1985). Although a large portion of medical school revenues were previously derived from research funds, a review of medical school financing demonstrates that a growing fraction of medical school revenues are derived from professional practice plans (Hughes et al., 1991). During the late 1980s the revenues from professional services began to exceed those derived from research sources (Figure 2-7) (Ahrens, 1992; Jolin et al., 1992).

Although junior faculty members are recruited with the expectation that they will develop creative lines of investigation, the pressures of starting an academic practice, building a referral base, and contributing to departmental coffers can be overwhelming (Applegate, 1990; Jones et al., 1985). Academic health centers have contributed to these pressures and problems by imposing expanded funding expectations on young physician-investigators. It is believed that these investigators can support themselves with clinical income while performing pilot research studies and until they gain grant support. This also reinforces the disincentive to pursue clinical research when funding appears tenuous and encourages young investigators to pursue more secure career opportunities in bench research.

The perception that laboratory-based research is more scholarly and leads more readily to promotion lures junior faculty away from patient-based research. Moreover, while NIH and industry provide substantial sums of money for large, multi-institutional clinical studies and clinical trials, the principal investigators

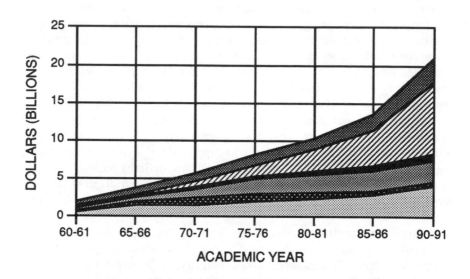

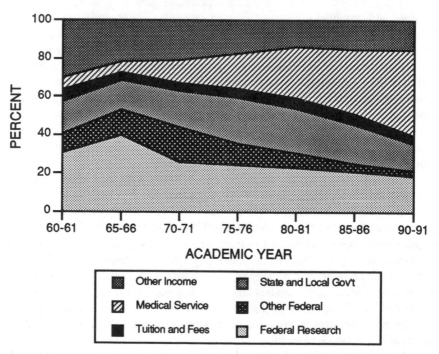

FIGURE 2-7 Distribution of sources of revenue for medical schools, 1961–1990. Top panel shows revenue sources in billions of 1990 dollars. Bottom panel shows the distribution as a percent of the annual total. (Source: Jolin et al., 1992.)

are, of necessity, generally well-established senior investigators. For a newly independent junior faculty member, the inability to compete successfully for NIH funding, identify a unique research niche, and develop one's research independence seem to be insurmountable obstacles (Cohen, 1991). In addition, the necessity to participate in multicenter projects that require a large team approach is unappealing. Moreover, it takes many months for scientific and human protection committees to review and approve a human study protocol before patients can be enrolled in a clinical study. The new congressional requirement for subgroup analysis of women and minorities will also increase the size and cost of each clinical trial as well as the difficulty of enrolling patients into each trial. The time required to initiate, implement, and publish a human study is thus prolonged and arduous, and the potential number of publications from these studies over a similar period of effort is perceived to be fewer than that for laboratory-based research. Therefore, junior faculty perceive that the best route to promotion is development of a laboratory-based research effort. Laboratory experiments with well-established controls often can be completed rapidly; determining the clinical correlates in a patient-based clinical study can take years. Consequently, clinical research publications are frequently case reports or descriptive reviews of patients (Cadman, 1993).

FACULTY TRACKS

Perceptions of second-class faculty status abound in both camps of the medical school faculty. Some physicians feel that their laboratory-based Ph.D. colleagues regard them as having inferior training in scientific methods and, therefore, as being less sophisticated scientists. At the same time, the Ph.D. community sometimes feels that it is perceived as second-class faculty by its physician colleagues, particularly those with a primary appointment in a clinical department. Even Ph.D.s in clinical departments feel that they are viewed as outcasts by their Ph.D. colleagues in the preclinical departments. Although it is nearly impossible to diminish these perceptions, no empirical data exist to support the conjecture that one group is superior to or more productive than the other in conducting research. Each clearly has unique contributions to make to expanding the knowledge base of medical science.

Institutions have dealt with these issues through different means. Some institutions have established multiple career tracks for the physician faculty to recognize their different scholarly contributions (Bickel, 1991; Bickel and Whiting, 1991). For example, the Department of Internal Medicine at the University of Michigan initiated a two-track system for tenurable clinical faculty that is intended to define the expectations of departmental faculty by the department's leadership (Kelley and Stross, 1992). In addition to the nontenurable, full-time clinical faculty, tenurable faculty are divided into physician-scientists and clinician-scholars. Although both groups are required to commit approximately 20 percent of their effort to teaching, the remaining time commitment is different for the two tracks. Physician-scientists are expected to commit the remaining 80 percent of their effort to research and receive departmental support for start-up, space, and personnel for initiating their research activities. Clinician-scholars are expected to spend 50 percent of their effort in the direct care of patients without a teaching component and 30 percent of their effort in research. Although clinician-scholars are not provided laboratory space, they do receive support for personnel, travel, computers, and other activities. The obvious advantages of a well-delineated multiple-track system are acknowledgment of the range of scholarly contributions that can be made by the clinical faculty and the fact that the expectations of performance and scholarship for all faculty groups are clearly defined at the outset.

Other institutions have remained committed to a single-track system, holding all faculty to the same academic standards for promotion. For example, Batshaw and others (1988) undertook an analysis of the single-track system at Johns Hopkins University School of Medicine to determine whether clinician-teachers were less likely to be promoted than the research-intensive faculty (Batshaw et al., 1988). The study concluded that there were no significant differences between the probabilities that clinical and research faculty would be promoted to either associate or full professor at Johns Hopkins University School of Medicine. Probably more significant was the fact that those who were promoted published nearly twice as many articles in peer-reviewed journals as those who were not promoted. No distinction was made between publishing clinical or basic science articles.

There is no easy way to change the perceptions about promotion and tenure. Each group has made significant contributions to building the knowledge base for medical care—basic scientists for their contributions in understanding fundamental biological processes, physician-scientists for translating new technologies to clinical practice, and clinician-scholars for their ability to implement new approaches based on sound scientific knowledge. Whether an institution has multiple tracks or not should not detract from the overall balance of objectives of the academic health center.

The committee believes that one avenue might be to encourage each group to gain an appreciation for the other's contributions. At least one institution, Tufts University School of Medicine, has implemented a course to provide Ph.D.s with the perspective of clinical sciences (Arias, 1989). The course is not intended to train Ph.D.s to become clinicians; its goal is to facilitate a dialogue between basic scientists and clinical investigators. Some professional societies are also adding symposia and instructional courses to the agendas of their annual meetings in an attempt to bridge the chasm between basic scientists and clinicians. For example, the American Federation of Clinical Research, the American Society for Clinical Investigation, and the American Association of

Physicians sponsor annual symposia on molecular biology for the nonmolecular biologist and clinical epidemiology and health services research for the novice. It is hoped that courses such as this will create a synergism from which new and exciting collaborations will ultimately flow. These types of linkages will become even more critical as the fruits of the biological revolution move toward human applications and the need to evaluate these new medical care practices grows.

COMPETING TIME DEMANDS

To reserve research time, an investigator must be able to garner research funds. To be competitive, an investigator must demonstrate competence in designing and conducting a research project. Even a small clinical study can require considerable funds and resources, including computers, data managers, research nurses, computers, and patients. Thus, protected time and a recruitment package, similar to those offered to junior laboratory-based investigators, must be made available to clinical investigators.

The ability to be a triple-threat (physician, teacher, scientist) may be limited in today's academic health care environment. Clinical faculty at all levels are required to maintain competence in their field of specialty or subspecialty to be board certified. The effects of the new policies regarding time-limited recertification recently implemented by many boards may have unintended negative consequences on clinical investigative careers. Clinical investigators need to be specialists in their areas of investigation and strive for academic recognition through scholarly contributions to the medical knowledge base. Recertification will require that a physician be competent in treating the broad spectrum of maladies in a particular subspecialty. However, this requirement seems to be in direct conflict with the goals of academic medicine, by which academically based physicians are frequently narrowly focused within the subspecialty in which they work to impart new knowledge about a particular disease or treatment thereof. Were they not so focused, it would be difficult to assess their scholarly contributions.

CLINICAL RESEARCH TRAINING

The training of clinical investigators has been fragmented and diverse (Levey, 1988). Many have had no specific research training other than the design and analysis of a research project during a subspecialty fellowship under the supervision of a mentor (Neinstein and Mackenzie, 1989; Burke, 1986). Some who are interested in epidemiology and outcomes assessment may have completed master's programs in public health either before or after obtaining their M.D. degrees. The model that many clinical investigators have followed, however, is one or more years of laboratory-based research. In the efficient transfer of technology from the laboratory to the bedside and in the development of laboratory-based research to study questions arising in the clinical environment, an understanding of laboratory investigation can be invaluable (Littlefield, 1986). Although this model has been effective in allowing physicians to gain basic skills in research design and hypothesis testing, its effectiveness in providing the requisite skills for clinical research is unknown. It is believed that laboratory experience, however, is inadequate preparation for designing and conducting clinical research, which has its own set of methods, techniques, and ways of posing and answering relevant scientific questions using humans subjects (Feinstein, 1985a and 1985b; Fletcher et al., 1982; Janowsky et al., 1986; Nathan, 1988; Stolley, 1988).

Physicians who are trained exclusively in laboratory techniques may not be appropriately prepared to design and execute clinical studies without further clinical research training in fields such as biostatistics, ethics, regulatory issues, patents and licensing, pharmacology, and medical economics or other bridging disciplines. NIH supports a myriad of training programs that are available to physicians in various stages of training. As elucidated in Chapter 4, however, the overwhelming majority of programs are directed toward laboratory research. A few programs focus on human research or clinical epidemiology, such as the Robert Wood Johnson Clinical Scholars program, but outcomes data from these programs are sparse. The problem may be circular, in that the paucity of funds, perceived or real, for human studies, in turn, places a low priority on clinical research training. Therefore, resources are not allocated and clinical research training programs are not funded.

MENTORING

The importance of mentors and role models in the training pathways for research scientists of all types cannot be understated (Cameron, 1981). Although the literature is laden with the educational and training needs for physicians pursuing research career paths, scant attention has been paid to the roles and influences of mentors, advisers, or role models. Each of these is believed to play a crucial role in stimulating individuals to pursue a particular career path, shaping the content of their training, socializing them in the research environment, and providing support and guidance in the formative stages of their career (Swazey, 1994). Whereas being a role model is largely passive, the development of a mentor-protégé relationship is a gradual, interactive process that builds on interpersonal relationships. Unfortunately, few empirical data exist on the effects of mentoring, and adequate elucidation of what constitutes effective relationships between a mentors and trainees, and the effects of mentoring on the developing clinical investigator have not been adequately addressed. Judith Swazey's white paper "Advisors, Mentors, and Role Models in Graduate and Professional Education: Implications for the Recruitment, Training, and Retention of Physician-Investigators" (Swazey, 1994), explores the nature of each of these relationships in shaping a clinical investigator.

When internal medicine faculty were asked what factors most influenced their career choice to be a physician-investigator, a mentor was considered among the most important (Levey et al., 1988). A vigorous evaluation of the components of a successful academic career confirms the value of a mentor. The study by Levey et al. (1988) documented that the supporting and nurturing roles of a mentor during the first few years of faculty member's research experience were critical for launching a productive career. In addition to providing ongoing supervision and training and introducing the junior faculty member to the mechanics of being a successful investigator, the most respected mentors also offered emotional support.

Although many agree that mentoring is a significant force shaping the careers of young investigators, there is little consensus in the literature on the roles or responsibilities of a mentor (Calkins and Wakeford, 1982). Vance (1982) has encapsulated the essence of a mentor as "someone who serves as a career role model and who actively advises, guides, and promotes another's career and training" (p. 10). As Swazey points out in her paper a broad range of qualities, characteristics, and functions is ascribed to mentors (Swazey, 1994). A mentor can function as a coach, counselor, teacher, advocate, protector, sponsor, guide, and confidant. To this end, a mentor's activities include teaching cognitive knowledge and technical skills; developing the protégé's intellectual abilities; providing advice, encouragement, and criticism; helping their protégé learn risk-taking behavior, effective communications skills, and institutional and professional skills; fostering involvement in research and scholarly productivity; and facilitating entry into postgraduate or initial career positions and career advancement (Swazey, 1994). Swazey summarizes a good or successful mentor as one who is self-confident, willing to share, patient, understanding, available and accessible, willing to commit time and emotion to the mentor-protégé relationship, influential in one's field, and genuinely interested in the professional development of the protégé. Conversely, mentors should not be overprotective or supervise too closely, be harshly harshly critical or focus on inadequacies, be manipulative, withhold information, take over projects, or exploit the protégé. In conclusion, an effective mentor knows when to encourage independence and derives personal satisfaction in providing assistance and advice to help shape the career of a trainee without the expectation of being a part of the published accomplishments.

LIFESTYLE ISSUES

Similar to individuals in other professional careers, physicians in training pursue various career paths with the expectation that they will have rewarding employment opportunities upon completion of their training. The pathway to being a successful clinical investigator is not an easy one. It requires energy, drive, ambition, devotion, initiative, entrepreneurship, individualism as well as team work, and plenty of hard work (Rahmitoola, 1990). In return, fair compensation is essential to afford adequate housing, provide for a family, and purchase a reliable automobile, particularly at the junior faculty level.

Many trainees and junior faculty, however, perceive the financial security of an academic career as ephemeral. For many who have incurred large educational debt burdens during college and medical school, the financial insecurity of an academic career serves as a disincentive for choosing this career path. Many believe that the large educational debt, the discrepancy between the incomes of academically based physicians compared with those of physicians in private practice, the difficulty of garnering competitive research funding from NIH and other sources for basic as well as clinical research, and obstacles to advancement in the academic community discourage trainees from pursuing academic career paths (Hughes et al., 1991; Institute of Medicine, 1988a). The implications of debt and career choices will be covered more thoroughly in Chapter 4.

CONCLUSIONS

In conclusion, the committee believes that there are numerous hurdles confronting clinical investigators at all levels of faculty career development. Recognition in the academic health center includes promotion, protected time, and financial support. The scholarship of the successful clinical investigator should be appropriately recognized in the academic setting. This includes recognition that the nature of the clinical investigator's research, the sources of the funding, and the journals in which investigators publish may differ substantially from those of fundamental investigators.

Leadership at all levels within these institutions must define their expectations of junior faculty and support them so that these young men and women can meet and exceed the expectations. Teaching and serving as role models, advisers, and mentors are important in attracting students to careers in clinical investigation. These faculty activities, therefore, must be recognized and rewarded.

In addition to well-trained and adequately funded patient-based clinical investigators, the successful execution of patient-based clinical research requires a suitable institutional infrastructure. Similar to newly independent, laboratory-based researchers, recruitment packages for clinical investigators should include protected time for setting up and conducting clinical studies as well as resources such as space, computer equipment, data management, and research support personnel.

University-based and research-intensive medical centers should develop mechanisms to achieve the optimal infrastructure to support inpatient- and outpatient-based clinical research. The features of such an infrastructure may include a clinical practice that is structured to deliver health care in a scholarly and investigative fashion and the integration of students, residents, fellows, and other health care professionals into human research activities. In addition, multidisciplinary facilities are required at universities to support core requirements for clinical research; these might include such elements as biostatistics, data management, and an opportunity to work with other health professionals. Creative start-up efforts through university mechanisms to establish core facilities that will seek continued funding through extramural sources represent important activities that should be strongly encouraged within the academic setting.

The committee believes strongly that the translation and application of advances in research to patient care require a strong partnership between academic institutions and industry. Facilitation of technology transfer by both parties is important and deserves special support. The relationship between faculty, the academic institution, and industry is changing dramatically and represents a new paradigm. This will require new standards in the definition and resolution of conflicts of interests at all levels in support of this change. Academia-industry relationships are covered more thoroughly in Chapter 5.

3

Clinical Research Funding and Infrastructure

About $22 billion (16.7 percent) of the estimated $132 billion currently invested in research and development (R&D) by all sectors in the United States is health related (National Institutes of Health, 1993b; National Science Foundation, 1992). The federal government is generally regarded as the primary sponsor of biomedical research, but, in fact, funding comes from a myriad of public and private sponsors, each with their own objectives or missions. During the 1980s, however, the portion supported by the federal government plummeted, decreasing from 59 percent in 1980 to an estimated 41 percent in 1992 (Figure 3-1) (National Institutes of Health, 1993b). The most notable change in this ratio over the past decade has been the growing contribution by industry, which has grown from 31 to 48 percent over the same period. Of the remainder, private nonprofit organizations supported about 4 to 5 percent, and state and local governments supported a small amount of health research.

Although less well appreciated, the contributions by the academic health centers themselves cover many of the costs of performing research (Commonwealth Fund, 1985). For example, many centers sponsor a variety of research activities with their own funds, such as covering the costs of starting up newly independent investigators, providing bridging funds for ongoing, high-quality research activities that fell just short of the funding level because of limited federal funds, and funding other projects that for various reasons may not or cannot be funded by other sponsors. Private philanthropy is not easily quantified, because it can be derived from a variety of private sources and large gifts or commitments to build research infrastructure may not be included in the accounting for research.

63

Also intertwined in this labyrinth of clinical research funding is the role of third-party payers. Although third-party payers, particularly Medicare, have underwritten some of the costs of medical education, the costs of experimental or investigational therapies have not generally been allowed as reimbursable, even though the results of clinical studies will define future standards for medical care. The growing concerns about cost-containment and a shift toward managed care are having an effect on what insurers will cover, even in the use of standard therapy (Antman et al., 1988 and 1989; Wittes 1987b). The committee is concerned that these coverage decisions might not be based on the best and most up-to-date information. Furthermore, cost-containment decisions might encourage the use of outmoded therapies rather than foster the timely introduction of truly novel or innovative therapies that could lead to long-term savings. Some feel that insurers and other third-party payers have a fundamental interest in and responsibility for supporting evaluative, patient-oriented clinical research to engage in coverage decisions and to facilitate the adoption of more cost-effective care (leaf, 1989; Newcomer, 1990). The total costs of clinical research cannot be shifted to insurers, but they are participants in providing care and should support and promote definitive studies that will define standards of care, assess the effectiveness of current therapies, and provide new effective therapies. Thus, the committee includes here a section on the roles and responsibilities of third-party payers.

Realizing how critical funding is to successful research careers, particularly the perception by clinical scientists of their inability to garner funds for patient-oriented studies, the committee devoted time to develop a clearer understanding of the research funding base. Many of the commissioned papers included some reference to the tenuous nature of research funding, and the committee sponsored an invitational workshop, "Clinical Research and Training: Spotlight on Funding," in June 1992. This chapter explores trends in research funding by the various sectors. Because of inadequate data collection methods by research sponsors, it was frequently impossible to disaggregate research funds devoted to patient-oriented clinical research from other research funds. When possible, however, the trends in funding for patient-related research are elaborated. Since academic research careers are closely intertwined with the investigator-initiated, peer-reviewed grant system in the Public Health Service, including the National Institutes of Health (NIH) (and previously the Alcohol, Drug Abuse and Mental Health Administration [ADAMHA]), the committee focused considerable attention on this process.

THE BIG PICTURE

Prior to World War II, health research was sponsored primarily by industry, academic institutions, and private individuals (Ginzberg and Dutka, 1989).

Following the war, policy changes initiated by Vannevar Bush, then head of the Office of Scientific Research and Development, began the surge of federal investment in university-based fundamental research. Bush and his colleagues formulated a set of proposals intended to sustain the nation's wartime research momentum and direct it toward civilian goals. These policies, outlined in his report to the President, "Science—the Endless Frontier" (Bush, 1945), proposed a coordinated federal policy of investing in research and the training of new researchers that would be driven by scientific merit rather than by political or geographical interests. This approach became the cornerstone of the peer-reviewed, academically based system now in place for federally sponsored, competitive extramural research grant programs. From the end of the war to the mid-1960s, the federal government invested heavily in health research and allocated resources to build health research facilities and to create programs to train health researchers (Institute of Medicine, 1990). Moreover, the synergism between federally sponsored research and research sponsored by industry and the private nonprofit sectors thrust the United States into the forefront of biomedical research.

In the 1960s, increasing allocations for the war in Southeast Asia and the Cold War buildup began to constrain the federal resources available for domestic programs, including health research. In the 1970s, the health research budget plateaued, and high inflationary pressures further reduced the purchasing power of research funds. Over the past decade, the nation's expenditures for health research have tripled when measured in current dollars. After adjusting for inflation, which was relatively low throughout the 1980s, this investment grew by 65 percent (Figure 3-1).

The health research enterprise has been highly successful, but the system has become increasingly stressed in recent years. The most significant reason is the concern over growing federal debt and recent legislation attempting to reduce the huge annual federal budget outlays. The 1980's policy of increased spending but decreased taxes has put the U.S. government in a precarious financial position and has mortgaged the country for many years to come. There are anticipated decreases in defense spending, but expectations for increased funding in other categories of the federal budget remain low. Recent attempts to reduce federal deficits have increased the competition for scarce funds for all federally financed programs. State funds and those from private-sector sources have been unable to compensate for the slower growth of available federal funds. The increasing competition among worthy projects has often resulted in concessions to short-term needs rather than longer-term investments. The combination of increasing research costs and increasingly constrained funding has sent shock waves throughout the academic research community (Lederman, 1991; Movsesian, 1990). The broad array of research sponsors and the decentralized nature of the research of thousands of individual investigators are responsible for the success of health research over the past half-century.

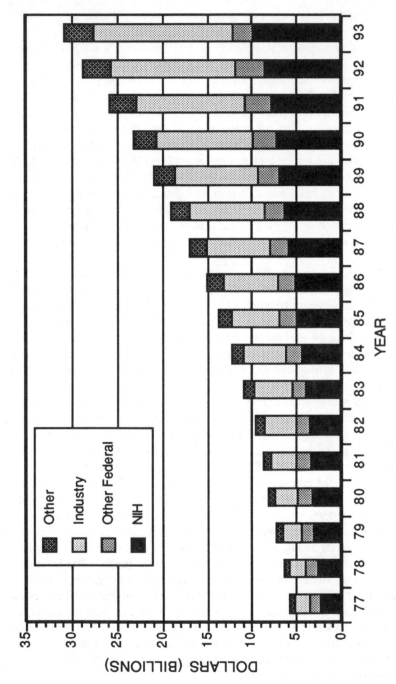

FIGURE 3-1 U.S. Support for health research and development by source of funds from 1977 to 1993. (Source: National Institutes of Health, 1993b.)

FEDERAL SUPPORT FOR HEALTH SCIENCES R&D

As a result of the postwar policy changes, the federal government became the largest single sponsor of health research, and programs that support health research can be found in numerous federal agencies (U.S. Congress, Office of Technology Assessment, 1991). About three fifths of these funds now come from programs in the U.S. Department of Health and Human Services (DHHS), including those in the Public Health Service (PHS) (Figure 3-2) (National Institutes of Health, 1993b). Within the PHS, NIH—which now includes the National Institute of Alcohol and Alcohol Abuse, the National Institute of Drug Abuse, and the National Institute of Mental Health—allocate the largest percentage of federal funds for health-related research (Figure 3-2). Research funds are also appropriated for the Centers for Disease Control and Prevention (CDC); the Health Care Financing Administration; the Health Resources Administration; the Food and Drug Administration (FDA); the Health Services Administration; the Office of Health Research, Statistics, and Technology; the Agency for Health Care Policy and Research; and the Office of the Assistant Secretary for Health in PHS. Other federal departments and agencies have budgets for health sciences research as well, most notably the Departments of Agriculture, Defense, Education, Energy, and Veterans Affairs and the National Science Foundation (see Figure 3-2). Even though some agencies have only a minimal role in sponsoring clinical research, they may require highly talented clinical investigators to carry out their mission, such as investigators at FDA and CDC. Thus, the committee sought to determine the fraction of federally sponsored research that involved human subjects.

National Institutes of Health

Of the nearly half of all financial support for health research that comes from federal sources, about three quarters is disbursed through NIH. The postwar policy decision to support fundamental research in academic institutions stimulated steady increases in NIH's budget (Figure 3-3). The most rapid growth in the NIH budget occurred between 1955 and 1965. From the late 1960s to 1980, budget growth for NIH leveled off. During the 1980s, however, congressional appropriations to NIH increased an average of 10 percent a year, resulting in a 2 percent per annum real growth in the NIH budget (National Institutes of Health, 1991). Many of the increases over the past few years can be attributed to the growth in funding for AIDS research. The new initiative for research into women's health issues has not yet stimulated growth in the NIH budget, but the Clinton administration and U.S. Congress have the opportunity to make these changes.

68

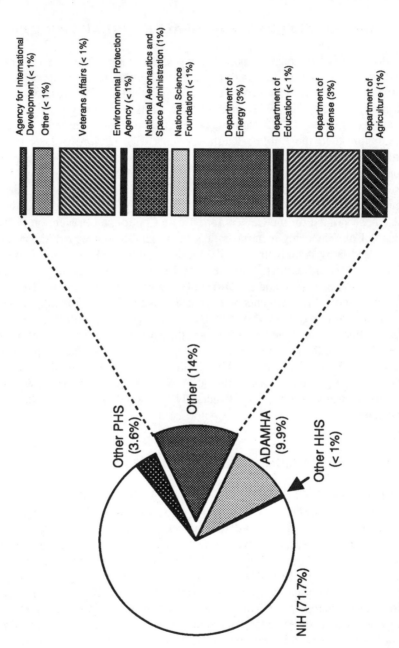

FIGURE 3-2 Source of federal support for health research and development by agency for 1992. (Source: National Institutes of Health, 1993b.)

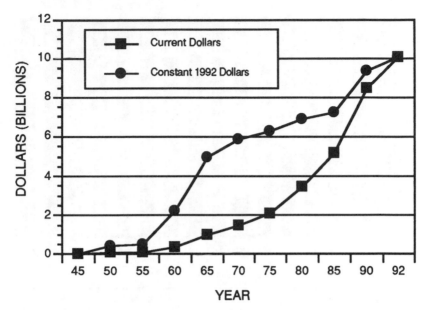

FIGURE 3-3 NIH appropriations from 1945 to 1992 in current and constant 1992 dollars. (Source: U.S. Department of Health and Human Services, Public Health Service, 1991e.)

Allocations among extramural and intramural NIH programs and program management have not changed significantly since the late 1970s (Figure 3-4). Only about 10 to 12 percent of NIH budget is allocated for research conducted intramurally. Nearly 80 percent of the NIH budget is allocated to extramural programs for research and training at universities and other research institutions both in the United States and abroad (National Institutes of Health, 1993b). Most of these extramural research funds are allocated through peer review processes for research grants and cooperative agreements. A small fraction of these funds are allocated for research contracts as well. Nevertheless, since the expansion of NIH extramural programs began in the mid-1940s, R&D grants have been, and continue to be, the cornerstone of NIH and ADAMHA extramural support for health research.

Intramural Research

Although the intramural research program at NIH includes a broad portfolio of activities such as basic research, training, communication of scientific findings, development of policies on biomedical research priorities, and

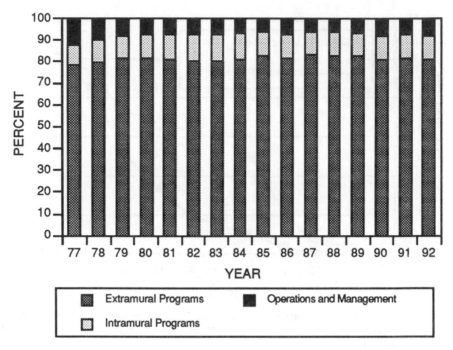

FIGURE 3-4 Allocation of the NIH budget from 1977 to 1992. (Source: National Institutes of Health, 1993b.)

translation of research findings into more effective medical care, the committee was most concerned about the research activities and training at the Warren Grant Magnuson Clinical Center. The clinical center was established in 1953 on the Bethesda, Maryland, campus of NIH to facilitate research using human subjects that could not be conducted at academic medical centers for various reasons (Ahrens, 1992). The clinical center currently has about 500 patient beds, or about 50 percent of all the research beds in the country. The remaining 50 percent are located throughout the country in academic health centers that are largely supported by NIH institutes and centers. Since its inception, the clinical center has served as a training ground for clinical investigators, many of whom are now on the faculty at academic health centers around the country. Resource limitations precluded the committee from undertaking a comprehensive assessment of the clinical center, but the committee drew upon several studies done in the 1980s that examined the structure of NIH (Institute of Medicine, 1985), the intramural program (Institute of Medicine, 1988b), and research at the clinical center (Ahrens, 1992; Institute of Medicine, 1987; National Institutes of Health, 1986).

There are two primary advantages for scientists who conduct research at the clinical center: (1) they do not have to compete for resources through the extramural peer review system and (2) they are not distracted from their research by obligations to teach or provide clinical services to the general public like their counterparts at academic medical centers are (Ahrens, 1992). Many criticisms of the intramural program have surfaced over the past decade suggesting that the quality of intramural research has declined. Some have suggested that peer review of the intramural research community is not as rigorous as that of the extramural research community. Further, it has recently been suggested that the organization of research groups has stifled cutting edge investigations. It has been argued, on the other hand, that scientific oversight within NIH is as rigorous for intramural research scientists as peer review is for the extramural research community. The intramural research budget has not grown in real terms over the past decade, and intramural research scientists are therefore competing internally for scarce resources. The clinical center has accredited training programs in some fields, increasing the teaching requirements of the staff physician-scientists.

Although the NIH campus served as a primary training ground for health scientists in the 1950s and 1960s, there were signs in the 1980s that NIH was beginning to have difficulty attracting and retaining scientists, including clinical investigators. During the 1980s, there was speculation that the intramural research program was not performing at the same level of quality demonstrated in the past. The relatively low government salary scales, noncompetitive fringe benefits, and the other bureaucratic constraints of working in a federal agency are thought to be contributory (Institute of Medicine, 1988b). It also has been postulated that the military draft may have been a driving force encouraging research-oriented scientists to pursue research training there during the mid to late 1960s.

In response to these concerns and to the suggestion that the intramural program could benefit by shifting to the private sector, the Institute of Medicine (IOM) conducted an in-depth review of the program in 1988 (Institute of Medicine, 1988b). The IOM study committee concluded that the intramural program has made, and continues to make, valuable contributions to understanding basic biological and disease processes. For example, an analysis by Ahrens of 36 physician-scientists at the clinical center revealed that intramural scientists publish more papers on both clinical and nonclinical research than their counterparts in medical schools do (Ahrens, 1992). Moreover, the first gene therapy protocols have been carried out at the clinical center.

Despite difficulties in effectively coordinating activities across institutes and responding efficiently to new challenges or crises, the IOM study committee concluded that the federated organizational structure of NIH has helped meet the nation's biomedical research goals. To maintain the intramural program's excellence and credibility and to improve in areas which it is deficient, the study committee recommended some changes in NIH administration as well as in the scope of responsibilities of scientific administrators directing the intramural programs (Institute of Medicine, 1988b).

Beyond the general problems associated with the intramural program, the clinical center presents specific problems because of its role and position in the federation of institutes. According to the an NIH report, the center has struggled with an identity problem (National Institutes of Health, 1986). In one sense, the center might be viewed as a hospital with all the requisite responsibilities associated with patient care. In another sense, the center appears to be a collection of the clinical research fiefdoms of the activities of each separate institute, where "The Clinical Center *per se* has very little power in determining its practical management, its clinical research program, or its fiscal decisions." (National Institutes of Health, 1986). Indeed, the clinical center budget is determined by the individual institutes on the basis of their research involvement and previous bed allocation. Although a medical board composed of the clinical directors from each institute help guide policy at the clinical center, some believe that an external advisory board should be constituted along the lines of the institute advisory councils to review protocols to ensure appropriate allocation of clinical center resources and an appropriate level of research activity for each institute.

Although the committee understands that there are problems with the physical infrastructure of the clinical center and intramural clinical investigators share the same career obstacles, the committee did not feel that it had enough information or insight to make recommendations concerning the intramural program. Furthermore, a recent report on the NIH intramural program by an ad hoc panel has proposed a new, yet smaller (about 200 bed) clinical center (Marshall, 1994).

Extramural Programs at NIH

R&D grants, particularly investigator-initiated research project grants (R01), are the cornerstone of the extramural research program at NIH. To more clearly understand the support base for clinical research, the committee felt that it would be useful to recap some of the problems and policy changes that have affected the entire extramural research community over the past decade. When possible, the committee's analysis focused on patient-oriented clinical research.

As growth in the NIH budget slowed during the mid-1970s, competition for grants intensified, and the number of new and competing renewal grants awarded by NIH fluctuated annually (Institute of Medicine, 1979; Seggel, 1985). Through the 1970s the number of funded new and competing proposals ranged from as few as 3,500 in 1976 to as many as 5,900 in 1979. The number funded annually did not follow any particular pattern, but depended on the cumulative grant portfolio and funds appropriated for a particular institute. These erratic patterns meant that even outstanding grant proposals often were not funded. Scientists began to feel that obtaining funding from NIH was unpredictable and had no regard for an investigator's previous research accomplishments or the significance of one's research. Moreover, the decreasing proportion of research grants being awarded to physicians raised concerns that the number of physician-investigators was declining and that measures must be taken to turn this situation around (Kelley, 1980; Thier et al., 1980; Wyngaarden, 1979).

The 1979 and 1980 reports by Institute of Medicine for the DHHS Steering Committee for the Development of a Health Research Strategy reexamined these concerns about the future of federal support for new and ongoing health research in light of impending federal budget constraints. The Steering Committee called for five-year plans and evaluative procedures to be established for all of the health-related agencies in DHHS and emphasized the need to stabilize the science base by making investigator-initiated research projects the first priority in NIH and ADAMHA research budgets (Institute of Medicine, 1979 and 1980). The 1979 Steering Committee report suggested that the minimum number of competitive research grant awards for fiscal year 1981 be 5,000 for NIH and 569 for ADAMHA (Seggel, 1985). Although NIH was able to fund the recommended number of new and competing awards, appropriations for 1981 allowed ADAMHA to fund only 284 new and competing awards that year—only half the recommended level. As a result, U.S. Congress and the executive branch agreed on a policy that specified the minimum number of new and competing grants NIH and ADAMHA would be required to fund each year—a "stabilization policy." Thus, establishing the number of new and competing proposals to be funded became an integral part of the federal budget policy that remained in place through fiscal year 1988 (Institute of Medicine, 1990).

The stabilization policy prevented erosion of the nation's scientific base by maintaining minimum annual numbers of investigator-initiated research grants. The total number of research project grants sponsored by NIH grew from 15,500 to 20,867 between 1977 and 1988. Research project grants increased from 51 percent of the total NIH extramural budget in 1978 to 67 percent in 1989 (Figure 3-5). Funding for research project grants grew from $2.5 billion in 1977 to $3.9 billion by 1989, when measured in constant 1988 dollars. Along with this growth, the expectation of funding may have encourged scientists to submit more grant applications, which increased from 14,142 in 1980 to 20,154 by 1990 (Figure 3-6) (National Institutes of Health, 1993b). It should also be noted, however, that the number of amended applications grew significantly over the same period and now makes up nearly 30 percent of the application pool. By 1987, the number of new and competing awards made annually reached a peak of 6,400 for NIH and 600 for ADAMHA.

Other forces were affecting the available pool of funds for scientists competing for funding in 1990. Despite added appropriations from Congress throughout the 1980s, the funds available were never adequate to fund fully the

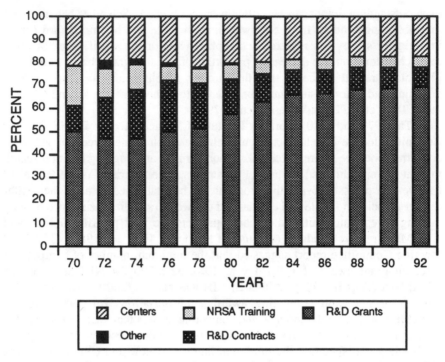

FIGURE 3-5 NIH extramural awards as a percentage of the extramural budget from 1970 to 1992. (Source: National Institutes of Health, 1993a.)

agreed upon number of awards. In order to comply, NIH and ADAMHA were forced into a policy of reducing ongoing research commitments (continuing awards for already approved and funded grants) as well as the amounts paid to new and competing awards in what is commonly referred to as "downward negotiation"—a recent practice for reconciling NIH and ADAMHA research grant commitments with annual appropriations by making across-the-board reductions in all grant awards. Although no negotiations between the scientist and NIH or ADAMHA actually occur, these budget "cuts" placed additional burdens on scientists; they were expected to perform the research outlined in their proposals with less than the recommended amount of funding.

Although NIH and ADAMHA were increasing the numbers of new and competing awards through the stabilization policy, another policy affected the pool of available funds. The research community felt that the average three-year award period for traditional research project grants (R01) was too short and did not allow sufficient time to achieve research goals or for long-term research program planning. Frequent renewals placed too much emphasis on the writing of grants

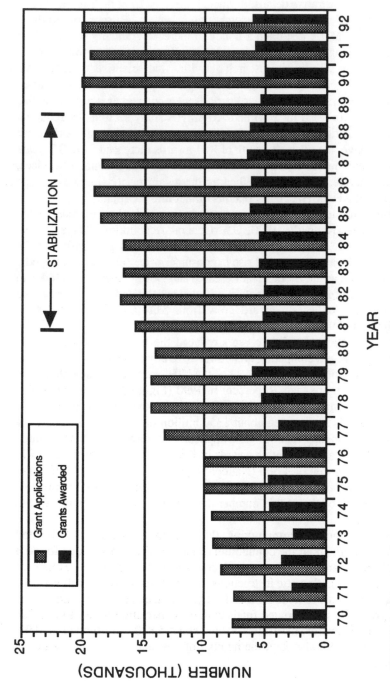

FIGURE 3-6 Number of new and competing continuation grant applications submitted to NIH and the number of grants awarded from 1970 to 1992. (Source: National Institutes of Health, Division of Research Grants.)

and attending to administrative details, distracted scientists from their research, and overburdened the review groups with competing renewals. Responding to these calls, NIH and ADAMHA instituted a policy to increase gradually the length of grant awards beginning in 1986. The intended result of increasing award periods was to provide more stability in research activities and scientists' careers and, perhaps, to discourage the number of multiple grant applications by individual investigators. In addition, longer award periods were viewed as a way to reduce the administrative workload for NIH and ADAMHA study sections by reducing the number of competitive renewal applications processed each year. As a result of this policy change, the average length of R01 awards increased from 3.3 years in 1980 to 4.1 years in 1990 (U.S. Department of Health and Human Services, Public Health Service, 1992c). Lengthening the award periods, however, also obligated NIH and ADAMHA appropriations further into the future.

The policy for lengthening award periods was linked to increasing the average award size (Kennedy, 1990, U.S. General Accounting Office, 1988). According to the U.S. Department of Commerce, the costs of performing health research outpaces the average annual rise in consumer prices and has developed a deflator index known as the Biomedical Research and Development Price Index to account for this difference. Even factoring in this accelerated cost increase, the average size of an R01 grant award grew from $114,6000 to $134,400 in inflation-adjusted dollars (1982 = 100) between 1980 and 1991. These accumulating obligations for future years reduced the funds available to meet annual targets of new and competing grant awards. Obligations for noncompeting continuations grew from 67 to 68 percent of the NIH extramural research budget in the mid-1980s to more than 76 percent in 1990 (Figure 3-7). Although this appears to be a small percentage shift, these growing obligations for noncompeting awards represented about $350 million that was not available for funding new and competing renewal grant applications. As a result, NIH awarded only about 5,400 new and competing awards in 1989, and dropped even further in 1990 to a devastating low of 4,600 (National Institutes of Health, 1993b). Not only were new and competing awards declining, but in 1989 the total number of grants dropped to 20,681, and this number dropped yet even further in 1990 to 20,316.

The House report accompanying the appropriations for 1991 cited congressional concern about the conundrum of increased appropriations for NIH but the declining numbers of new and competing awards (U.S. House of Representatives, 1991). Specific instructions were relayed to NIH to roll back the average length of awards to no more than four years. In an attempt to buttress the system, Congress also appropriated funds with the expectation of reaching 6,000 new and competing awards; nevertheless, only about 5,800 were funded in 1991. Appropriations for 1992 also kept the number of new and competing awards at about 5,800.

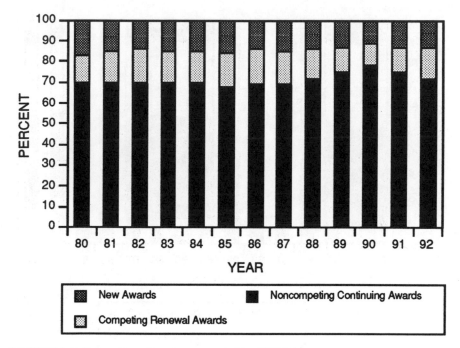

FIGURE 3-7 Percentage of amount awarded by NIH for competing and noncompeting grant awards from 1980 to 1992. (Source: National Institutes of Health, Division of Research Grants.)

The annual budget process for fiscal year 1993 was peculiar in its own right. For the first time in more than a decade, the tables were turned between the President's budget request and congressional appropriations. Standard protocol throughout the 1980s was a presidential budget request for NIH that just slightly exceeded the previous year's appropriations. Subsequently, Congress would add to the request, giving NIH an increase that would cover inflation plus a small amount more. Unlike previous years, however, the President requested a large increase in the NIH budget for 1993. Congressional appropriations were far below the President's request and barely kept the NIH budget ahead of inflation. As a result, new and competing awards were about 5,800 in 1991 and 6,000 in 1992. With extreme budget pressures on the federal government, it is not clear how the annual budget ritual will be played out over the next few years.

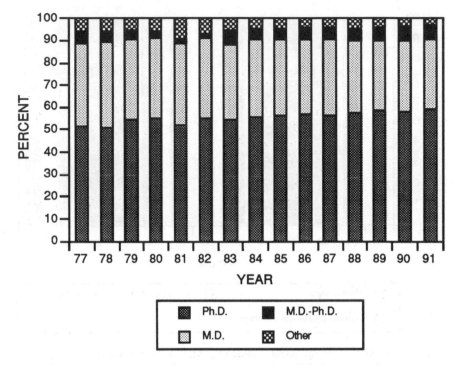

FIGURE 3-8 Degrees of principal investigators on traditional research project grant (R01) applications indicating the use of human materials or human subjects. (Source: National Institutes of Health, Division of Research Grants.)

Setting Program Priorities Through Peer Review

Over the past two decades, much attention has been focused on the success rates of physician-scientists in peer review competition for NIH and ADAMHA research grants. The clinical research effort was measured by the number of clinicians (physician- or dentist-scientists) obtaining grant support in the 1950s and 1960s. More than 50 percent of all current research project grant applications for studies using human subjects or materials are led by a Ph.D. as the principal investigator (Figure 3-8), and thus, the proportion of applications from M.D. principal investigators is decreasing (Vaitukaitis, 1991). This imbalance is slightly offset by a growing proportion of principal investigators with M.D. and Ph.D. degrees.

Applications, Awards, and Success Rates Although annual awards for new and competing grants from NIH have hovered between 5,000 and 6,000 throughout the 1980s, the number of applications grew from 14,142 to 20,154

TABLE 3-1 Distribution of All NIH Grant Awards by Degree of the Principal
Investigator for Selected Years from 1970 to 1987

Year	Total Number Of Grants	Number of Grants (Percent of Total)		
		M.D.s	M.D.-Ph.D.s	Ph.D.s
1970	11,683	4,289 (36.7)	693 (5.9)	5,993 (51.3)
1975	13,899	4,485 (32.3)	797 (5.7)	8,017 (57.7)
1980	19,325	5,555 (28.7)	852 (4.4)	12,283 (63.6)
1985	22,271	5,807 (26.1)	808 (3.6)	13,725 (61.6)
1987	24,384	6,393 (26.2)	904 (3.7)	15,589 (63.9)

Note: The numbers in the table do not add up to the totals nor do the percentages
add up to 100 because a small number of awardees hold degrees other than those
listed in the table.
Source: Reprinted, with permission, from Healy (1988), p.1059. Copyright 1992
by The New England Journal of Medicine.

between 1980 and 1990, far exceeding the ability of NIH to fund even a
reasonable fraction (Figure 3-6).

In 1970 the fraction of grant awards to M.D. principal investigators was
36.7 percent, with 51.3 percent going to Ph.D.s and 5.9 percent going to M.D.-
Ph.D.s. Although the number of awards to M.D.s increased (along with the
overall number of NIH grants), the fraction to M.D.s declined to 26.2 percent and
the fraction to M.D.-Ph.D.s declined to 3.7 percent by 1987. There has been a
concomitant rise in the number of awards to Ph.D.s who garner about two thirds
of grant awards (Table 3-1).

The committee examined the success rates among the three groups for all
research grants and for those involving human subjects or materials. In neither
comparison was there an appreciable difference in success rates among the groups.
Thus, perceived differences in the quality of grants among the various groups are
not substantiated, even when the proposal involves research on humans or human
materials (Figure 3-9).

Costs of Human Studies The costs of performing clinical research are
higher than those for performing preclinical research (Kimes et al., 1991).
Whatever the reasons, grant awards that indicate the use of human materials or
human subjects are consistently larger than other grants (Figure 3-10).

Peer Review More than 2,000 scientists are involved in the NIH peer
review system (National Institutes of Health, 1992b). This unique system, in
which nongovernment scientists are entrusted with public monies for distribution

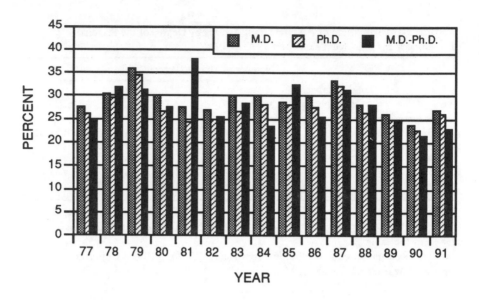

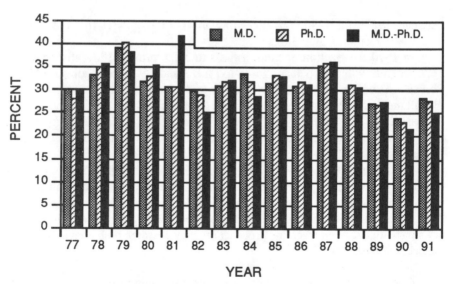

FIGURE 3-9   Success rates of M.D.s, PH.D.s and M.D.-Ph.D.s for competing traditional research project (R01) grant applications indicating the use of human materials (top panel) or human subjects compared to those not using human materials or subjects (bottom panel) from 1977 to 1991.   (Source: National Institutes of Health, Division of Research Grants.)

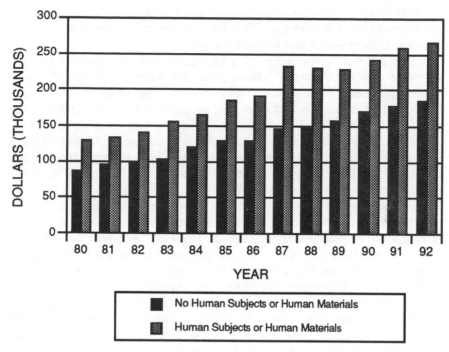

FIGURE 3-10 Average award size of NIH research project grants comparing awards for studies using human materials or human subjects with those awards for studies not using human materials or subjects. (Source: National Institutes of Health, Division of Research Grants.)

to their colleagues for the pursuit of scientific knowledge, is considered the best in the world. The committee believes that these scientists should be commended for giving their time to support a system built on public trust. Nevertheless, many concerns have been aired about peer review of grant applications for both preclinical and clinical research.

Studies involving patients pose special methodologic challenges that are not encountered in laboratory bench research. In bench research, the subjects of the experiment are selected to ensure that they are virtually identical. In clinical research, by contrast, the populations under study, even in studies involving identical twins, are never truly identical. Whereas in bench research experiments are conducted in such a manner that everything other than the experimental maneuver is applied to the control group, many aspects of clinical research studies cannot be controlled. Moreover, there are fewer constraints on how the results from bench studies can be assessed (i.e., isolation of cellular material, euthanasia of animals, ex vivo studies). In clinical studies, the outcomes must be assessed in whole patients who agree to participate, and most importantly, the process of measurement must do no harm. Therefore, human research appears to be less scientific to those accustomed to bench research.

The potential consequence of a bias against clinical research is a less favorable review for studies involving patients when compared with bench studies. Since only 20 percent of all initial review group members are physicians familiar with the care of patients, this is of particular concern (National Institutes of Health, 1992b). These concerns have arisen, in part, because of a lack of specific guidelines for grant application referral or assignment to study sections, lack of guidelines for study section administrators (i.e., different study sections employ widely differing strategies), and the lack of oversight of any of the review process and constitution of study sections.

Several reviews of the peer review system have been performed (the most recent in 1991), but the problems mentioned have not been resolved to everyone's satisfaction (National Institutes of Health, 1992c,d). Although the committee could not undertake an analysis of the competency of reviewers for assessing patient-oriented research, it is clear that the number of M.D.s on study sections is very low (U.S. Department of Health and Human Services, Public Health Service, 1986, 1992b). It is also perceived that the M.D.s who are on study sections are oriented more toward basic science than clinical research. Whether this is a cause of inadequate review cannot be substantiated. Furthermore, the number of women and minorities on review panels is not representative of their participation rates in the scientific community, and very few from these groups are M.D.s (National Institutes of Health, 1992b).

The study sections were originally constituted along the lines of scientific disciplines. With minor exceptions, the study sections are suitably constituted to review basic science grant applications. Few, however, focus specifically on human biology or studies involving human subjects. Concern has been expressed that this put clinical research at a disadvantage in the review system. The only data available on the distribution of priority scores for grant applications reveal only minor differences between nonhuman research and research indicating the use of humans or human materials (Figure 3-11). However, NIH has no means of separating applications proposing the use of human materials from those directly involving human subjects. Furthermore, since the content of grant applications is confidential, the committee was unable to perform its own analysis on grant applications. Nonetheless, it is believed that the perception of a bias may have influenced investigators to withold applications.

Funding Clinical Research

The preceding discussion addressed concerns about all extramural funding by NIH (and previously ADAMHA). The committee is expressly concerned about

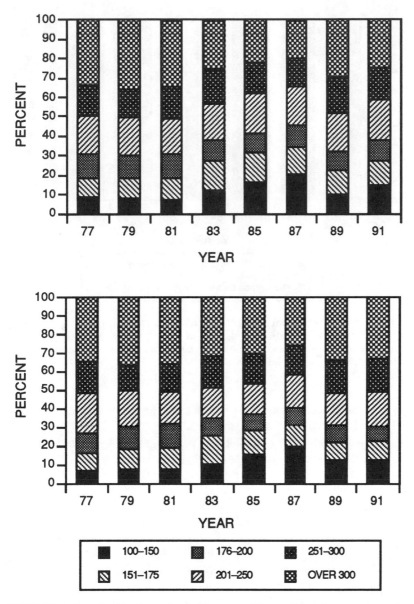

FIGURE 3-11 Distribution of priority scores for traditional research project grant (R01) applications comparing those indicating the use of human materials or subjects (top panel) with those applications not indicating use of humans or human materials (bottom panel). (Source: National Institutes of Health, Division of Research Grants.)

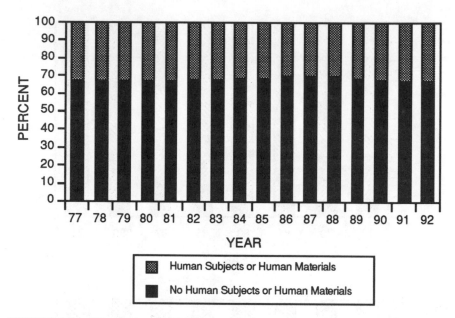

FIGURE 3-12 Distribution of NIH competing traditional research project grant (R01) applications comparing those indicating the use of human materials or subjects with those applictions not indicating use of humans or human materials. (Source: National Institutes of Health, Division of Research Grants.)

the fraction of extramural research funds allocated for clinical research, more specifically, funds for patient-oriented clinical research.

Almost every inventory of clinical research supported by NIH in the past has been troubled by ambiguity about what clinical research is, who is performing it, and how much funding is provided (Ahrens, 1992; Institute of Medicine, 1988a; Wyngaarden, 1986). Earlier studies have relied on either the fraction of grants requiring institutional review board (IRB) approval or the number of principal investigators with clinical degrees (M.D., D.D.S., D.O., and the like) who win grant awards. Some analyses cross-link these two measures to arrive at an estimate of clinical research. Although these estimates can be used as surrogate measures of clinical research activities, the committee was concerned that such measures do not accurately portray the amount of clinical research activity that directly involves interactions with human subjects. As indicated in Chapter 1, clinical research can have various meanings to different audiences. The committee agrees with a broad definition encompassing a wide spectrum of research activities, but elected to focus on career pathways leading to patient-oriented clinical research. The next section explores these measures of clinical

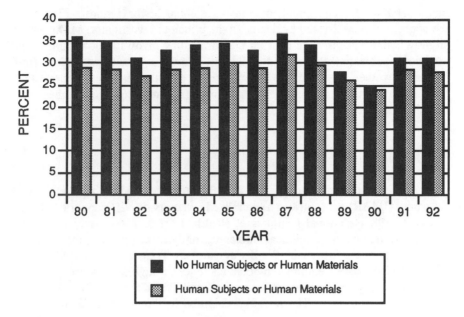

FIGURE 3-13 Success rates of traditional research project grant (R01) applications comparing those indicating the use of human materials or subjects with those applications not indicating use of humans or human materials. (Source: National Institutes of Health, Division of Research Grants.)

research and presents the committee's analysis of a sample of R01 grants indicating use of human subjects or materials.

IMPAC Data

As indicated previously, the number of new and competing research project grant applications submitted to NIH grew from 14,142 in 1980 to 20,154 in 1990. Throughout this period, the fraction of grant applications indicating that the studies intended to use human subjects or materials has remained remarkably constant, at about one third (Figure 3-12) (Vaitukaitis, 1991). However, this is based on the human subject box on PHS grant application form number 398, which includes both proposals for studies that actually involve human subjects and proposals that are exempt under IRB rules for research on human materials such as body fluids, pathological specimens, or certain observational human studies. Nonetheless, the trends in the applications are useful.

Over the past decade, the trend in award rates for grant applications involving humans have been parallelled those grant applications not involving humans, but have been a couple of percentage points lower (Figure 3-13). When the applications are divided by degree of the principal investigator, M.D.s have a slightly higher success rate than Ph.D.s for studies involving both human and nonhuman subjects (Figures 3-14 and 3-15). However, grant applications from M.D.s for studies not involving humans have a slightly better success rate than grant applications for studies involving humans (Figure 3-16). Again, these data include all IRB reviewed clinical research.

OMAR Data

After a hiatus of several years, the NIH Office of Medical Applications of Research (OMAR) reestablished a centralized inventory of NIH-supported clinical studies in 1985 (National Institutes of Health, 1992a). This provided a single source of information on clinical studies, partially in response to the reporting requirements of the Stevenson-Wydler Technology Transfer Act of 1980. Thus, OMAR collects data from the individual institutes through the representatives of the Coordinating Committee on Assessment and Transfer of Technology at the end of each fiscal year. The working definition for their data collection is the following:

> A clinical study is a research study undertaken with nine or more human subjects to evaluate prospectively the diagnostic/prophylactic/ therapeutic effect of an intervention (drug, device, regimen, or procedure) used or intended ultimately for use in the practice of medicine or the prevention of disease. The term "clinical study" does not include registries, epidemiological surveys, or epidemiological studies conducted retrospectively (National Institutes of Health, 1992a).

More details about the data collection and analysis are provided in OMAR's annual reports. The committee felt that it was instructive to show the tabulation of OMAR data and recap the significant findings (Table 3-2). From 1986 and 1987 the number of clinical studies supported by all institutes (except the National Cancer Institute [NCI] and the Division of Research Resources [DRR]) grew by nearly 11 percent, from 1,133 to 1,272. At the same time, OMAR reported that funding for clinical studies grew by more than 27 percent, from $381 million to $501 million. Unfortunately, the OMAR data are not current, and longitudinal comparisons are difficult to unravel.

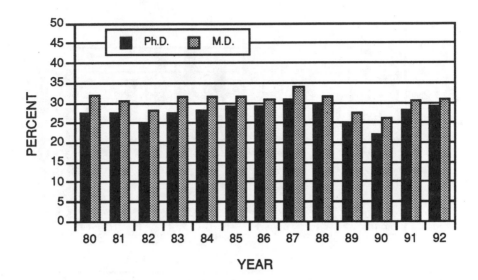

FIGURE 3-14 Success rates of traditional research project grant (R01) applications for those studies indicating the use of human materials or subjects for M.D.s and Ph.D.s. (Source: National Institutes of Health, Division of Research Grants.)

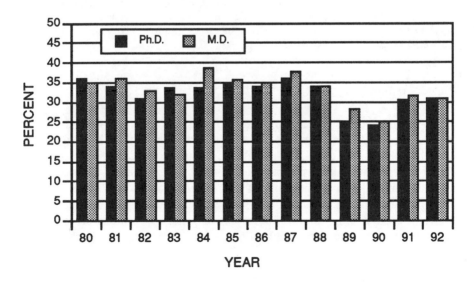

FIGURE 3-15 Success rates of traditional research project grant (R01) applications for those studies not indicating the use of human materials or subjects for M.D.s and Ph.D.s. (Source: National Institutes of Health, Division of Research Grants.)

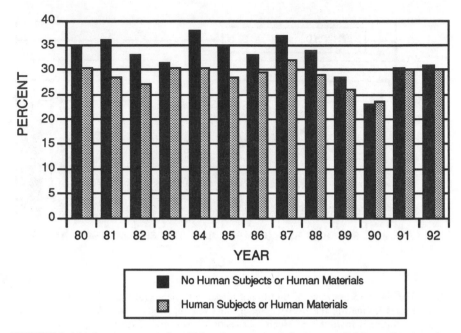

FIGURE 3-16 Success rates of traditional research project grant (R01) applications by M.D.s comparing studies not indicating the use of human materials or subjects with those that use human materials or human subjects. (Source: National Institutes of Health, Division of Research Grants.)

Ahrens' Analysis

Ahrens reported on his longitudinal analysis of abstracts from a random sample of 557 R01 grant awards selected from the years 1977, 1982, and 1987 (Ahrens, 1992). His classification scheme included six separate categories of clinical research in addition to nonclinical research. He concluded that nonclinical research declined from 49 percent of the 1977 sample to about 43 percent of the 1987 sample. The sample sizes, however, were small (less than 2 percent of all R01s for each year). Moreover, abstracts of grant applications are often not representative of the entire application, nor reflective of the work actually performed.

CRISP Data

NIH maintains an information system on Computerized Retrieval of Information on Research Projects (CRISP), which is supported by PHS. As can

TABLE 3-2 NIH Support for Human Studies for Fiscal Years 1985–1987 as Reported by the NIH Office of Medical Applications for Research.

Item	FY 1985	FY 1986	FY 1987
Number of studies with support[a]	1,112	1,133	1,272
Total obligations for fiscal year			
• NIH subtotal[a]	$243,627,000	$251,661,000	$345,790,000
• NCI	$117,470,428	$107,430,356	$128,391,447
• NCRR[b]	$15,969,811	$21,560,887	$26,735,913
• Total	$377,067,239	$380,652,243	$500,917,360
Average cost per study each year[a]	$219,089	$222,119	$271,847
Total number of patients, all studies (projected)[a]	445,397	493,279	562,165
Average number of patients (projected) per study[a,c]	417	477	431
Average cost per patient per study per year[a,c]	$615	$555	$744

[a] Excluding the National Cancer Institute (NCI) and the National Center for Research Resources (NCRR).
[b] The National Center for Research Resources was formerly the Division of Research Resources.
[c] Excludes a single study with a sample size in excess of 100,000.
Source: National Institutes of Health, 1990.

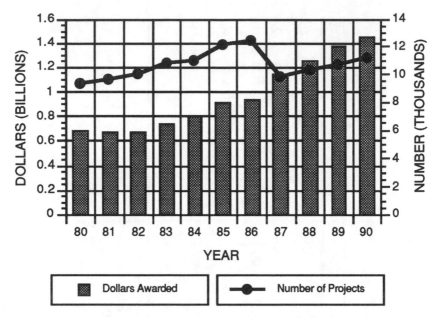

FIGURE 3-17 Results of a search of the Computerized Retrieval of Information on Research Projects (CRISP) system linking the term "clinical" with "human" showing the number of projects and subprojects (on P01s) and the dollars awarded, 1980–1990. (Source: National Institutes of Health, Division of Research Grants.)

be expected, most of the research projects are from NIH (and formerly ADAMHA) including some information on intramural research. Abstracts for each research project are entered into the database with data elements on funding, awarding institute, awardee, awardee's institution, and so forth. Author abstracts are used when possible; otherwise, abstracts are prepared by writers. CRISP files are indexed and search headings are established to be similar to those used for MEDLINE.

Thus, in an attempt to find another measure to determine the level of support for patient-oriented clinical research, the committee asked NIH staff to perform a search linking the terms *human* with *clinical* on research supported by NIH from 1980 to 1990. The results of that analysis are shown in Figure 3-17. These data show that support for human or clinical research grew from $682 million in 1980 to $1,458 million in 1990. When adjusted for inflation, this represents 19 percent real growth. Over the same period, the number of projects and subprojects (from P01s) increased from 9,370 to 11,127.

The CRISP database uses research project abstracts to codify the research. Primary, secondary, and tertiary key words for each abstract are entered by NIH staff—not by the grant author. Thus, the search strategy is based on subjective coding of research projects. When abstracts are missing, they are prepared by writers. Moreover, abstracts frequently provide too little information to determine the actual scope of a research project, and there is no apparent avenue for recording a change in scope by the investigator in the database. Finally, the award amounts entered into the CRISP system are the initial awards by the institute and are not corrected for administrative adjustments including downward negotiation.

Committee's Analysis

The committee recognized the extreme variability and ambiguity in the aforementioned analyses or measures of clinical research. Since the committee focused on patient-oriented research, it wanted to ascertain what fraction of NIH grants that indicated the use of human subjects or materials were actually for patient-oriented clinical research. Because this data element is not captured in any present database, the committee developed a strategy to categorize a random sample of R01 grant awards. Because the committee felt that grant abstracts were unreliable, it chose to perform the analysis using the actual grant files from each of 11 institutes. Data from the National Institute of Dental Research and the National Center for Nursing Research were considered by their respective task forces and were not included in the analysis. Six grants from the National Institute of Environmental Health Sciences were excluded because their files are retained in Research Triangle, North Carolina. Also, since the study was coordinated through the Office of the Deputy Director for Extramural Research at NIH and began in early 1992, the former ADAMHA institutes were not included. Nonetheless, the committee believes that the sample was representative of investigator-initiated grants.

Of the 16,313 R01s that were active in fiscal year 1991, 14,535 were reviewed by IRGs in the Division of Research Grants. Of the latter, in 4,284 or about 30 percent, the human studies box was checked (referred to from now on as IRB positive). The committee estimated that a sample size of approximately 10 percent, or 430 grants, for studies involving human subjects or materials would be sufficient to estimate the fraction of grant awards for studies that actually involve interaction with human subjects.

There were 114 regular and ad hoc IRGs that reviewed IRB-positive grants that year. Many of these IRGs infrequently review grant applications for studies involving humans, that is, less than 25 percent of grant awards resulting from a respective study section review are IRB positive. At the same time, some IRGs frequently review grant applications for studies involving humans. Since a straight random sample across all IRGs would raise the possibility that the sample could be drawn from study sections that only occasionally review IRB-positive grants, or, more likely, from IRGs that review mostly IRB-positive grants, the committee developed a sampling strategy to ensure that IRGs with

TABLE 3-3 Grouping of 1991 R01 Grant Awards Reviewed by NIH Division of Research Grants Initial Review Groups (IRGs) by Prevalence of Institutional Review Board (IRB) Indicator

Quartile	Prevalence of IRB Positivity (%)	Number of Study Sections	Number of R01 Awards	Number of IRB+ R01s	Average Proportion IRB+ (%)
First	0–25	51	7,836	875	11
Second	26–50	40	4,596	1,825	39
Third	51–75	11	1,227	760	62
Fourth	76–100	12	876	824	94
Total		114	14,535	4,284	29

Source: National Institutes of Health, Division of Research Grants.

both high and low numbers of IRB-positive grants were evaluated. Thus, the IRGs were placed into four quartiles as shown in Table 3-3. The denominator of interest for this analysis was the 4,284 grants that indicated the use of human subjects or materials. To ensure that the sample represented IRGs that reviewed many IRB-positive grants as well as those that reviewed few IRB-positive grants, a random sample of 100 grants was selected from the first and fourth quartiles. The second and third quartiles were combined, and a sample of 250 grants was selected. Thus, the overall sample was 450, or slightly more than 10 percent of all IRB-positive R01 awards. Because of missing files or unavailable data, 446 grants (10.4 percent of the 4,284 human grants) were actually reviewed. The sample also included representative grants from each of 11 institutes. Table 3-4 shows the target number for review in each group and the actual number read.

Rather than develop an elaborate scheme for classifying the grants, the committee sought to simplify the strategy by using the following categories of research:

1. **Fundamental research** seeks to answer fundamental questions about the nature of biology through a broad range of basic and clinical research. Most of these studies involve nonhuman materials, although some may involve human materials. Any of these studies may eventually lead to major improvements in the prevention or cure of disease, but for the purpose of this analysis the committee sought to distinguish fundamental research from the two categories described below.

2. **Human research** is the portion of clinical research in which patients serve directly as the research subjects, often referred to

as *patient-oriented* or *patient-related* research. For example, this category of clinical research includes research activities such as the characterization of normal and diseased human function; evaluation of new diagnostic, therapeutic, or prognostic techniques, approaches, and devices; evaluation of existent practices or technology in standard practice; and phase I–IV drug trials. Thus, this category of research activity has direct application to the prevention, diagnosis, treatment, or cure of disease in the individual or group of individuals under study; rehabilitation (including quality of life issues) of the patient; or study of human pathophysiology. Furthermore, it involves direct, "hands-on" evaluation of the human subject.

    3. **Epidemiologic research** investigates the circumstances under which disease occurs in populations. It seeks factors that cause disease such as environmental exposures, personal habits, genes, viruses, and the like. Epidemiologic studies both describe the distribution of disease in populations (rates over time and between places) and analyze disease risk determinants. Such research is the source of many ideas about the causes of disease, factors that determine high risk for development of disease, and methods to promote the prevention or control of disease.

Using these categories, the committee sought to unravel the ambiguity of the grant categorization process that lumps all human research together. Thus, this scheme allowed the committee to focus on that portion of clinical research—true human research—that was the central theme of this study.

    With the cooperation of the grants managers in each institute, the complete grant files were obtained and available for the analysis. The data were collected in a manner that kept all personal identifiers confidential. The grants were classified according to the three categories of research listed above. Because many grants may have components of human research combined with other experiments, it was necessary to estimate the proportion of effort and funding committed to each category in increments of 10 percent. The committee recognized the potential pitfalls of subjectively estimating percent effort when two or more categories of research were involved.

    The results of the analysis are shown in Tables 3-4 and 3-5. Interestingly, 186, or 41.6 percent, of these grants were for fundamental research, as described above in the first category—fundamental research. Of these, 46 did not involve human subjects or materials at all, and another 85 had more or equal amounts of nonhuman research than human materials research. Of the 227, or about 50.8 percent, that involved some human research, 161 were classified as category 2 (human subject research) and 66 were combined fundamental and human research. The remaining 33 grants were in epidemiology. If these data are representative of the entire 4,284 grants for studies involving human research, then 2,180 grants or

TABLE 3-4 Results of Classification of IRB-positive R01 Awards Reviewed by NIH Division of Research Grants Initial Review Groups (IRGs)

Quartile	Number of Awards					
	Fundamental Research	Human Research	Fundamental and Human Research	Epidemi-ology	Target Number	Total Number
First	65	18	12	0	100	95
Second and third	119	78	51	4	250	252
Fourth	2	65	3	29	100	99
Total	186	161	66	33	450	446

Source: National Institutes of Health, Division of Research Grants.

TABLE 3-5 Proportion of Each Quartile Composed of IRB-positive Grant Awards

Quartile	Fundamental Research	Human Research	Fundamental and Human Research	Epidemi-ology	Total Number
First	0.684	0.189	0.126	0	0.999
Second and third	0.472	0.309	0.202	0.015	0.998
Fourth	0.020	0.656	0.030	0.292	0.998

Source: National Institutes of Health, Division of Research Grants.

about 51 percent of the IRB-positive awards would involve interactions with human subjects.

Next, the proportions of each category of research were determined for each group to derive the stratum-specific proportions that are presented in Table 3-6. Multiplication of these proportions by the number of awards that are IRB positive in each stratum gave an estimate of overall human research in relation to the denominator of 14,535. Thus, the committee concluded that 1,504, or 10.4 percent, of the 14,535 R01 grants active in 1991 were purely for studies involving human subjects; an additional 657, or 4.5 percent, had combined fundamental (human and nonhuman) and human subject research; and less than 2 percent involved human epidemiology. To extrapolate these findings, roughly 84 percent of the R01 grant awards support nonhuman research.

TABLE 3-6 Estimation of the Total Number of Patient-Oriented R01 Research Grant Awards from IRB-Positive Data

Quartile	Fundamental Research	Human Research	Fundamental and Human Research	Epidemi-ology	Total Number
First	599	165	110	0	875
Second and third	1,220	799	522	38	2,579
Fourth	16	540	25	241	822
Total	1,836	1,504	657	279	4,275

Source: National Institutes of Health, Division of Research Grants.

The committee is fully aware of the potential pitfalls in this type of analysis. For example, it could be argued that most of the R01 grants for studies involving human subject are reviewed by panels convened by the respective institute rather than IRGs in the Division of Research Grants. Indeed, about 1,800 R01 grants active in 1991 were reviewed by IRGs convened by the institutes; nearly 800 R01 grant awardees indicated the use of human subjects or materials. Because institute review panels are often convened to review grant applications submitted in response to requests for applications, the committee felt that they were not a representative sample of unsolicited, investigator-initiated grant proposals. Another potential gap is human research that is supported by program project awards (P01). It is believed that these large, multifaceted projects frequently include a human research component. Many of these proposals are reviewed by institute review groups as well. The committee did not have the time or the resources to analyze these awards. Program projects, however, are only a small portion of the extramural research budget compared with the R01 portion. Although the committee cannot draw conclusions from these data on the total amount of human research funded by NIH, this exercise demonstrated that the present classification is not useful for accurately determining the fraction that is truly human research. Lastly, this analysis was performed only on grant awards. As mentioned above, analysis of grant applications is not possible, but Cuca has reported on the bias of getting clinical research grants funded through the peer review system (Cuca, 1983; Cuca and McLoughlin, 1987), and Friereich (1990) and Friedman et al. (1991) have examined similar problems specific to cancer research.

R&D Centers

NIH supports nearly 600 centers designed to consolidate related research efforts and resources into a single administrative and programmatic structure. About 100 of these are special resource centers for animals or biotechnology resources. The remaining 500 are specialized centers (P50), center core grants (P30), comprehensive centers (P60), and general clinical research centers (GCRCs) (M01).

Centers, whether they are funded by NIH or an institution's own funds, can serve as vital institutional resources for multidisciplinary research. The funds provided through grants to centers from NIH are to be used for salaries of key staff, operation of shared resources and services, and center administration. These funds also may be used to recruit new talent to the center, to fund investigators who previously have not obtained competitive peer-reviewed federal funding, to provide interim research support for center investigators, and to obtain new shared resources. Although the committee did not perform a detailed analysis of the NIH program for centers, they commissioned Charles Pak of the University of Texas Health Sciences Center to write a paper on the value of the GCRC program, particularly its potential role in training patient-oriented investigators (Pak, 1994), and drew from the 1989 IOM report on the NCI cancer centers program (Institute of Medicine, 1989a).

General Clinical Research Centers The GCRC program, begun in 1959, was designed to support a clinical research infrastructure located within academic medical institutions around the country. Thus, the program was perceived as an extension of the Warren Grant Magnuson Clinical Center located on the NIH campus in Bethesda, Maryland. To this end, a typical GCRC is rather like a miniclinical center that occupies an area in a hospital through a contractual agreement (Ross, 1985). Unlike the Magnuson Clinical Center, which is organized as a collection of the individual institutes' clinical research arms to reflect their own disease orientation, the GCRCs were intended to have a general research orientation that cuts across disciplinary lines and serves all departments.

The goals of the program are the following: (1) to make available to medical scientists the resources that are necessary for the conduct of clinical research; (2) to provide an environment for studies of normal and abnormal body functions and for investigations of the cause, progression, prevention, control, and cure of human disease; (3) to provide an optimum setting for controlled clinical investigations; (4) to encourage collaboration among basic and clinical scientists, to encourage, develop, and maintain a national corps of expert clinical investigators; (5) to serve as an environment for training other health professionals in clinical research; and (6) to provide resources in which advances in basic knowledge can be translated into new or improved methods for patient care (U.S. Department of Health and Human Services, Public Health Service, 1991a).

Although commonly a designated part of a hospital, each GCRC is designed to support areas within academic medical centers dedicated to patient-related research. These centers can be composed of specialized inpatient and outpatient facilities, laboratories and equipment, and mainframe computers, and the facilities are staffed by specialized personnel, such as biostatisticians, computer systems managers, research nurses and dieticians, and research laboratory technicians. For example, an inpatient clinical research center is a self-contained unit with its own research beds, administration, nursing staff, laboratory, metabolic kitchen, and computerized data analysis facility. Outpatient units are commonly contiguous to the inpatient facility and are becoming an important complement to the center, just as large segments of the medical profession are moving toward ambulatory care.

Center funding is provided through a competitive grant program by the National Center for Research Resources. The principal investigator named on the grant is usually a dean, thus cutting across departmental affiliations. The program director, however, is responsible for administering the grant (even writing the grant proposal) and the day-to-day management of the center, including supervision of the center-supported staff and facilities. The program director is supported by an advisory committee that reviews proposed research protocols for use of the center. Although the GCRC grant supports the research infrastructure for center studies such as room and board for subjects, nursing, and some laboratory support, individual investigators are responsible for securing funding for specialized procedures or their own research.

One estimate suggests that nearly 5,000 research projects involving as many as 7,000 investigators are currently under way in GCRCs (Pak, 1994). The range of topics, in decreasing order of number of projects, include endocrinology, maternal and child health, immunology, cardiovascular disease, diabetes, gastroenterology, cancer, kidney disease, genetics, aging, hypertension, and arthritis.

The program was initiated in 1959, and the first eight centers with 133 patient beds were established in 1960. The number of GCRCs and patient beds grew rapidly, reaching a peak of 1,137 beds in 1967 and 93 centers in 1969 and 1970 (Ahrens, 1992). Through the 1970s the number of centers dropped to 75, and the number of beds declined to 600. The GCRC no longer funds centers in terms of patient beds; rather, funding is based on inpatient bed-days and outpatient visits. There are currently 74 centers nationwide supporting about 130,000 inpatient bed-days and 200,000 outpatient visits.

Although funding for the GCRCs increased from $103 million in 1986 to $127 million in 1992, the program did not realize an increase in 1993. Moreover, much of the growth over the past few years can be attributed to increases in funding for human immunodeficiency virus (HIV) research, which accounted for $13 million in 1986 and grew to $24 million in 1992. The non-AIDS portion of the GCRCs has thus not kept up with inflation.

The committee is concerned about the future of the GCRCs because they are logical sites for bridging what many believe is a widening gap between laboratory research and human studies. The GCRCs represent a nationwide resource that could be used to increase the number of scientific advances that are translated to the bedside, as well as to continue to advance the understanding of human pathophysiology. Furthermore, GCRCs have supported a Clinical Associates Program (CAP) for several years. To expand this training function, the centers might serve as unique sites for mounting a training program for medical students and residents who choose to perform patient-oriented research (the CAP program will be covered thoroughly in Chapter 4, on clinical research training). GCRCs might also serve as an important interface between industry and academia, and these attributes will be discussed in Chapter 5.

Other Centers Many of the individual institutes support specialized or comprehensive centers such as NCI's cancer centers and the multiarthritis centers of the National Institute of Arthritis and Musculoskeletal and Skin Diseases. This committee did not assess each institute's portfolio of centers, nor did it make a judgment of their value. Much controversy has surrounded the support of centers over the past several years, in part because of the difficulties in obtaining individual investigator-initiated grants. Although this commmittee also places the highest value on investigator-initiated grants, it also believes that the conduct of human research requires infrastructure and resources that can be efficiently provided through centers. Understandably, funding for centers that have become obsolete or unproductive should be terminated, but new ones can be devised to meet new research challenges.

Centers for Disease Control and Prevention

The mission of the Centers for Disease Control and Prevention (CDC) is to assist state and local health authorities and other health-related organizations decrease the spread of communicable diseases, protect the public from other diseases or conditions amenable to reductions, provide protection from certain environmental hazards, improve occupational safety and health, and disease prevention. CDC is also responsible for licensing clinical laboratories engaged in interstate commerce, conducting foreign quarantine activities aimed at preventing the introduction of disease into the United States, and developing scientific criteria for occupational health hazards. About nine tenths of CDC's budget is allocated to the nonresearch portion of its mission, predominantly through block grants to states.

Of the $982 million appropriated to CDC in fiscal year 1989, only about 10 percent ($100.6 million) was obligated for health research. In constant 1988 dollars, research funds at CDC grew from $56.6 million to $95.5 million between 1984 and 1989. Increases were greatest in fiscal years 1987 and 1988, when research funds grew by 18.8 and 26.8 percent, respectively, in constant dollars. These increases coincided directly with the increasing national emphasis on research into HIV infection.

The National Institute of Occupational Safety and Health (NIOSH) is a research arm of CDC. NIOSH conducts research; develops criteria for occupational safety and health standards; and provides technical services to government, labor, and industry, including training in the recognition, avoidance, and prevention of unsafe or unhealthful working conditions and the proper use of adequate safety and health equipment. Through these activities, NIOSH tries to reduce the high economic and social costs associated with occupational illness and injury. Obligations for research funded by NIOSH grew only slightly between 1984 and 1987, and they declined in the following two years. Of the $70.4 million appropriated to NIOSH for fiscal year 1989, $24.7 million was committed for research, and about $10.1 million was obligated for training.

CDC has been a leader in the nation's efforts to prevent and control the spread of HIV infection, managing a comprehensive HIV prevention program that includes surveillance; epidemiologic and laboratory studies; and prevention through information, education, and risk reduction. Appropriations for AIDS activities for fiscal year 1989 were $382.3 million—39 percent of the CDC budget. The research portion of this allocation was $44.6 million, for epidemiologic and laboratory studies to determine the natural history of the disease and to gain more knowledge about the transmission of HIV. Research funds allocated to other parts of CDC have grown much faster than those to NIOSH

Another part of the CDC, the National Center for Health Statistics (NCHS), is responsible for collecting, maintaining, analyzing, and disseminating statistics on the health, illness, and disability of the U.S. population and the effects of these factors on the U.S. economy. Although this function is not classified as research, there is a large component of epidemiologic studies for the developmednt of databases. NCHS also is responsible for collecting nonhealth data on the numbers of births, deaths, marriages, and divorces in the United States. For fiscal year 1989, $49 million was appropriated to NCHS.

Agency for Health Care Policy and Research

The Agency for Health Care Policy and Research (AHCPR) was established in 1989 as a focal point for health services research in the PHS. Whereas its predecessor, the National Center for Health Services Research, focused on general health services research, which is the study of the organization, structure, and financing of health care, AHCPR also had a mandate to develop and support research on the quality, appropriateness, and relative effectiveness of clinical intervention. The need, as expressed by Congress, was to reduce inappropriate variations in practice; to reduce, where possible, the uncertainty and lack of information often faced by clinicians and physicians; and, most important, to empower the patient to be a more informed participant in the decisionmaking process (Agency for Health Care Policy and Research, 1992). AHCPR is also in the forefront of developing the field of primary care research (U.S. Department of Health and Human Services, Public Health Service, 1991c, 1991d). As this country attempts to shift the emphasis of medicine to primary care and produce primary care physicians, a sound scientific primary care research base will be necessary. Although the research portfolio of AHCPR spans a broad spectrum of health services research, the committee focused on the portion that involves patient interactions that lead to improved medical practice.

AHCPR's Medical Treatment Effectiveness Program (MEDTEP) seeks to improve the effectiveness and appropriateness of health care through improved understanding of outcomes and alternative interventions (U.S. Department of Health and Human Services, Public Health Service, 1991b). Clinical management of a given condition can be quite variable throughout the country. The outcomes of the available strategies are often equally variable. Thus, MEDTEP is a multifaceted program composed of the following four interrelated components designed to assess the relative effectiveness of alternative strategies for treating common clinical conditions:

1. the development of databases;
2. the conduct and support of research on outcomes, effectiveness, and appropriateness of health care services and procedures;
3. the development of clinical practice guidelines; and
4. the dissemination, assimilation, and evaluation of research findings and clinical practice guidelines.

Although all these areas are vital to improving health care, the committee focused on the second area—the conduct and support of research on outcomes, effectiveness, and appropriateness of health care services and procedures. One of MEDTEP's unique contributions is the focus on common conditions; its relevance to all patients with a given condition (including those with comorbidities) and all providers caring for these patients; and its broad definition of clinical success, which includes symptom relief, quality of life, functional status, patient satisfaction, and costs (Agency for Health Care Policy and Reaearch, 1992).

Although earlier studies analyzed large claims databases to understand differences in the clinical management of given conditions, MEDTEP supports a small number of clinical effectiveness trials on selected conditions identified by Patient Outcomes Research Teams (PORTs). Unlike the efficacy trials commonly supported by NIH and the pharmaceutical industry, these effectiveness trials will focus on clinical outcomes that occur under ordinary conditions. Each of the PORT projects includes an elaborate five-year program encompassing synthesis of the research on a condition (using meta-analysis), acquisition and analysis of primary and secondary data, development of clinical recommendations, dissemination of findings, and evaluation of the effects of the findings on clinical practice. A sample of PORTs already under way include prostate disease, low back pain, acute myocardial infarction, cateracts, total knee replacement, ischemic heart disease, biliary tract disease, pneumonia, type II diabetes, hip fracture and replacement, prevention of stroke, and delivery by cesarean section and other obstetrical procedures. Clinicians trained in outcomes or effectiveness methodologies are critical to the success of the PORTs. Of the 12 PORTs, 10 are run by clinicians, 1 is run by an economist, and 1 is run by a mathematical statistician. Eventually, AHCPR will support Medical Treatment Effectiveness Research Centers on Minority Populations and a pharmaceutical outcomes program. There are also opportunities for cross-agency collaboration. For example, AHCPR supplemented a clinical trial on otitis media funded primarily by the National Institute of Child and Human Development to collect extra data on the quality-of-life dimensions to the research as well as to track patients not accepted into the trial.

AHCPR had a budget of $120 million in fiscal year 1992. The MEDTEP line accounted for approximately $67 million of the total. Of this, $44 million was allocated for grant and contract research, including interagency agreements with other Public Health Service components. The remainder of the $67 million supports the development of clinical practice guidelines, training through the National Research Service Award (NRSA), dissertation awards, and other programmatic functions of the agency (Raskin, 1992).

With respect to NRSA training, AHCPR's annual budget is relatively small, amounting to approximately $3 million when compared with NIH's $300 million annual training budget. These funds support about 95 individuals through either institutional or individual awards. Of those, about 42 are M.D.s in training; a significant percentage of this number are primary care physicians. AHCPR also supports approximately 20 to 25 predoctoral dissertation awards.

U.S. Department of Veterans Affairs

Historically, the U.S. Department of Veterans Affairs (VA), previously known as the Veterans Administration, has provided health care to veterans through a network of 172 hospitals and centers nationwide. Approximately 130 of these units have medical trainees and about 100 have formal agreements with medical schools. The VA provides financial support for 8,350 residents and interns—nearly 13 percent of the trainees in the United States. In addition, Congress appropriates R&D funds to the VA to conduct studies pertaining to veterans' health or using veteran patient populations. The VA research program sponsors investigations across a broad spectrum of health research, including basic and clinical sciences, health services (outcomes, cost-effectiveness, and technology assessment), applied research, and rehabilitation and prosthetics (Smith, 1992a).

VA has several attributes that make it a good resource base for clinical research. First, patient recruitment for clinical investigations is easier for VA than for NIH. Second, the costs for the standard medical care portion of clinical investigations are charged to health care delivery funds rather than research dollars, so that only the marginal costs of the research consume research appropriations— a potential model for non-VA research as well. The clinical trials conducted by VA may have a far-reaching impact on research performed by other federal agencies. VA also is exploring ways to enhance its position as a resource base for clinical investigations by more open cooperation with private industry (Institute of Medicine, 1989b).

Recognizing this unique niche for conducting health research, the research management in the VA has developed a new mission statement that emphasizes clinical research, particularly clinically derived research as well as clinically relevant research:

> To develop and conduct research representing a continuum of programs—biomedical research, health services research, and prosthetics and rehabilitation—which integrates the clinical needs and research inquiries to enhance the quality of health care delivery to veterans (Smith, 1992b).

The VA R&D budget is a separate line item in the federal budget and is divided into the following three major categories: (1) medical research, (2) rehabilitation research, and (3) health services R&D. In fiscal year 1993, VA was appropriated $232 million to support about 1,500 programs (Smith, 1992a). About 75 percent of the budget supports investigator-initiated biomedical research. The VA research budget, however, has not increased over the past decade when measured in constant dollars (Figure 3-18) (U.S. Department of Veterans Affairs, 1991). Flat budgets and growing research costs have negatively affected the numbers of projects that can be supported, particularly in the medical portion of the research budget (Figure 3-19) (Smith, 1992b; U.S. Department of Veterans Affairs, 1991). Nevertheless, over the past few years the rehabilitation research component has shown a gradual increase, and health services research has shown a tremendous surge in funding. Eight percent of the research budget is directed toward VA cooperative studies (multihospital clinical trials).

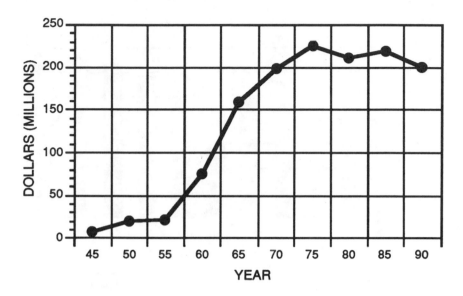

FIGURE 3-18 Appropriations for reseach in the U.S. Department of Veterans Affairs, 1945–1990. (Source: U.S. Department of Veterans Affairs, 1992)

Although the VA research budget is not very large when compared with that of NIH, it should be noted that salaries for clinical investigators, facility support, and so forth are derived from other portions of the VA budget. If those costs are added in, the budget might approach the equivalent of $500 million (Smith, 1992b). Moreover, if the NIH-funded research being performed in VA facilities is included, the VA research budget approaches the equivalent of $900 million. Although VA is able to leverage a significant amount of research with its modest budget, it is under the same budget pressures as other science agencies competing for scarce resources. For example, the average cost of an investigator-initiated grant in 1987 was $60,000; by 1992, the average cost had increased to $90,000. This growth reflects solely the increasing costs of performing research because salaries and overhead are not included.

All VA-sponsored research is conducted intramurally. About 80 percent of the investigators are clinicians who administer care to veterans at VA medical centers. Eligibility criteria in the VA research system require that applicants for an investigator-initiated grant must have a five-eighths appointment within the VA (Smith, 1992b). This requirement is an attempt to ensure that the investigators are clinicians who are involved in patient care.

Approximately 10 percent of the VA research budget is allocated for career development at all levels (Smith, 1992b). This includes limited salary support for some levels of training for young physician-investigators. Generally, salary

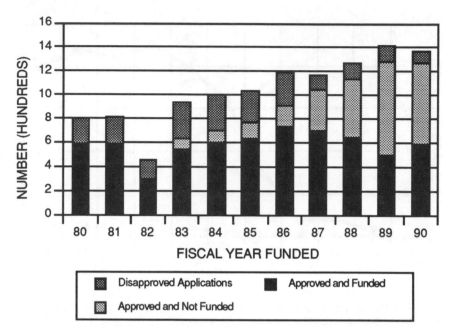

FIGURE 3-19 Disposition of competing research grant applications undergoing merit review for the U.S. Department of Veterans Affairs, 1980–1990. (Source: U.S. Department of Veterans Affairs, 1992)

support for established VA investigators is covered with nonresearch funds. To encourage careers in clinical research, VA is developing a career development program that will cover salaries and provide a small amount of research support. The salaries and positions are then transferred to individual VA hospitals. This program is available for the entire spectrum of clinician-investigators—from those directly out of their residency programs to very senior investigators.

Another new program under development emphasizes the collaboration between the VA research program and academic research through research fellowships. These fellowships would be available to postresidency physicians who would be eligible for fellowships supported by their academic institution, with a contribution from the VA research program of $3,000 to $10,000 a year.

The VA is very concerned that its research program is in jeopardy, however (Smith, 1992a, b). As a percentage of total VA appropriations, the research budget declined from 3.5 percent in 1970 to 1.5 percent in 1993. In the past two years, only budget transfers from the U.S. Department of Defense have kept the VA research budget ahead of inflation. VA believes its programs, particularly the career development program, are in a fragile funding situation. It appears that VA will not be able to fund any new programs at all—no new career development and no new investigator-initiated awards—and only about a third of continuing competitive renewals will receive funding.

U.S. Department of Education

The National Institute on Disability and Rehabilitation Research (NIDRR) is part of the Office of Special Education and Rehabilitative Services in the U.S. Department of Education (U.S. Department of Education, Office of Special Education and Rehabilitative Services, 1991b). The Rehabilitation Research and Training Centers (RRTCs) are the largest program. Although much of the focus of the RRTCs is on vocational strategies, some support is provided to physicians and allied health professionals for research in rehabilitative medicine. The budget of the NIDRR was $65 million for fiscal year 1993.

U.S. Department of Defense

The U.S. Department of Defense (DOD) conducts health research vital to national security. Three branches conduct intramural and extramural health research: (1) the U.S. Army Medical Research and Development Command (USAMRDC), (2) the Directorate of Life Sciences in the Air Force Office of Scientific Research, and (3) the Life Sciences Programs Directorate of the Office of Naval Research (Institute of Medicine, 1990). While the three branches conduct a significant amount of health sciences research, there is no reliable estimate of how much is performed on human subjects.

Of the three branches, USAMRDC receives the largest allocation of DOD funds for military health sciences research—about 80 percent of the total DOD health sciences research budget. In fiscal year 1989, $252 million was appropriated. The USAMRDC conducts mission-oriented medical R&D designed to support the soldier in the field. This program supports research on increasing efficiency of soldiers by improving instrumentation and new medical knowledge in the following areas: (1) military disease hazards, including infectious diseases, biological warfare defense, and AIDS; (2) combat casualty care, including shock, wound healing, and craniofacial injuries; (3) medical chemical defense; and (4) army systems hazards.

The Directorate of Life Sciences in the Air Force Office of Scientific Research has a health-related research budget much smaller than that of USAMRDC. In 1989 allocations for health research were only $17.1 million. These funds support research in several areas of neuroscience, experimental psychology, toxicology, visual and auditory psychophysics, radiation biology, and cardiovascular physiology.

The Office of Naval Research funds health research through the Life Sciences Programs Directorate. In fiscal year 1989, $24.4 million was allocated to biological and medical sciences and $11.5 million was allocated to cognitive and neural sciences. The 1990 budget had only slight increases for the biological and medical sciences—to $25.3 million—and an increase $13.7 million for the cognitive and neural sciences.

Although the committee is aware that the armed services may not be heavily involved in medical research on human subjects, some research areas may fall into the purview of the armed services. For example, the armed services has supported human studies on vaccines and therapies for tropical diseases. New opportunities are becoming available for the armed services to expand their clinical studies in several areas; for example, funding was recently made available for breast cancer. The Surgical Task Force of this committee has also recommended that the military examine potential involvement in treatment strategies for trauma at established civilian trauma centers, which might expand the knowledge base for treating trauma received on the battlefield (see Appendix C).

NONPROFIT ORGANIZATIONS

Throughout the twentieth century, private nonprofit organizations have played a critical role in funding health sciences research. Many early private foundations were established to benefit particular institutions or to address specific social or health problems with assets generally derived from an individual's or a family's gifts. During the twentieth century, voluntary health agencies, which are also referred to as operating foundations, have proliferated. In addition, a special type of nonprofit organization—the medical research organization—has developed. Each type of organization differs in its mission, governance, and mechanisms of support. Although these organizations make up a limited portion of all health sciences research support, they are vital to the nation's medical research enterprise because of their flexibility and their dedication to curing human disease and suffering.

NIH estimated that private nonprofit organizations contributed about $1,196 million (or about 4.3 percent of the total), to health R&D in 1992 (U. S. Department of Health and Human Serevices, Public Health Service, 1992c). This figure, however, probably underestimates the role of philanthropy in health sciences research by excluding endowed professorships and donations for facilities and equipment. Another estimate has placed philanthropy at nearly one-quarter of a typical institution's budget for biomedical R&D (Boniface and Rimel, 1987).

Foundations

Although federal investment in health sciences research has eclipsed that of foundations since World War II, foundations still play a vital role in the research enterprise. Few foundations conduct in-house research, because most believe that support for extramural research and research infrastructure provides the most efficient use of funds. Private foundations currently provide a great variety of support mechanisms for health sciences research and use their resources to support new areas of investigation or to augment federal funding. Common categories of foundation support include individual research project grants, predoctoral and postdoctoral fellowships, equipment grants, payment of publication expenses, special library collections grants, and sponsorship of conferences or workshops. Although some foundations support research and research training for physicians and other health professionals, it is unclear how much is being invested in patient-oriented research or clinical research training. Nonetheless, foundations, have provided crucial support in filling gaps in the research agenda that have not been addressed appropriately or profitably by government or industry.

The mechanisms for setting priorities and making funding decisions vary among foundations (Institute of Medicine, 1990). In some instances, funding decisions are made through personal contacts or because of a foundation's interest in a specific disorder. Large, independent foundations may form advisory committees to determine areas of emphasis; proposals may also be subjected to a peer review process similar to that used by NIH. Smaller foundations may not plan program initiatives; instead, they may fund the best unsolicited proposals received in a given time period. The extent of foundation support for health sciences research varies from year to year, depending on the relative timing of costly initiatives.

Voluntary Health Agencies

Voluntary health agencies (VHAs), such as the American Cancer Society and the American Heart Association, play critically important roles in advancing research in their areas of interest. VHAs (often referred to as operating foundations) are private charities supported primarily by public donations. In addition to grants for research and training, these organizations also support activities that include public awareness and education, patient referrals, continuing education for health professionals, and lobbying to increase federal funding for disease-specific research. Now, perhaps over 200 national and regional VHAs actively support health research, and many of VHAs were founded by the families and friends of individuals suffering from a given disease.

The six largest VHAs (in revenues) are, in descending order, the American Cancer Society, the American Heart Association, the March of Dimes-Birth

Defects Foundation, the Muscular Dystrophy Association, the National Easter Seal Society, and the American Lung Association. These six organizations reported combined expenditures for disease-related research of more than $250 million in 1988 (Institute of Medicine, 1990). Because these organizations rely on voluntary contributions, they often are unable to make long-term commitments to research efforts such as multiyear clinical studies. They are effective, however, in responding rapidly to new research initiatives and providing resources to scientists to develop new lines of investigation.

VHAs also can play a critical role in the early stages of scientific career development. Through funding mechanisms such as fellowships and career development awards, these organizations attract young researchers to a specific field and provide them with research funding before they are able to compete successfully for federal support. Grant awards from these organizations commonly range between $20,000 and $50,000.

The effects of the lobbying activities of VHAs cannot be overstated. These organizations have been instrumental in increasing public awareness of the need to fight particular diseases and in soliciting grass-roots support for more federal research funds. They also have been very influential in establishing new institutes at NIH focusing on specific diseases and sets of diseases.

Medical Research Organizations

Medical research organizations (MROs) are unique in the portfolio of nonprofit support for research and research training. MROs are required by law to spend 3.5 percent of their endowments annually on medical research in conjunction with a hospital. The largest MRO, with assets estimated to be more than $6 billion, is the Howard Hughes Medical Institute (HHMI). In recent years HHMI has become the largest single private nonprofit contributor to biomedical research, with 1992 expenditures estimated at $281 million—a total greater than the expenditures of many NIH institutes. The J. David Gladstone Foundation Laboratories for Cardiovascular Disease, which is affiliated with the University of California at San Francisco, is another example and has assets estimated at $118 million.

HHMI traditionally has established large laboratories, with core groups of investigators in universities and hospitals around the United States to facilitate interaction with the larger research community. Investigators are appointed for fixed terms of three to seven years, with full funding provided for faculty and technician salaries as well as research expenses. Investigator productivity is evaluated through research conferences, annual progress reports, and site visits. Recently, HHMI has initiated a program to support individual investigators at institutions that do not have a core HHMI laboratory. This program will expand

HHMI support from approximately 180 investigators in its 30 core laboratories to approximately 250 at more than 40 institutions over the next few years.

HHMI's program is restricted to a few selected areas of research: cell biology and cell regulation, genetics, immunology, neuroscience, and structural biology. A 10-member medical advisory board has ultimate responsibility for the quality of the research program, and scientific review boards comprising scientists in each of the five areas oversee work in their respective fields. Although the HHMI program is highly regarded for its contributions to biomedicine and support for physician-scientists, its role in supporting patient-oriented clinical investigations is less clear. Physicians supported by HHMI may have clinical interests and may conduct clinical investigations, but the research portfolio of the institute is directed at preclinical research. Furthermore, although HHMI is sufficiently large to make major contributions in its selected areas of research, it does not seek to replace the central role of NIH in any field.

In addition to its research portfolio, HHMI has undertaken a broad program to strengthen science education from the precollege to the postdoctoral stages. The graduate science education program funds several levels of graduate training. For instance, doctoral fellowships in the biological sciences (60 yearly) provide predoctoral students with a stipend and cost-of-education allowance for three to five years; medical student research training fellowships (up to 60 a year) are modeled after HHMI's Research Scholars Program, supporting students for a year of research training at any U.S. academic or research institution. HHMI began the Undergraduate Science Education Program in 1988 to award grants to strengthen science education and research in private undergraduate colleges and increase the number of students, especially minorities and women, pursuing careers in the biomedical sciences. The program recently has been expanded to selected public universities.

INDUSTRY

Before World War II, industry funded more than half of all health sciences research in the United States (Boniface and Rimel, 1987; Ginzberg and Dutka, 1989). After the war, industry's support, although still increasing, was outpaced by the investment of the federal government. Since the early 1980s, however, industry has been playing an increasingly important role in health sciences research, focusing primarily on product development. The kinds of industries engaged in health sciences R&D include biotechnology firms and manufacturers of pharmaceuticals, medical devices, and instruments. These industries tend to be very research intensive, and R&D investment is measured as a percentage of sales. For example, DiMasi et al. (1991) have estimated that it costs more than $230 million for a pharmaceutical firm to bring a new drug to market.

Understandably, corporate research focuses mainly on applied research and product development that moves products to market rather than on the undirected disease-oriented research or fundamental basic biology familiar to NIH. Pharmaceuticals, biologicals, and medical implants all require human studies to reach the market; therefore, clinical investigators and manufacturers need to work together closely to ensure that testing proceeds efficiently and under the strictest scientific methodology. Development and testing requirements for investigative new drugs or devices probably account for these large R&D expenditures (Battelle, 1991, Fletcher, 1989). Also, high levels of research investment have been attributed in part to the commercial potential for biological products such as genetically engineered insulin (Institute of Medicine, 1990). In 1991 industry contributed an estimated $13.5 billion to health research, accounting for about 48 percent of the total national investment in health research (Figure 3-1) (National Institutes of Health, 1993b).

In the past, a great deal of research was performed "in house" for proprietary reasons, and industry relied on university research programs to develop basic knowledge and scientific talent. In addition, pharmaceutical firms, and now biotechnology firms, generally contracted with clinicians in academic centers to test compounds in all phases of clinical trials. During the 1980s these established paradigms of academic-industry and industry-government relationships began to shift. Rapid advances in science and changes in the tax code encouraging R&D investment and technology transfer have prompted many special linkages among industry, government, and academic scientists (Witt, 1991). Shared interests in specific problems have helped to create some industry-sponsored cooperative basic research programs located in universities (National Academy of Sciences, Government-University-Industry Research Roundtable, 1986). Industry has also been working closely with NIH to develop numerous therapies, particularly new drugs to fight HIV infection. Although most regard these new linkages favorably, they can create problems of conflict of interest from the level of individual investigators to that of the research institutions themselves. Some of these unique relationships between industry and academic scientists are elucidated in Chapter 5.

The shifting policies of the health insurance industry and Medicare is another problem confronting manufacturing industries that require human testing to bring their products to market. The move toward cost-containment has driven many employers to shop for health plans that provide a certain level of care at the lowest cost to themselves and their employees. More and more employers are choosing to provide managed health care as the only option. Although managed health care can potentially reduce the costs of health care in the short term, its effects on innovation through drugs, devices, and procedures have not been fully realized (Holmes, 1992; Laetz, 1991; Leaf, 1989; Moody, 1992; Telling, 1992). As the debate over ways to contain the rate of growth of health care intensifies in

TABLE 3-7 Distribution of U.S. R&D Expenditures for Ethical Pharmaceuticals by Function, 1991

Function	Amount ($ million)	Percent
Clinical evaluation phases I, II, III	1,555.0	26.7
Biological screening pharmacologic testing	984.2	16.9
Synthesis and extraction	570.8	9.8
Pharmaceutical dosage formulation and stability testing	447.4	9.4
Toxicology and safety testing	407.7	7.0
Process development for manufacturing and quality control	425.2	7.3
Clinical evaluation: phase IV	233.0	4.0
Regulatory, IND and NDA preparation, submission and processing	192.2	3.3
Bioavailability studies	151.4	2.6
Other	757.1	13.0
Total	5,824.0	100.0

Source: Reprinted, with permission, from Pharmaceutical Manufacturers Association (1993). Copyright 1993 by the Pharmaceutical Manufacturers Association.

the next few months and years, clinical research must be perceived as a vital part of the U.S. health care system and crucial for improving health.

The costs of pharmaceutical innovation are high. DiMasi et al. (1991) have estimated that it took 12 years and, on average, $231 million (1987 dollars) to bring a new drug to market for drugs tested in humans between 1970 and 1982. Throughout the 1980s, the pharmaceutical industry increased expenditures for R&D above that of the annual increases for R&D allocated to NIH. While the average industrial investment in R&D by industry is about 5 to 6 percent of gross income, pharmaceutical firms invest a high level in R&D expenditures in relation to sales—for example, 13 percent in 1987.

The distribution of R&D expenditures varies by company and type of research. The National Science Foundation reports that nearly 80 percent of industrial R&D is development, about 15 percent is applied R&D, and basic research accounts for only 5 percent (National Science Foundation, 1988b). There is another way to view investment; that is, approximately one third of a pharmaceutical firm's R&D investment is devoted to discovery and new product development, one third is spent on existing product improvement and expansion of current business, and one third is directed toward process improvement for defending current market shares of products (Institute of Medicine, 1990). Whatever the measure or matrix of investment, a large portion of pharmaceutical R&D is spent on clinical evaluation of drugs in phases I through IV of clinical evaluation (Table 3-7).

Biotechnology is one subcategory of industrial biomedical R&D of particular importance to this committee (Blumenthal et al., 1986a, 1986b). The ability to synthesize proteins and peptides, new biological approaches to drug delivery such as the use of liposomes to encapsulate drugs, and other biological advances are rapidly expanding opportunities for finding and testing new biological therapies (Telling, 1992). The private sector, however, is not the exclusive investor in biotechnology. Whereas the federal government, primarily NIH, has been the primary source of R&D funds for biotechnology, the commercial markets for new biologicals is encouraging increased investment in biotechnology by industry. NIH reported that nearly 22 percent, or $1.02 billion, of its 1988 R&D budget was allocated to research on developing biotechnology techniques or employing the biotechnology (Institute of Medicine, 1990). The size of NIH investment in biotechnology reflects the importance of molecular and cellular biology in biomedicine.

CLINICAL RESEARCH AND THIRD-PARTY PAYERS

A chapter on the resources of funding for clinical research would not be complete without a discussion of the contributions to clinical research by third-party payers. In the United States, the relationship among insurers, subscribers, employers, and providers is unique. For many with employer-based health coverage, the employer establishes the contract of coverage, the employee pays part of the premium for the health coverage that the employer has established, and the third-party payer is the steward of the funds. The policy for those with federally supported coverage, such as Medicare or Medicaid, has been not to cover investigational or experimental therapies. The sad irony is that the 35 million or more people who have no health care coverage have more freedom to enroll in clinical studies or receive experimental therapy because they have no stake in who pays, and no third party questions their decision.

Unfortunately, very little is known about the amount of support actually contributed by third-party payers. There are no databases that track this investment, and in many instances, it is believed that the less known, the better. Another variable in this equation is the amount of unreimbursed care provided by hospitals and medical centers for individuals enrolled in clinical studies or trials; for example, those covered under Medicare. The committee was clearly aware of the problems of assessing the level of involvement of third-party payers in clinical research, but it felt strongly that the relevant policy issues should be explored. Thus, while this section is short on data, it draws upon presentations by executives from the insurance sector given at the workshop "Clinical Research and Training: Spotlight on Funding" (see Appendix D).

An unwritten understanding previously promoted, or at least did not discourage, the participation of patients in clinical studies or trials in which third parties contributed patient care costs, whether or not they were cognizant of it. For example, an extra computed tomography scan or other test might be performed to collect longitudinal data, and the claim would be covered without question. Changes in health care coverage in the past 15 years—with the emphasis on reigning in costs by cutting hospital stays and other care not proven to be cost-effective or efficacious—have altered this fragile relationship. The move to prospective payment based on diagnostic-related groups may also have affected the enrollment of patients in clinical studies. With computerized technology, third-party payers are able to scrutinize how patients are being treated and question why they should be supporting experimental studies. Government programs, both Medicare and state Medicaid programs are having the same difficulties that the science agencies are experiencing—scrambling for scarce resources in the federal budget. The for-profit private insurers must be equally concerned with covering the soaring costs for standard therapies and paying dividends to shareholders. Even the nonprofit insurers like Blue Cross and Blue Shield must be concerned with balancing their cash flow. Thus, most third-party payers probably believe that clinical research falls far outside of their boundaries of responsibility.

Old therapies that may or may not be effective are not being adequately assessed, and new medical technologies and therapies are evolving very rapidly. At the same time, biomedical scientists are becoming increasingly sophisticated in understanding the biological bases of disease processes and the heterogeneity of patient populations. This synergism stokes the engine for even more scientific inquiry to define more precise fits between treatments and specific patient populations, not only for the good of science, but certainly for the benefit of the patients. Coupled to this is the public's expectation for increasingly sophisticated health care with cascades of tests and procedures and without concern for how the costs will be covered. Patients with incurable diseases also expect to have access to the best possible care or optimal therapy—even if that involves enrolling in a clinical study for testing an unproven therapy. Viewed purely on a cost basis, standard therapy may be the least expensive in the short run. A well-designed clinical trial, however, may uncover an improved therapy to reduce morbidity or mortality and, it is hoped, improve quality of life, despite the high initial costs. The conundrum that has arisen is that an adversarial situation has developed between the patients and their doctors, on the one hand, and the patients and the third-party payers, on the other, because the affected parties cannot agree on what portion of clinical investigation is reimbursable (Newcomer, 1990).

The bottom line is that reimbursement of costs is essential. Someone must ultimately pay for the costs associated with experimental therapy as well as the costs of standard medical care, whether it is the federal government (Health Care Financing Administration, NIH, and the like), the third-party payers, the institutions, or other sponsors of research. Following the paradigm of the past, clinical investigtors expected that insurers would reimburse the costs of legitimate care associated with sponsored research of the highest quality. At the same time, it was believed that the sponsor of the research should bear the cost associated with the research. Nevertheless, it is frequently difficult to separate the care costs from the research costs, and most of the disagreement focuses on this gray area. This is particularly evident in the treatment of cancer, where almost all treatment is some form of experiment, often using class C (cancer) drugs or combining two or more types of therapies (Antman et al., 1988; Wittes, 1987b).

Another point of contention is the refusal by a payer to allow reimbursement for any care if a covered patient is enrolled in a study Wittes 1987b and 1988). Patients, however, are suing their insurers to allow them to enroll in clinical studies and receive coverage for both the standard care and the experimental therapy, especially when standard therapies are not much improved over no treatment. Although this puts pressure on third-party payers to cover the costs associated with the standard care and those associated with the experimental therapy, moving these controversies into the courts may not be the best way to encourage participation in clinical research. After prolonged legal procedures, as well as high legal costs for the patient and the patient's family, the decision is usually left in the hands of a jury, which is unlikely to have the requisite expertise in experimental medicine. The result fails to serve good medicine, appropriate patient care, or sound reimbursement policy. Furthermore, it ties up everyone's time and resources and prolongs the potential benefit a patient might receive from the investigational therapy. A better route would be to have clinicians, in collaboration with payers, make sound decisions based on clear clinical research data about whether to provide care under an experimental protocol.

One example of growing cooperation among the affected parties is the use of autologous bone marrow transplantation for treating metastatic breast cancer. This is a developing technology that is costly, effort-intensive, and somewhat toxic, but it has shown some promise over standard therapy. Briefly, it consists of harvesting autologous bone marrow from a patient, administering very high doses of chemotherapy or radiation therapy to inactivate the metastatic cells, and then reconstituting the normal hematopoietic elements from the harvested bone marrow. Hospitalization is necessary for anywhere from a few days to several weeks, and the cost for such treatment has been in the range of $75,000 to

$150,000 per patient. That this therapy is available is a tribute to the sponsors of fundamental research, including the National Cancer Institute, the American Cancer Society, and the American Leukemia Society. More interesting, however, is the paradigm for supporting a large, multicenter clinical trial on the therapy. After losing several suits forcing various payers to cover the costs of this therapy, a coalition of third-party payers, including some of the individual Blue Cross and Blue Shield plans, have agreed to fund a demonstration project in which they will accept some responsibility for paying the clinical care costs associated with these particular national studies. This may signal a new paradigm for sharing the costs of clinical research in which payers, clinical investigators, and patients all cooperate to further understanding of novel and innovative therapies.

Third-Party Payers' Perspective

It has become increasingly necessary for plans to serve their subscribers while striving for access to quality health care at an affordable price. Inextricably bound to those objectives are the processes of technology assessment and coverage determination. Medical technology committees, frequently including physicians and subscribers, have become increasingly sophisticated and have established sets of criteria to guide coverage, including cost-effectiveness, legal, ethical, and cultural differences, and distributive justice (Whether the technology is available to all subscribers.). These criteria have been delineated after some years of study to help determine when a technology has reached a stage at which it is no longer considered investigational and can be accepted as eligible for coverage. Once the criteria have been satisfied and the committee has determined that a critical mass of evidence is available to show that a procedure or technology is established as standard care, most will agree that it is eligible for coverage determination (Leaf, 1989). The bigger concern, however, appears to be over who should pay for the initial studies to collect the requisite primary data and how the data should be collected, shared, and analyzed (Antman et al., 1988; Wittes 1987b). For example, FDA approval of a drug or device for a given condition often, although not always, meets the criteria for coverage (Wittes, 1987a).

Another problem arises, however, when an approved drug is used to treat a disease for which it is not approved (off-label use) (Moertel, 1991; U.S. Government Accounting Office, 1991). In some instances, there may be compelling evidence that a particular drug is effective, but the pharmaceutical manufacturer does not choose to add this information to the label because of the costs associated with additional FDA approval or the short time remaining on a sole-source patent. Patients and the provider are often left with few options. At the same time, third-party payers see their role as that of gatekeepers preventing overutilization and expansion of technology beyond its intended use or the continued use of outmoded technology. This scenario presents a serious gap in the U.S. system of who should pay for what. For example, pharmaceutical patents are time-limited. When an already approved therapy shows promise for another condition and a manufacturer is unable or unwilling to cover the costs associated with gaining approval for the use of the drug in the treatment of that other condition, who should pay for the investigations? Should the government allocate funds for the trials? Should the third-party payers be obligated to participate? Would a coalition of all concerned parties resolve this conundrum?

During the early 1980s, a modification of coverage determination was designed to cover certain therapies that were not yet established, but had demonstrated promising success rates at particular institutions—selective coverage. For example, a payer might determine that a procedure in the hands of skilled physicians looks promising and would cover the associated costs at a particular medical center (for example, the early days of heart transplantation). Thus, a body of evidence might have accumulated demonstrating a procedure had positive outcomes and that it might no longer be considered investigational when performed at that institution. Although this late-stage coverage is appreciated, many resources that were not reimbursed were consumed to reach this stage.

Third-party payers are also concerned about the proliferation of clinical trials for any one condition. Because many of these trials are investigator initiated, one might find five or six different research groups, each treating patients on a different protocol for the same disease. Depending on the available patient populations, many of these trials might not be able to accrue enough patients to achieve statistical validity. Moreover, the third-party payers may not be able to determine which ones should be covered and which ones should not. Another problem cited is the varied perspectives of the investigators, even those collaborating on one project. By the time one gets through compromising with 5 or 10 very aggressive investigators, each one altering the study design in his or her own way, a study may be misguided and not answer the originial question, or perhaps answer questions that were not very germane about the disease in question to society as a whole. These difficulties are not very appealing to insurers and make them disinclined to sponsor clinical studies.

Involvement in Study Design and Data Analyses

If third-party payers are to become significant collaborators in clinical studies and trials, their roles in experimental design and data analysis should be fully elucidated. As a stakeholder, the question arises as to how much of a role the insurer should have in creating the study design. Would it constitute a conflict of interest if an insurer supports a study with a design that could be potentially biased at the outset because of company participation? How can participation be assured without compromising the scientific validity of the investigation?

Data Sharing and Analysis

Once a third-party payer decides to support a study, another question arises; that is, how much access should they have to the data? On the one hand, the insurer will have access to the claims data, from which it could draw certain conclusions. On the other hand, how much access to the scientific data should the insurer be allowed? Again, as a stakeholder, the third-party payer probably believes that it should have complete access to medical information on patients covered under its policies. In the appropriate conduct of randomized clinical trials, however, the study is blinded and the codes cannot be broken until the statistical considerations are met. Other types of clinical studies may warrant other arrangements of data sharing.

In addition to the issues surrounding access of data by the third-party payers, access to third-party payer databases by investigators also raises several issues. The insurers maintain the massive databases required for accounting purposes in the U.S. health care system. Such data bases could be utilized for continuous evaluation of medical practice. Studies of such data might not only provide a sounder basis for reimbursing new and experimental interventions but also could allow reevaluation of older, potentially obsolete or ineffective technologies that should no longer be employed. Numerous deficiencies in these databases, however, preclude this use. For example, each insurer has a claim form that collects and codes information differently. Without a standard type of data collection, comparison of data sets from different sources becomes impossible. Moreover, many of the claims data are probably not complete enough to draw conclusions about the effectiveness or outcomes of different therapies.

Possible Solutions

From the perspective of third-party payers, direct funding of clinical research is not possible. Viewing themselves as custodians of subscribers' funds, they do not have the reserves or the authority to devote resources to underwriting all clinical research, particularly that in which a third-party payer has a commercial interest. However, as custodians of those funds, third-party payers make coverage decisions that affect the health and well-being of their subscribers. Thus, payers have an obligation to find out what works and what does not. Nevertheless, possible solutions that will serve the interests of all parties can be developed without allowing costs to continue to soar (Antman, 1989; Wittes, 1988). The committee believes that high-quality care at a reasonable cost can be retained, while at the same time advancing new and unproven therapies that could potentially improve quality of life.

Much can and should be done to ensure, encourage, and enhance the cooperative investment of time and interest that all parties have in clinical research, clinical research training, and the responsible utilization of new approaches to the diagnosis and treatment of disease. New approaches must encourage, not discourage, the responsible use of emerging technologies and therapies and the development of new uses for accepted interventions. To increase the quality of life and the effectiveness of health care, all parties need to foster continued innovation, not only in academic and industrial research laboratories but also at the bedside.

There must be a true partnership that meets the goals and expectations of all participating parties and ensures the timely and cost-effective application of the findings of clinical research or the application of new technologies. Meaningful partnerships and coalitions need to be created. These coalitions could include not only university academic health centers but also private foundations, federal and state agencies, the pharmaceutical and biomedical technological industry, and those in the health insurance industry. For example, an interdisciplinary, interorganizational group could be created to help establish guidelines and provide recommendations for the use of, and payment for, therapies that have gone beyond the early investigational phase or for therapies over which there is a degree of controversy. Membership for such a group could be drawn, for example, from the Institute of Medicine, the Agency for Health Care Policy and Research, NIH, the health insurance sector, health-related private foundations, and representative consumers. This group would develop and maintain guidelines and criteria and decide what new procedures, therapies, or devices should or should not be reimbursable. One form of cooperation might be to adopt a uniform policy of paying for experimental therapies for all patients on approved protocols by NIH. Another might be to establish a diagnosis-related group-style prospective payment system that would ensure that adequate numbers of patients were enrolled in a trial to answer a question with adequate statistical power.

The potential advantages of increased cooperation are obvious. By working together rather than through the courts or other judgmental bodies, the committee believes that the appropriateness and effectiveness of care for patients can be improved. Improved outcomes for patients may result in economic savings for the patients and the payers. Thus, knowledge of how best to provide care will be expanded and transmitted to a broad base of qualified providers and, of great importance, to the next generation of practitioners. Of course, any changes need to occur in a climate that recognizes that the resources for health care are under greater stress and pressure than in any other time in U.S. history, whether it be in the academic health centers, pharmaceutical and biotechnology industry, or the insurance industry.

MODELS OF COOPERATION

Undeniably, the U.S. system of health research has been highly successful largely because of the unhindered ability of investigators to pursue intriguing and pertinent questions ranging from very fundamental basic biology to clinical studies requiring the participation of human subjects. Previously, the separation of who should pay for what was of little concern because of plentiful resources and fairly well-established areas of responsibility. Simplistically, NIH and other federal agencies funded investigator-initiated human studies and other clinical studies deemed necessary by advisory bodies or Congress to fill gaps in certain areas, industry has been motivated by the potential for profits and clinical studies are driven by regulatory concerns, the insurance industry may or may not cover certain aspects of investigational care, and academic health centers and hospitals have underwritten significant portions of unrecovered clinical research expenses out of their own reserves. With the growing attention to health care cost-containment and increasing constraints on the federal research budget, however, the committee fears that fundamental human research may be inadvertently squeezed out of the research portfolio. Clearly, the potential for return on investment continues to be a strong incentive for industry to sponsor clinical trials of test substances, chemical or biological. A large amount of the knowledge base upon which new therapeutic agents may be founded, however, is derived from investigator-initiated preclinical research and studies of human biology and disease that are likely to have no immediate or long-term commercial interest. Thus, the committee believes that new models of cooperation among all parties with a vested interest in health care are necessary for continued progress in human research to further improve modern health care.

To explore these opportunities for increased cooperation among industry, government, academic health centers, and third-party payers, the committee sought examples in other scientific areas to serve as models or prototypes. One notable example is SEMATECH, which was formed during the 1980s in response to the intense international competition in the semiconductor industry. SEMATECH is a consortium of U.S. semiconductor manufacturers working with government and academia; it sponsors and conducts precompetitive cutting-edge research in semiconductor manufacturing technology for U.S. manufacturers. It was originally created out of a concern that the U.S. manufacturers were losing market share and may be forced out of the global market altogether, therefore risking the national security if the U.S. military were reliant on foreign manufacturers for vital computer chips.

The annual budget for SEMATECH is $200 million—far above the ability of many firms to shoulder independently. Half of the budget is raised through corporate memberships, with a ceiling of $15 million to prevent single-company domination and a floor of $1 million. The remaining $100 million is provided through the U.S. Department of Defense through the Advanced Research Projects

Agency. The funds are used to conduct research at SEMATECH by staff and scientists from the member companies. SEMATECH also awards research contracts to small semiconductor research firms and universities.

For member companies to conduct cooperative research through such consortia, they must file for antitrust exemptions with the U.S. Department of Justice. Whereas SEMATECH may appear to be an anomaly in U.S. R&D sector, more than 380 such filings have been recorded. In sum, SEMATECH serves as one prototype that could be duplicated in the health research arena to support fundamental human research (precompetitive) and clinical research training.

In the policy arena, the Government-University-Industry Research Roundtable (GUIRR) of the National Academy of Sciences is a forum of senior-level government science managers, leaders in industrial research, and leaders in university leadership who meet to discuss broad science policy issues affecting all groups. The formation of GUIRR is unique in its own sense because it required approval by the White House Office of Management and Budget to allow senior government managers to meet in closed sessions with industry leaders. Although by its charter GUIRR is prohibited from making recommendations, it serves as a unique forum for science policy discussions and a means to bridge gaps among the federal government, industry, and the academic community.

Some health fields are already taking the initiative to assemble funds through consortia of industry and private philanthropy to promote research and training in specific areas. For example, the Alliance for Aging Research has proposed a National Geriatrics Development Fund to create Leadership Centers in Geriatrics at various academic medical centers with geriatric medicine programs. The Alliance, with the support of the Commonwealth Fund, hopes to raise matching funds from industry and nonprofit foundations to carry out this mission. Awards will be made through a peer-reviewed competition.

Although business as usual has brought the United States to the pinnacle of health research, the committee feels that new paradigms for research cooperation and support are warranted. The committee believes that models of cooperation that could be applied in the arena of human research already exist. All parties—industry, academia, government, and third-party payers—need to recognize that clinical research is not someone else's responsibility, but is the collective responsibility of all. One proposal would be to form an alliance or consortia of all parties, similar to SEMATECH, so that critical, fundamental human research can be supported to the benefit of all parties and, most importantly, improve the health of the U.S public. Thus, funds from government, industry, third-party payers, nonprofit organizations, special interest groups, and academia could be pooled and available for peer-reviewed competition to close gaps of knowledge in particular areas or provide special emphasis in others deemed appropriate or urgent.

CONCLUSIONS

The committee concluded that patient-oriented clinical research is supported by a diverse, yet interlocking network of federal agencies, industry, and private nonprofit organizations that share many common goals. Of these, the federal government is the single largest sponsor of health research in the United States. Of the more than $75 billion the federal government invested in R&D during fiscal year 1993, nearly $11 billion was health related. Contributions by health-oriented corporations are roughly equal in magnitude, but they are devoted largely to product application developments rather than fundamental discovery research. Contributions by private nonprofit sponsors favor fundamental discovery research, generally in somewhat restricted fields of interest, but represent only about four to five percent of the total U.S. investment in health research.

In light of this investment and the continuing budget limitations, the scientific community must reexamine its resource base to improve its effectiveness and efficiency. Federally sponsored health research by the various agencies is generally mission oriented. Whereas NIH is the primary agency that disburses federal health research funds for investigation into fundamental biological discovery, other agencies such as VA and AHCPR are key players in health research, particularly patient-oriented research. Thus, the committee emphasizes that all types of health research expand the boundaries of knowledge for improving health care and should be considered crucial parts of the realm of health research.

Although industry has been playing an increasingly important role in health research, focusing primarily on product development, it relies heavily on university research programs for fundamental knowledge (both basic and clinical) and talent. Cooperative ventures between universities (or government) and industry provide a unique mechanism for sharing knowledge and for technology transfer, a central policy of the federal government for increasing U.S. economic competitiveness.

Foundations, voluntary health agencies, and other nonprofit organizations have played a very important role in sponsoring health research. The committee believes that these organizations have been particularly helpful by providing crucial support in filling gaps in the nation's research agenda and sponsoring new initiatives. Although the federal government rapidly eclipsed the investment by these organizations following World War II, these organizations have continued to supply a steady stream of research dollars. These funds are used for individual research projects, supporting career development awards in specific research fields, equipment, facilities, and various programs of knowledge dissemination. The committee anticipates that these organizations will continue to provide support for the health sciences.

The health insurance industry also is a stakeholder in the realm of clinical research. Third-party payers need to recognize their responsibility to subscribers and society as a whole for improving health care. The committee does not imply that insurers should foot the entire costs for experimental or investigational therapy, but that they should work with the medical scientific community to determine what works and what does not.

To facilitate cooperation to uncover new knowledge about human disease and improve health care, the committee recommends the formation of an alliance that will bring all parties with a vested interest to the table in support of patient-oriented clinical research. New paradigms of cooperation are warranted to continue to improve the health of the U.S. public.

4

Training Pathways

A generation ago medical research was conducted largely by physicians, most of whom had little formal training in science (Smith, 1989). Clinical investigation was focused on disease and disease processes and was conducted largely at the patient level. Advances in cell biology and molecular genetics are bringing investigators closer to discovering how genes direct and influence normal human development as well as disease. Developments in areas such as neurobiology, immunology, and developmental biology present new challenges for designing and testing innovative treatments and preventions. Furthermore, new methodologies for assessing the outcomes of current and new medical technologies are evolving rapidly. Rigorous clinical research training is required to ensure valid results, inferences, and conclusions to improve health care practices. Yet, there is a growing concern that too few people are being trained to conduct sophisticated studies on the advances presented by these new developments in science and technology (Kelley, 1988; Martin, 1991).

Numerous criticisms have been leveled at the U.S. system of undergraduate and graduate medical education, including a growing divergence between patient needs and physician training; excessive emphasis on research and service in research-intensive universities at the expense of teaching; poor integration between the preclinical and clinical components of medical education; changes in hospital-based clinical training and the move to more ambulatory care, as a reult of which trainees are unable to observe the entire course of disease; and a teaching style that fails to engender the development of faculty role models or imbue students with problem-solving skills and positive attitudes for lifelong learning (Cantor et al., 1991; Goodman et al., 1991). Moreover, along with the growing

123

complexities of the U.S. health care system and its burgeoning problems, medical students are expected to become increasingly compassionate and caring as well as more aware and knowledgeable about patients' insurance coverage, case law, and ethics.

Dentistry, nursing, and other health professional groups also encounter barriers to clinical research careers that may or may not be similar to the barriers found in medicine. For example, unlike medicine, where there is extensive graduate medical education, the dental school curriculum is designed to prepare dentists who can practice dentistry upon graduation—after four years of graduate education. The dentistry curriculum thus combines didactic course work and clinical skills development during those four years, which brings into question the amount of time that dental students can commit to developing research skills (Appendix A). Although nurses, pharmacists, and allied health professionals generally acquire their clinical practice skills at the undergraduate level, most acquire their research skills in doctoral programs. In the past, many of these doctoral programs have been in other fields, such as education or psychology. New doctoral programs in nursing and allied health disciplines are being created, however (Appendix B; Selker, 1994).

The committee did not have the expertise to judge the effectiveness or the quality of programs in dentistry, nursing, and the allied health professions. The committee therefore sought input from the appropriate professional groups through task forces, commissioned papers, or written comments. Most groups felt that there were obstacles in the training pathways leading to careers in patient-oriented clinical research. Some of these were seen as peculiar to a given profession, whereas others were viewed as generic to all health care groups. The complete task force reports on dentistry and on nursing and clinical psychology can be found in Appendixes A and B, respectively, and the background paper by Dr. Selker elaborates on clinical research in the allied health professions (1994). Where appropriate, however, the concerns of those groups will be noted in the text.

The committee believes that health care professionals in all fields should be well-versed in the sciences underpinning the practice of health care. Sophisticated scientific and quantitative preparation empowers health care practitioners to pose insightful questions about human biology and behavior, to retrieve and critically analyze information for use in solving clinical problems, and to remain open to unexpected new possibilities. The diverse responsibilities in the various professional groups engaged in clinical research require that they have different kinds and levels of educational and scientific backgrounds. Unlike doctoral programs, in which the goal is to train highly skilled research scientists, the primary goal of health professional schools is to blend the scientific knowledge base with clinical skills to prepare highly qualified and competent practitioners of health care. In a health care environment in which health care knowledge and technology are accelerating rapidly and new discoveries are reported almost daily, preparing health practitioners who are well-grounded in the biological, social, behavioral, information, and quantitative sciences becomes ever more challenging. Clearly, all health care professionals should have a firm grasp of the traditional biomedical sciences as well as the social and behavioral sciences (Association of American Medical Schools, 1992b; Greenlick, 1992). Newer interdisciplinary biological sciences such as molecular biology, molecular genetics, and neuroscience, as well as increasingly sophisticated quantitative methods in areas such as medical effectiveness research, are also expanding the boundaries of knowledge for health care.

To begin to analyze the many perceived obstacles in the pathways leading to clinical research careers at the professional school level, the committee posed several generic questions:

- Is the present system for clinical research training inadequate?
- What does society want and expect students to know?
- Are professional schools organized to meet these goals?
- Are the faculty and administration committed to change?
- Are resources available for effecting change where changes are needed?

To approach these questions, the committee developed a list of issues that were addressed by the subcommittees examining issues affecting clinical research careers in the precollege and undergraduate periods, during graduate education, and during postdoctoral training. The committee examined the recruitment into scientific careers and the retention of those interested in pursuing research careers. Clearly, issues that affect students early are the quality and quantity of hands-on research experiences that are directly related to resources and quality of teaching. If students are unprepared or "turned off" to science and mathematics early in the educational process (that is, during their education from kindergarten through grade 12 [K–12]), should mechanisms be developed to change the environment and inspire interest in these fields? The influence of role models and mentors throughout the education and training pathway also have an effect on decisions to pursue scientific careers (Cameron, 1991). As students move into college, some of the same factors concerning quality of scientific curricula apply, but other factors can also affect their career choices, including income potential, job availability and security, and economic factors. Extensive length of training, accumulating educational debt, absence of quality research experiences and funding for research training, lack of time for engaging in research activities, lack of effective mentoring, and other lifestyle factors are some of the factors confronting health professionals who are interested in graduate education and postgraduate training (Applegate 1990; Smith, 1989). Furthermore, the demographics of the United States are changing, and the committee recognizes that changes in the education and training environment must be sensitive to gender and cultural differences and encourage increasing numbers of these groups to pursue research careers. Thus, this chapter examines the barriers and obstacles to research careers throughout the education and training pathway. Many of the issues confronting individuals are generic to all scientific careers, while some are specific to clinical research careers. The distinctions will be noted where applicable. It should be noted, however, that the committee has been hindered in its analyses by the extreme lack of outcomes data for research training programs and for factors affecting career choice.

Although the audience for this report might question the relevance of K–12 science experiences and their relationship to clinical research careers, the committee felt that it was important to reemphasize obstacles throughout the entire education and training pathways for clinical investigators. All too often, reports of this nature focus too narrowly on the late stages of training and neglect the earlier stages of education that influence the pool from which scientific talent will be drawn. Because each successive level of the training pathway relies on the preparation of the talent pool of the previous level, the committee felt that it would be productive to examine obstacles to scientific careers, particularly clinical investigative careers, from kindergarten to the achievement of a career as an established scientist.

The first portion of this chapter presents an overview of existing efforts to stimulate interest in careers in the sciences and health professions among students of all ages. Particular attention is paid to activities that involve or encourage students to become interested in scientific investigation. Because the committee membership did not have professional educators at the K–12 levels or at the undergraduate level, they chose to draw upon the work of others who have considered this issue. Among the sources relied on were *Educating Scientists and Engineers: Grade School to Grad School* (U.S. Congress, Office of Technology Assessment, 1988a); *Nurturing Scientific Talent: A Discussion Paper* (National Academy of Sciences, Government-University-Industry Research Roundtable, 1987); *Fulfilling the Promise: Biology Education in the Nation's Schools* (National Research Council, 1990); and *By the Year 2000; First in the World* (Federal Coordinating Committee for Science, Engineering and Technology, Committee on Education and Human Resources, 1991). To supplement these sources, the committee commissioned a paper by Marcia Matyas formerly of the American Association for the Advancement of Science, "Early Exposure to Research: Opportunities and Effects" (Matyas, 1994) from which this section of the report draws heavily.

The following sections of the chapter closely examine what is known, or not known, about professional education and training for careers in clinical investigation. These sections are supplemented by excerpts from the workshop "Clinical Research and Research Training: Spotlight on Funding" (Appendix D) the task force reports (Appendixes A, B, and C), and commissioned papers on training programs of the National Institutes of Health (NIH), models for postdoctoral clinical research training, the influence of resident review committees and certification boards on research training, and mentoring.

DEMOGRAPHICS

The committee recognizes that the recruitment and retention of scientists and health professionals into careers as clinical investigators must reflect the changing demographics of the United States (U.S. Congress, Office of Technology Assessment, 1985). Unlike nursing, which has been dominated by women, scientists and academic physicians in the past have characteristically been white males. Women now constitute nearly half of all medical students in U.S. medical schools and earn slightly more than a third of all life sciences doctorates (National Research Council, 1987b, 1991). The picture is not as hopeful for African Americans, Hispanics, and native Americans, who remain underrepresented in research and medicine (National Research Council, 1987a). This is of considerable concern because by the turn of the century, one third of the children living in the United States will be members of minority groups. These demographic data indicate that special efforts are needed to recruit members of these groups to pursue careers in patient-oriented clinical research (Robert Wood Johnson Foundation, 1987).

KINDERGARTEN TO COLLEGE

The decision to pursue a career in the sciences or health professions is the result of the interaction of many educational, psychosocial, and environmental factors. Exposure to science and mathematics instruction beginning in elementary school profoundly influences career choice (Federal Coordinating Council on Science, Engineering and Technology, 1991). Most commonly, school-age children get their first exposure to science by conducting hands-on experiments in the classroom. Other factors not directly related to the formal educational process are important as well. For example, many decisions to pursue a career in the sciences are the result of personal characteristics, such as positive motivation and good study habits. The expectations of parents, teachers, and peers; adequate mentoring; the presence of career opportunities; good occupational status; and job security also clearly play a role. Students can also be influenced by their participation in informal science experiences offered through museums or youth clubs (Matyas and Malcom, 1991). The committee believes that life experiences and the quality of science education during the formative years have a profound effect on the future talent pool from which highly capable clinical investigators will be drawn at later stages of the education pathway.

Classroom Experience

There are some 45 million students and 2.5 million teachers in the nation's 60,000 public and 40,000 private elementary and secondary schools. Because of the diversity of schools, school districts, and local control over education, the quality and effectiveness of science and mathematics education can be equally diverse. With the exception of a few magnet science high schools with the stated goal of fostering greater interest in scientific careers, most schools and school districts cannot or do not emphasize one subject area over another.

Although hands-on science activities are an ideal way to stimulate student interest in science, for a variety of reasons, many students are not introduced to these kinds of science experiences. For one thing, most students have only minimal exposure to science-related instruction. According to one national survey of teachers, an average of only 18 minutes a day is devoted to science in grades kindergarten–3; in grades 4–6, the average exposure is 29 minutes (Weiss et al., 1989). Far more time is spent teaching mathematics and reading. When hands-on or laboratory activities are used in the classroom, they are seldom truly experimental. More typically they are "cookbook" activities, with prescribed outcomes designed to illustrate specific phenomena. Students rarely have the chance to develop their own hypotheses, design and execute experiments, and draw conclusions.

Teachers are probably the most critical ingredient in a young person's education. Good teaching can inspire students and foster intellectual pursuits by promoting interest in the subject matter, comprehension, and perseverance. Poor teaching can stifle learning, leading to student disinterest and complacency. According to the Federal Coordinating Council on Science, Engineering and Technology (FCCSET) Committee on Education and Human Resources (1991), less than one third of the nation's elementary, middle school, and high school math and science teachers meet coursework standards established by their own professional organizations. Elementary school teachers often are expected to teach science and mathematics, yet they have taken little or no course work in these subjects. High school math and science teachers are less likely, on average, than teachers in other fields to have concentrated in their primary teaching field during college (Federal Coordinating Council on Science, Engineering and Technology, 1991). As a group, teachers at each grade level are more likely to rely on didactic methods than hands-on experimentation, small-group problem solving, or demonstrations.

Not only is it difficult to recruit highly talented teachers with science backgrounds but it is also difficult to retain the highly skilled teachers already in the system. Although teacher salaries grew nearly 25 percent in real terms from 1983 to 1988, budget cutbacks at the federal, state, and local levels over the past few years have forced many public school teachers to forgo salary raises or even to take reductions in compensation and benefits. It has been estimated that for every science or math teacher entering teaching for the first time, 13 leave the profession (Federal Coordinating Council on Science, Engineering and Technology, 1991).

Educational quality also is heavily dependent on the availability of resources—including not only money but also up-to-date texts and instructional materials. Teacher morale declines as these professionals are asked to do more with increasingly inadequate resources and outdated instructional materials. Furthermore, most schools do not have adequate equipment or facilities to allow routine laboratory experimentation. This is especially true in elementary and middle schools. For K–12 teachers, inadequate facilities, lack of materials for individualized instruction, and insufficient funds for purchasing equipment and supplies were among the problems most often cited as "serious" impediments to teaching science.

Science Fairs and Competitions

In contrast to the classroom experience, science fairs and competitions often provide valuable exposure to research. Although many science fairs accept nonexperimental projects, it is becoming increasingly common to require students to conduct background research, develop a hypothesis, and conduct a series of experiments to prove or disprove the hypothesis. The International Science and Engineering Fair and the Westinghouse Talent Search are among the largest such initiatives in the United States.[1]

Another forum for student involvement in research is the American Junior Academy of Science, which allows high school students to present their research at the annual meeting of the American Association for the Advancement of Science. Publications such as the *Journal of High School Science Research* and the *Journal of Student Research* provide high school students with the opportunity to publish their studies. Although these programs and activities involve thousands of students each year, their focus is almost exclusively on high school students. Despite this progress, the majority of U.S. students finish their precollege years without having had a significant research experience (Matyas and Malcom, 1991).

For many precollege students, the primary opportunity to engage in hands-on science activities comes through informal experiences, such as visits to science museums, or participation in youth organizations, such as Boy Scouts of the USA, Girl Scouts of the USA, Girls, Inc. (formerly Girls Clubs of America, Inc.), and church groups (Matyas and Malcom, 1991). Parents can also facilitate

---

[1] Both the International Science and Engineering Fair and the Westinghouse Talent Search are conducted through Science Service, Inc., Washington, D.C.

TABLE 4-1 Science Classroom Activities Used by Teachers During Their Most
Recent Science Lesson by Grade Level, 1985–1986

Science Classroom Activity	Percentage of Classes		
	K–6	7–9	10–12
Lecture	74	83	84
Discussion	87	82	80
Demonstrations	52	42	44
Hands-on or laboratory materials	51	43	39
Use of computers	2	5	5
Working in small groups	33	35	36
Doing seat work from textbook	31	45	35
Completing supplemental work sheets	38	44	37
Assigning homework	28	54	52

Source: Weiss, 1987.

these activities at home by providing toys and materials that encourage
exploration and experimentation.

Specific Initiatives

A number of programs have been designed to give precollege students
experience with hands-on, inquiry-based science. A few engage students in actual
research projects (Table 4-1). For the most part, programs that involve students
in research are targeted at the high school level and reach limited numbers of
students.

Student research experiences also can be indirectly affected by programs
aimed at improving the science literacy of teachers and parents. In-service
programs, for example, can help teachers acquire knowledge of content and
teaching methods to incorporate laboratory components into the science
curriculum. Workshops can inform teachers and parents about research
opportunities that allow children to become involved, either directly with an
individual researcher or through a formal program.

Effecting Change

On the positive side, there is evidence that science and mathematics education is receiving increasing attention by policymakers at many levels. Among the goals established in 1989 by the nation's governors for improving the U.S. educational system, for example, was that U.S. students become first in the world in science and mathematics achievement by the year 2000 (Federal Coordinating Committee for Science, Engineering, and Technology, 1991). Subsequently, the FCCSET established strategic objectives for improving students' preparation in the sciences and mathematics.

Concern about a future shortage of scientists and engineers has spurred expanded federal investment in an effort to increase student interest in science, mathematics, and engineering. In fiscal year 1992, federal agencies participating in the FCCSET Committee on Education and Human Resources[2] requested that nearly $180 million be spent on student opportunities and incentives. This reflects a 56 percent increase over 1990 budget levels. An additional $100.5 million was requested by the Department of Defense for Reserve Officers' Training Corps scholarships, many of which go to students majoring in science or engineering.

It is difficult to estimate the level of financial commitment to science education by colleges, universities, industry, and professional societies. It is the committee's sense, however, that there has been an overall increase in both funding for and activities related to enhancing precollege science education.

Federal Programs

Certain federal agencies offer students the chance to gain research experience through summer apprenticeship programs. These programs usually enroll students in grades 10 through 12. A number of agencies conduct Saturday academy programs, which run during the academic year. The NIH's Biomedical Research Assistant Saturday Scholars program, for example, involves 90 junior and senior high school students in hands-on laboratory activities on Saturday mornings. NIH has also initiated a new program called the Science Education Partnership program to encourage careers in the biomedical sciences. The National Oceanic and Atmospheric Administration also sponsors a Saturday academy for junior and senior high school students (Matyas, 1994).

---

[2] FCCSET includes the Departments of Agriculture, Commerce, Defense, Education, Energy, Health and Human Services, Housing and Urban Development, Interior, Justice, Labor, Transportation, and Veterans Affairs and the Environmental Protection Agency, National Aeronautics and Space Administration, National Science Foundation, Smithsonian Institution, and Barry M. Goldwater Foundation.

A new NIH program, the Biomedical Preparatory School, gives high school students course credits for time spent in agency laboratories. Under the U.S. Department of Defense's Junior Science and Humanities Program, some 10,000 high school students annually participate in regional meetings where they present their research findings. The National Science Foundation's (NSF's) Young Scholars Program, which targets minority students, lets students work side by side with researchers (National Science Foundation, 1990). In 1992, approximately 8,000 students participated in the program. NSF also encourages minority student involvement in research through its Summer Science Camps and Comprehensive Regional Centers for Minorities.

Nonfederal Programs

There is also a significant nonfederal attempt to provide research experiences to precollege students. The *1992 Directory of Student Science Training Programs for Precollege Students* lists 428 such programs, almost all of which are implemented at or by colleges and universities (Science Service, Inc., 1991). A small number of programs are hosted by science museums; industrial and professional societies participate only rarely in such efforts.

Summary

Although some attempts are being made to increase students' interest in science and mathematics, current initiatives fall short in a number of respects. Most science education efforts function more to retain students already in the science career pipeline than to recruit new entrants. In general, the younger the student, the less intensive the research experience is likely to be. The number of students who participate in such activities is relatively small compared with the number of students at the early high school level who are interested in a science or engineering career. In 1977, among 7 million high school sophomores, roughly 730,000 expressed an interest in a future career in science or engineering. The kinds of programs described here, however, have the capacity to serve less than one third of these students. To tap into the larger pool of interested students, additional ways of involving students in research activities are needed, as is greater involvement of the public and private scientific communities.

RESEARCH EXPERIENCES FOR UNDERGRADUATE STUDENTS

In many respects, undergraduate education and training in the United States rival or surpass those of comparable educational systems in most other countries around the globe. The U.S. research enterprise, which depends heavily on the flow of talented undergraduates into academic and industrial laboratories, is also one of the strongest in the world. For all of its strengths, however, U.S. higher education, particularly in the sciences, is facing numerous challenges. Rising tuition costs, for example, present significant barriers for many high school students hoping to enroll in college. Of particular concern, however, is that students who do gain entry into the higher education system appear to be showing less and less interest in studying science and mathematics (U.S. Department of Education, Office of Educational Research and Improvement, 1991; Lapoint et al. 1989). The proportion of college freshmen planning to major in the two subjects dropped by half between 1966 and 1988, from 11.5 to 5.8 percent (Green, 1989).

There is also evidence of considerable attrition into other fields among undergraduates who initially show an interest in the sciences (Hewitt and Seymour, 1991). Although 70 percent of business majors and more than 60 percent of education and social science majors earned their baccalaureate degrees in four years (Cooperative Institutional Research Program, 1982), fewer than 40 percent of students initially majoring in biology received their degrees; the remainder either obtained non-science degrees or dropped out of college. The committee believes that few, if any, students who are turned off to science at the time they enter college will pursue research careers.

At the undergraduate level, it is government and academia that are most involved in encouraging student involvement in science. To a lesser extent, professional societies encourage student interest in science-related studies through scholarship and research internships. Industry supports student research activities through scholarships and cooperative and summer internship programs. Most industry-supported programs, however, target students interested in engineering and the physical sciences rather than the life sciences (Matyas and Malcom, 1991).

Institutional Programs

Academic institutions are strong sponsors of student involvement in research. Often these efforts are part of the regular curriculum. For example, many liberal arts colleges require students to conduct a research project as part of their graduation requirements. Some institutions have programs specifically intended to encourage student participation in ongoing faculty research projects.

Many such efforts were catalyzed by federal initiatives, such as the National Science Foundation's now-defunct Undergraduate Research Program.

Like precollege programs, research opportunities for undergraduate students are often available during the summer months. One example of a successful program is the Summer Undergraduate Research Fellowships (SURFs) at the California Institute of Technology (1991). More than 1,300 students have participated in SURFs since its inception in 1979. Students work on a research project throughout the 10-week fellowship and then present their findings at a scientific meeting. More than 20 percent of SURF recipients have been coauthors of papers published in peer-reviewed scientific journals.

Among other similar academic initiatives is Carnegie Mellon University's Undergraduate Research Associates Program, which places strong emphasis on research participation among women and minorities, and the University of Kentucky College of Medicine Employment Opportunities Program, which provides research and work activities in medicine and a variety of other health fields including nursing, dentistry, and hospital administration (Matyas, 1994).

Federal Programs

Most federal programs that support student research activities do so through either summer research experiences or cooperative ventures in which the student alternates work at a federal research facility with formal course work at a college or university. Table 4-2 provides a partial list of the programs currently operated or funded by the federal government (Matyas, 1994). Many are focused on the needs of underrepresented minorities, women, and people with disabilities.

The National Institute of General Medical Sciences (NIGMS) sponsors the Minority Access to Research Careers (MARC) program, a major component of which is the Honors Undergraduate Research Program. Since 1977, the MARC Honors Undergraduate Research Program has provided tuition and stipend support to over 2,700 junior and senior honors students at predominantly minority institutions. Among its other goals, the MARC Honors Undergraduate Research Program strives to prepare minority students to compete for entry into graduate programs in the biomedical sciences. To date, the majority of students participating in the program have majored in the biological sciences (Garrison and Brown, 1985). A 1985 Institute of Medicine (IOM) evaluation of NIH's MARC Honors Undergraduate Research Program found that over three quarters of former MARC students went on to enroll in or complete graduate or professional studies. Thus, there is a strong indication that the MARC Honors Undergraduate Research Program promotes minority student enrollment in graduate or professional schools.

It is worth noting, however, that NIGMS's MARC Honors Undergraduate Research Program has had some unintended, albeit positive, results. Although

TABLE 4-2 Selected Federal Agencies Sponsoring Undergraduate Research Programs

Federal Agency	Program
U.S. Department of Commerce	National Institute of Standards and Technology (NIST) Student Cooperative Program (work/study) and Student "Q" program (summer co-op)
U.S. Department of Defense	Science and Engineering Co-op Program
U.S. Department of Energy	Minority Undergraduate Training for Engineering Careers (MUTEC)
	Galludet University Program (summer)
	Research Partnership Program (year-round)
	Minority Access to Engineering-Related Careers
	Science and Engineering Research Semester
U.S. Department of Health and Human Services	Minority Access to Research Careers (MARC) Honors Undergraduate Research Training Program
	Minority Biomedical Research Support Program (MBRS)
U.S Department of Interior	Minority Participation in Earth Sciences
U.S. Department of Justice	Forensic Science Research and Training (FSRTC) Summer Intern Program
Environmental Protection Agency	Minority Research Apprentice Program
	Cooperative Education Program
	Federal Junior Fellowship Program
National Aeronautics and Space Administration	Baccalaureate Cooperative Education Program
	Advanced Design Program
National Science Foundation	Research Experiences for Undergraduates (REU)
	Research Careers for Minority Scholars
	Engineering Senior Design Projects to Aid the Disabled

Source: Matyas, 1994.

the program was initially designed to encourage minority students to pursue Ph.D.s in the biomedical sciences, it has proven to be an excellent recruitment tool for bringing minority students into the medical profession. Only about seven percent of the undergraduate students who participate in MARC ultimately receive a Ph.D. MARC students often receive bachelors and even masters' degrees in the sciences or, more often, M.D. degrees, instead of pursuing a Ph.D. In a 1985 IOM evaluation of the program, over 40 percent of MARC Honors Undergraduate Research Program participants who went on to graduate or professional schools were training to be physicians (Institute of Medicine, 1985). Preliminary findings from a 1992 review of the MARC program are similar (Matyas, 1994). It is unclear, however, how many of these minority physicians have joined the faculty ranks or have become clinical investigators in other employment sectors such as government or industry.

The NSF's Research Experiences for Undergraduates (REU) program, begun in 1987, is designed to provide undergraduate students with hands-on research experience. It has many of the same objectives as NIGMS's MARC Undergraduate Research Honors Program, including encouraging undergraduates to attend graduate school in the sciences or engineering. During its first three years, REU supported 11,000 students, over half of whom attended predominantly undergraduate institutions. A 1990 evaluation of NSF's REU program revealed similar findings (National Science Foundation, 1990). Among one group of students, for example, participation in REU increased the proportion of students planning to acquire a master's or doctorate degree from 75 to 92 percent. Nearly 70 percent of participants enrolled in graduate school immediately following graduation.

In 1989, NIH initiated a similar program, Research Supplements for Underrepresented Minorities, to allow scientists with active NIH grants to add a minority high school student, undergraduate student, graduate student, or postdoctoral fellow to their research teams. Since its inception, the program has supported over 650 minority researchers.

There are also a number of federal initiatives that, through their support of academic institutions and faculty, indirectly buttress the undergraduate research experience. Within the Public Health Service, the NIH Minority Biomedical Research Support program has provided resources to over 90 minority colleges and universities to allow state-of-the-art research by faculty and students. The former Alcohol, Drug Abuse, and Mental Health Administration (ADAMHA) supported a program, Minority Institutions Research and Development Programs, that provided support for the "enhancement of existing research infrastructure" (Federal Coordinating Committee for Science, Engineering and Technology, Committee on Education and Human Resources, 1991).

Similarly, the NSF has a series of initiatives—the Faculty Enhancement Program, the Research in Undergraduate Institutions Program, and the Instrumentation and Laboratory Improvement Program—intended to increase the number and quality of research experiences for undergraduate students. NSF also sponsors efforts to improve the research infrastructures at predominantly minority institutions: Comprehensive Regional Centers for Minorities, Alliances for Minority Participation, Research Improvement in Minority Institutions, and Minority Research Centers of Excellence.

Program Shortcomings

Programs intended to stimulate interest in research among undergraduate students suffer from a number of shortcomings. Efforts to recruit and retain underrepresented groups more often than not are focused on engineering, not science (Matyas and Malcom, 1991). In addition, the majority of such initiatives target minority students rather than women, people with disabilities, or the general student population. According to one study, less than 10 percent of efforts by colleges and universities to recruit students interested in science specifically target women (Matyas and Malcom, 1991). More significant perhaps is that the kinds of initiatives geared to attract women undergraduates are less likely to involve opportunities for scientific research.

Special efforts to encourage students with disabilities to participate in science and engineering activities are extremely rare. More often than not, funds are provided to support individual students' laboratory or research activities. With funding from NSF, the American Association for the Advancement of Science is developing a six-school model program for recruiting the disabled, the Access to Engineering program. The committee is unaware of any similar effort to draw the disabled into medical research careers.

When majority and minority groups are taken as a whole, academic institutions and federal agencies are most likely to facilitate the involvement of students in nonengineering research activities. These programs, however, tend to involve highly motivated and high-achieving students in their sophomore and junior years who already have made a commitment to a science or engineering career. In many instances, the programs act more as vehicles of retention or affirmation than of recruitment.

Finally, although many programs involve students in biomedical research, rarely do precollege or undergraduate students participate in patient-oriented clinical research. NSF sponsors a program, Bioengineering and Aiding the Disabled, in which senior undergraduate engineering students design a piece of equipment to assist a person with a disability. NIH's Research Supplements for Underrepresented Minorities supports minority students or postdoctoral fellows involved in clinical research. Through its Explorer Post program, the Centers for Disease Control and Prevention recruits students ages 14 to 21 to attend lectures, go on field trips, and participate in basic and clinical research activities (Matyas, 1994). In addition to these federal initiatives, there are a few programs scattered in various academic institutions that expose students to clinical research, but a full inventory of these programs has not been made.

Assessing Program Effectiveness

To determine whether programs that expose students to the world of research encourage them to pursue research careers, one needs to know what the goals of the effort were and whether those goals were matched to appropriate activities. Goals may be specific or general, long range or short term. In all but the most exemplary programs, well-defined, measurable goals are lacking (Malcom, 1983). Many programs appear ineffective because their goals are set either too high or too low.

Even if a program appears successful in meeting its objectives, without a means to measure that success it is difficult for sponsors to decide whether continued investments are worthwhile. Studies of precollege and undergraduate programs designed to recruit and retain women or minorities in the sciences and engineering have found that less than half the programs did any formal studies of effectiveness (George et al., 1987, Lockheed et al., 1985, Malcom, 1983; Matyas and Malcom, 1991). Part of the reason for this poor record is that sponsors traditionally have budgeted only a small fraction of program monies for program evaluation. More recently, however, sponsors have begun to encourage and even require more extensive program evaluation and outcomes assessments.

Results obtained by those programs that have conducted formal evaluations indicate that the effects of early research experiences appear to have been positive. For example, in a number of studies examining precollege intervention programs, the integration of content knowledge with hands-on, inquiry-oriented laboratory activities, especially over a period of several years, was one of the critical characteristics of an exemplary program (George et al., 1987; Lockheed et al., 1985; Malcom, 1983; Matyas and Malcom, 1991).

In summary, although evaluations of research experience programs are not regularly completed, the evaluations that do exist suggest that these strategies are effective in encouraging high-achieving students who are already interested in science or engineering to continue their studies. There are strong classroom data and isolated programmatic data indicating that early research experiences may also have a positive effect on students who have average or poor academic skills and moderate or low interest in science or engineering careers (Kyle, 1984; Massachusetts Institute of Technology, 1990; Office of Technology Assessment, 1988a).

Designing Effective Programs

By establishing clear and measurable goals, selecting program activities that are proven effective for the target group, and designing and implementing an evaluation plan, effective new programs can be established with relative ease. It is important for program directors to approach program design and evaluation as a research problem whose results are used to assess what is and what is not working, to refine strategies, and to continue testing as the program is implemented in future years. These are the hallmarks of an effective program.

Establishing Specific Goals

The goals of a program intended to interest students in the sciences should be clear and measurable. Is the goal of the program to facilitate students' pursuit of research careers in science? Will it distinguish between students who are interested in pursuing an M.D. as opposed to a Ph.D.? Will the program focus only on specific science fields? These are some of the questions that must be considered as a program's goals are established.

Goals should also identify the program's target group, taking into consideration such features as student age, race, and academic achievement level. For example, if the goal of the program is to confirm the research career goals of students who are already high achievers and highly motivated, research experiences that occur late in the undergraduate period will be beneficial. If one of the goals is to entice students who may have little natural interest in research, then earlier research experiences—starting in the precollege and early undergraduate years—will be more effective.

Selecting Appropriate Strategies

There should be a clear match between the goals of the program and the activities of the participants. To identify the best activities to include and strategies to use in a program, a number of factors should be considered, including the age group of the participants, the timing of the program (summer, academic year, or year-round), and the available funding.

Activities and goals also should be matched to available funds. For its Summer Science Camps, for example, NSF budgets $100,000 for residential programs and $60,000 for commuter programs. Approximately 60 students participate in the average four-week session. If students are required to pay a fee for participation, financial aid should be offered. A common mistake made by new programs is to scale back activities to match the available funds without modifying the program's goals accordingly. In cases such as this, the goals are not met—not because the program itself was ineffective but because the goals did not reflect the actual scope or scale of the program effort.

Designing an Evaluation Plan

The design of an evaluation plan should begin when the program goals are being set and the activities are being selected. Program directors often make the mistake of waiting until the program is well under way before considering evaluation, only to realize that they have missed the opportunity to assess changes in attitudes, perceptions, motivation, and interest.

Most careful evaluations include both formative and summative components. Formative evaluation provides feedback to the program staff about how well individual program components are working. For example, students may complete an evaluation form addressing the application process, a particular seminar series, or program social functions. Summative evaluations attempt to assess the overall impact of the program. This information may be provided by exit interviews or surveys of participants and, more importantly, by later surveys to identify the long-term impact of the program on the studies and careers of its participants.

Characteristics of Successful Programs

Programs designed to encourage precollege and undergraduate students to pursue careers in the sciences—particularly in clinical research—will be successful only if their component activities and the strategies for carrying them out are effective. A number of studies have attempted to define the characteristics of successful programs (George et al., 1987; Lockheed et al., 1985; Malcom, 1983; Matyas and Malcom, 1991) (see box Characteristics of Successful Programs). When designing such an initiative, it is important to discover as much as possible about other similar efforts. Much can be learned by contacting those in charge of ongoing programs.

A number of institutions have moved from sponsoring isolated programs to implementing a set of articulated activities designed to "pump" students through the science and engineering "pipeline." One example of this coordinated approach is the Comprehensive Regional Center for Minorities (CRCM) at the University of Puerto Rico. Under CRCM, more than a dozen regional college and university campuses provide exposure to science and engineering for precollege and undergraduate students, K–12 teachers, and college and university faculty (George, 1991).

A similarly integrated strategy has been adopted by the University of Kentucky College of Medicine Education Outreach Center, which sponsors

---

CHARACTERISTICS OF SUCCESSFUL PROGRAMS

- Hands-on research experience including, if possible, an extramural research opportunity at another institution
- Extensive one-on-one interaction with a faculty member who can guide the student's research experience and act as a mentor
- Opportunities for students to live on campus or near the area where research takes place
- One-on-one interaction with faculty members and graduate students, including faculty and students who "look like" the participants in their race, ethnicity, gender, or disability
- Academic sessions (if included) that focus on enrichment rather than remediation
- Heavy emphasis on the applications of science and mathematics and on careers in those fields
- Long-term (multiyear) involvement of students
- Peer support system based on joint projects, classes, and social activities
- Parental involvement (especially for precollege programs) and support from the community of teachers and counselors
- Absence of educational inequities based on gender, race, ethnicity, or disability
- A strong program director and committed and stable (low-turnover) staff that shares the program's goals
- A stable, long-term funding base with multiple funding sources, including the host institution
- Financial support for participants, including such things as program fee waivers, stipends, or scholarships
- Sufficient time to actively recruit and identify program participants
- valuation, long-term follow-up, and careful data collection
- The integration into the institution's regular activities of program elements shown to encourage student participation in research

---

programs for K–12, undergraduate, and graduate students; partnerships and research programs for teachers; and community outreach efforts, such as a science telephone hotline for student questions and a computer bulletin board, Science Spoken Here.

The progression from single, one-time programs to coordinated, longer-term efforts is an important step toward structural reform, institutional commitment, and line-item budgets, which are among the goals of most intervention efforts.

Conclusions

Although crucial data are lacking, the committee believes that research experiences during the precollege and undergraduate years can have a strong and positive impact on students' interest in and commitment to future studies and careers in the sciences. Feedback from more than 30 years of involving students in laboratory research has provided important information about what does and what does not work in such programs. Much of this information is being put to use in the hundreds of research-experience programs currently being implemented by federal agencies, colleges and universities, industry, and others.

At the same time, the efforts made to date serve only a small segment of the students who are interested in science as a possible future career. Not all of these students are currently achieving high grades, but many have the potential to do so. There is a much larger population of students who also need to feel the excitement and satisfaction of participating in research activities. Reaching these students will require work on a number of levels.

First, programs currently proven to be effective should be used as models for expanding existing efforts. Second, new program models, which serve the needs of the "second tier" of students, should be developed (Tobias, 1990). NIH's Biomedical Preparatory School, which is geared to a diverse group of students, including those with less-than-perfect academic records, is a good example of this strategy. This should not be perceived as a lowering of standards to reach the second tier; rather, programs should be developed to encourage academic achievement and inspire these students to pursue health professional and clinical investigative careers.

Finally, there need to be systemic changes in science education at both the precollege and undergraduate levels so that research is not a special activity for only a few select students during a few weeks in the summer. Research should be embedded in the science curriculum so that the skills that every young toddler knows—generating hypotheses, designing and conducting experiments, and drawing conclusions—are not lost from the repertoire of learning skills but are formalized and reinforced throughout the precollege and undergraduate years. Programs should also be developed to foster clinical research training. Such exposure could include participation in data collection or other activities in clinical research.

HEALTH PROFESSIONAL SCHOOLS

Although much of the preceding discussion might be considered generic to all scientific and preprofessional careers, this section examines factors that affect students in the health professions. Because the task force reports on dentistry and on nursing and clinical psychology are appended to the report (see Appendixes A and B, respectively), readers will be referred to those appendixes for specific information pertaining to those professions.

Physician-Scientists

To examine the human resource pool for clinical research in medicine, it will be useful to review the numbers and demographics of applicants and matriculants to medical schools since World War II. Following the war there was an immediate jump in the number of applicants, from about 12,300 in 1943 to more than 21,500 in the late 1940s, probably resulting in part from the Servicemens Readjustment Act of 1944 (Ahrens, 1992). Although the number of applicants surged, the number of those accepted into medical school during the same period grew only slightly, from approximately 6,500 to 7,400. By the mid-1950s the number of applicants dropped to about 15,000 a year with about 8,000 accepted.

In 1958, the Bayne-Jones report was released (U.S. Department of Health and Welfare, 1958). That report called for more physicians and more medical schools to train them. Two years earlier, the Health Research Facilities Act authorized a Public Health Service (PHS) program to expand the capacity and improve the quality of the nation's medical research facilities (Institute of Medicine, 1990). Thus, between the mid-1950s and the mid-1970s the number of medical schools grew from 83 to 114. Over the same period, the number of available slots in medical schools nearly doubled from about 8,000 to 15,000. The number of applicants grew as well, from 15,000 to a peak of about 42,600 in 1974 (Jonas et al., 1992). From 1974, the annual number of applicants declined steadily until the 1988–1989 academic year, when 27,671 students applied for about 17,000 slots in the nation's 126 medical schools. Since 1980 the number of students accepted has hovered around 17,200. The decline in applicants changed the applicant/acceptance ratio over this period. Whereas the ratio was 2.83 applicants for each slot in 1974, the ratio had dropped to 2.10 by 1980 and reached a low of 1.56 in 1988 (Ahrens, 1992; Tudor, 1988). Actual first-year enrollments over the same period have been slightly lower, hovering between 16,800 and 17,200, and annual graduating classes have fluctuated between 15,300 and 16,300 nationwide (Association of American Medical Schools, 1992a).

The fairly level number of enrollments throughout the 1980s combined with a decline in the numbers of applicants raised concern in many sectors about the quality and preparedness of medical school applicants. The proportion of students with 3.5 to 4.0 grade point averages declined slightly, from 46.6 to 43.7 percent between 1987 and 1989, but grew to 46.2 percent by 1991. This drop in the percentage of first-year enrollees was accompanied by a concomitant rise in the percentage of students entering with B and C averages. These concerns, however, have been neither confirmed nor denied. The number of applicants rose again over the ensuing two years, to about 33,300, and the applicant/acceptance ratio rebounded to nearly 1.94. Of the entering 1991 class, 7.3 percent had master's or doctoral degrees.

Women did not begin entering medical schools in large numbers until the late 1970s. For example, women constituted only 12.8 percent of applicants in 1971 but grew to 31.8 percent 10 years later. In 1991, 41.1 percent (13,700 of 33,301) of the applicant pool were women and 58.9 percent (19,601) were men. Although the percentage of women in the various medical schools covers a wide range—from a low of 23 percent to a high of 71 percent—about 39.8 percent of the 1991 first-year class were women. Data on the grades and class standings of the women entering medical school show that the overall quality of the applicants has been maintained (Jonas et al., 1992).

The race and ethnicity of medical students have changed remarkably over the past decade as well (Jonas et al., 1992). Ten years ago, only about 16 percent of first-year students were members of minority groups. The class entering medical school in 1991 was made up of almost 30 percent racial and ethnic minorities. Although this demonstrates a dramatic change on the surface, progress by the subgroups shows startling differences. For example, the proportion of Asians and Pacific Islanders has grown from 5.1 percent of the entering class in 1982 to nearly 16 percent of the entering class in 1991, thus exceeding their representation in the general population. At the same time, the proportion of students from all other minority groups has increased only slightly. Because enrollments have remained level, the growing numbers of women and minority students have been realized with a concomitant decrease in the number of white, non-Hispanic men. The decline in the number of white males applying to medical school may suggest that other more favorable career options are competing with medicine.

What's Wrong with Medical Education?

Although the previous discussion examined the quantitative aspect of the physician talent pool, the committee was concerned about the qualitative issues for encouraging medical students to pursue research careers, particularly clinical investigative careers. A recent survey of medical students, house staff, and junior faculty at the University of California, San Francisco, revealed three commonly perceived disadvantages to an academic career involving research: (1) reduced research funding; (2) the culture and politics of research, including bureaucracy and sexism; and (3) decreased emphasis on clinical care and relevant health issues. Personal barriers included decreased funding and competition for scarce resources, too much competition for positions, and the clash of family commitments with a career that provides insufficient leisure time (Martin, 1991). Furthermore, there is general consensus that the difficulty of simultaneously maintaining competency in both science and medicine requires that time be set aside for training in both (Smith, 1989). Students perceive the conflicting demands of research and clinical care and have a growing sense that it is impossible to do both well (Martin, 1991). In addition, career decisions involving two professionals married to each other often work against the decision to enter research training or a research career.

Thus, the committee posed several questions about the effectiveness of medical education in promoting clinical research careers.

- What is wrong with medical education as it pertains to inspiring clinical research careers?
  - Are the expectations of medical students clearly delineated by the faculty?
  - What are the barriers to research participation during medical school?
- Can change be effected during medical school to encourage participation in clinical research?

It was clearly stated in the introduction to this report that research is a social and political process that requires communication, interpersonal relationships, and scientific exchange to uncover new knowledge about natural phenomena. To approach the answers to these issues affecting medical education as it pertains to clinical research training, the committee examined factors affecting medical students and residents such as curriculum, student indebtedness, role models and mentors, available time for conducting research, and enculturation into clinical research environments. For many, these issues overlap with those of medical students choosing to engage in preclinical research activities as well.

UNDERGRADUATE MEDICAL EDUCATION

As early as 1910, the Flexner Report highlighted the importance of basic science for medical education (Flexner, 1910). Twenty years ago, the charge was made that medical students were becoming scientific illiterates, and observers continue to bemoan the lack of analytical skills being taught to ensuing classes (Ahrens, 1992). Consistent with reports that medical students are less scientifically skilled is the impression that they are also less scientifically inclined. Thus, two critical questions must be asked. First, is the medical school science curriculum and science culture adequate for preparing physicians to be scientifically literate and enthusiastic about science? Second, is there something about science as a career that is a far more powerful influence on career choice than any exposure to science? The answers to these questions require a variety of approaches if there is to be an increase in the supply of physician-scientists.

In 1988, the IOM's study *Resources for Clinical Investigation* concluded that there are a number of reasons why clinical research has lost a great deal of its appeal for physicians in training. These include the large debt borne by recent

M.D. graduates, the discrepancy between the incomes of clinical investigators and those of their colleagues who have chosen to enter the more lucrative pathway of private practice, the increasing difficulty clinical investigators experience in getting funds for their research from NIH and other sources, and uncertainties about advancement in the academic community, where accomplishments in laboratory research come sooner and, consequently, are often held in higher regard than those in clinical investigation (Institute of Medicine, 1988a). Six years later, few of these reasons have disappeared, although the validities of some, such as the debt burden, have been called into question.

Medical School Science Curriculum and Culture

Today, medical education centers on the accumulation of an ever-increasing number of facts. Medical students are measured by their ability to recount these facts, often at the expense of enhancing their analytical skills. According to some analysts, even though current students know many more facts, they have little appreciation of the scientific method that was employed to develop this knowledge base and have minimal skills in analyzing clinical science questions (Bishop, 1984; Bryan, 1992; McManus, 1991). Possibly because the thrust of the medical school curriculum is directed toward the accumulation of facts to prepare practicing physicians, many believe that it offers few opportunities for developing analytical skills. At the very least, schools should provide each student with an opportunity to have a first-hand experience with the variability of biological and clinical data, to learn how to formulate a testable hypothesis, to endure the tedium of data collection, and to organize and interpret results (Segal et al., 1990). This should be required not only of those choosing research pathways but of all medical students to ensure that they become informed and analytical consumers of published reports in peer-reviewed journals (Reigelman et al., 1983).

Thirty years ago teachers in the preclinical sciences were expected to give lectures and monitor student learning activities during laboratory exercises. Laboratory exercises have been vastly reduced in modern medical curricula and lectures are now distributed more widely among specialists. In one medical school, for example, first-year medical students were lectured by 136 different faculty members, and second-year students were lectured by 183 different teachers (Abrahamson, 1991). A decade ago, NIH Director James Wyngaarden maintained that "one of the casualties of [the] new medical curriculum has been the simulated research-laboratory experiences common to many basic-science courses" (Wyngaarden, 1979, p. 1258). Medical students are not receiving the laboratory experiences necessary to understand the scientific method, and they are rarely exposed to scientists as role models who can provide consistency in both the learning and the practice of science. The result is that not only are there fewer physicians trained and capable of conducting research but there are also a smaller number of physicians capable of critically evaluating the medical research literature. The number of physicians training in research has not kept pace with the growth in the physician population (Institute of Medicine, 1989d).

Numerous studies have called for reform. Fewer didactic lectures, more small-group teaching, increased supervision of students learning clinical skills, and more interdisciplinary efforts that emphasize making basic science relevant to the clinical practice of medicine are among the efforts under way in the nation's medical schools (Association of American Medical Schools, 1984, 1992b; Jonas et al., 1991). Few schools, however, have a specific curriculum requirement for research.

A number of schools are experimenting with an alternative curriculum. Rush Medical College in Chicago instituted a problem-based curriculum in 1984 in response to a set of perceived problems in medical education, including the following:

- an emphasis on fact memorization over problem-solving and reasoning skills,
- limited instruction in assessing the medical literature in the preclinical curriculum,
- an overcrowded schedule of lectures and laboratory sessions, frequently coupled with poor attendance by students,
- limited direct orientation of basic science education to a clinical career,
- a need to instruct students more clearly on habits of lifelong learning, and
- a need to more fully develop appropriate professional attitudes and practices (Goodman et al., 1991).

A similar statement was made in the Association of American Medical Colleges report, *General Professional Education of the Physician and College Preparation for Medicine*, which again stressed the pitfalls of lecturing (Association of American Medical Colleges, 1984). Yet, there remain strong perceptions that even with reform in the medical school curriculum, the barriers to a satisfying research career remain significant enough to be a disincentive for many. Moreover, although many efforts are under way to improve the medical school curriculum, it is not clear whether research skills have been included as part of the overall goals of these changes. If they are included, it is not clear what the measures of effectiveness for research preparedness are in these new curricula.

TABLE 4-3 Career Choice Preference by Medical School Graduates from 1989 to 1991

M.D. Graduates' Preferences (First Choices) for Career Activities	1989 Graduates		1990 Graduates		1991 Graduates	
	No.	Percent	No.	Percent	No.	Percent
Full-time academic faculty Appointment:						
Basic science teaching and research	146	1.30	152	1.30	132	1.20
Clinical sciences	3,223	28.80	3,341	28.80	3,104	27.10
Salaried basic scientist:						
Basic medical sciences	16	0.10	21	0.02	22	0.02
Clinical sciences	36	0.03	30	0.03	29	0.03
Clinical Practice:						
Private clinical practice	6,254	56.00	6,560	56.50	6,365	55.70
Salaried clinical practice	1,251	11.20	1,247	10.70	1,442	12.60

Source: Beran, 1994; Graduation Questionnaire, Association of American Medical Colleges. Washington, D.C.

Research Interests of Medical Students

Some evidence points to a decrease in interest in postgraduate research activities among medical school graduates. For example, a graduation questionnaire administered by the Association of American Medical Colleges queries senior medical students on their preferences for career activities, including their desire to engage in research. Consistently, less than 1 percent indicate that becoming a salaried research scientist is their first choice (Table 4-3) (Beran, 1994). Just slightly over 1 percent indicate a preference for a full-time academic faculty appointment in basic science teaching and research. These results are not surprising; this probably represents a fraction of students who have, for some reason, chosen to pursue research careers rather than patient care.

Far more fourth-year medical students—27 to 28 percent—indicate a preference for a full-time academic appointment in clinical science rather than basic science. It should be noted, however, that an appointment in clinical science or a clinical department does not directly translate into a preference for a clinical research career. When asked to estimate the degree of involvement in research anticipated during their medical careers, between 13 and 15 percent indicate significant involvement (several years set aside for full-time research or 25 percent or more of a continuous career devoted to research pursuits) (Table 4-4) (Beran, 1994). Approximately 40 percent note that they anticipate involvement

TABLE 4-4 Degree of Involvement in Research Activity During Career as Indicated by Graduating Medical Students, 1989–1991

Expected Extent of Research Involvement	1989 Graduates		1990 Graduates		1991 Graduates	
	No.	Percent	No.	Percent	No.	Percent
Exclusively	28	0.3	34	0.3	43	0.4
Significantly involved (several years set aside for full-time research or more than 25 percent of continuous career devoted to research pursuits)	1,708	15.3	1,669	14.4	1,480	12.9
Somewhat involved (one year or less than 25 percent of continuous career)	4,529	40.5	4,655	40.1	4,646	40.6
Limited involvement (e.g., occasional participation in clinical trials)	4,084	36.5	4,405	37.9	4,291	37.5
Not involved	649	5.8	81	0.7	672	5.9

Source: Beran, 1994; Graduation Questionnaire, Association of American Medical Colleges. Washington, D.C.

in research (one year or less than 25 percent of a continuous career), and about 37 percent anticipate limited involvement (occasional participation in clinical trials).

On the positive side, a separate survey reported that physician-scientists most enjoyed the intellectual environment of research and the freedom that came with it, as well as the opportunities to teach. What they least liked were the pressures of time and the need to succeed, lack of support from superiors, and financial concerns (Martin, 1991). Thus, the perceptions of those who might pursue research accurately reflect the perceptions of those who presently conduct research.

Research Participation by Medical Students

When to undertake research training remains a point of controversy if one chooses to become a clinical investigator. Although some studies have questioned whether medical school research experiences are a factor in generating more physician-scientists (Woods, 1979), most would agree that research experiences during medical school are influential in encouraging some, if not total, research involvement during the medical career (Davis and Kelley, 1982; Segal et al., 1990). Another issue is whether the overall good of training more scientifically literate physicians is sufficient (with the increased likelihood that this will result in more physician-hours in research) or whether new and innovative efforts should be made to encourage more physicians to dedicate their careers to research (Bishop, 1984).

There is concern that most medical residents are hesitant to begin a research activity because of their lack of knowledge about the career possibilities in research and also because of a deficiency in basic research skills (Martin, 1991). Thus, some individuals are already "lost" to research if they have not been exposed before they begin their residencies. If research experience during medical school is a reasonable predictor of postgraduate research activity, the opportunity to take time off for research during medical school or during the first full year following receipt of the M.D. degree has the potential to encourage more physicians to pursue research pathways than programs providing brief research experiences during the residency and fellowship years.

To remedy this situation, some have suggested that there be a period of research prior to or during medical school in order for the student to decide whether he or she enjoys the activity and is good at it (Smith, 1989). Several studies have indicated that medical students who have been exposed to a research experience during their medical education are more likely to engage in research during their postgraduate years (Davis and Kelley, 1982; Jennett, 1988; Paiva et al., 1975; Segal et al., 1990). Some medical schools (for example, Duke, Yale, Case Western Reserve, and the University of Pennsylvania among others) have implemented programs in which medical students are encouraged or required to take one year off from medical studies to participate in research. To the committee's knowledge, the students in these programs have not been tracked in any systematic fashion to determine whether they have continued to pursue research activities.

In addition to funding training programs, which will be discussed below, another serious constraint confronting medical students who choose to engage in research is time. It has been estimated that M.D.s spend less than 50 percent of their time in the laboratory during research training, compared with nearly 75 percent for Ph.D.s (Martin, 1991). This can jeopardize the quality of the research experience. The first two years of the standard medical curriculum are crammed with course work and the learning of facts. The third year is generally filled with clinical rotations to introduce students to the various specialties that often influence their career choices. Time permitting, some students choose to do a research elective. The summers between the second and third or the third and fourth years are often the only significant blocks of time available for a serious commitment to research. The length of time available, however, is often two to three months or less. The focus on obtaining a residency position during the fourth year preoccupies students, although this period also is used for research electives.

Even when students choose to engage in research, the committee believes that most choose to perform studies in the laboratory rather than patient studies. Laboratory experiments that are frequently predesigned or already under way with the possibility of publication at the end of the research period are particularly attractive to students. Some research experiences allow students to develop their own hypotheses and to test them. Nonetheless, these opportunities are valuable from the standpoint that the students are surrounded by the culture and socialization of research. Furthermore, the student has a reasonable expectation of presenting the findings at a regional or national meeting and possibly publishing in a peer-reviewed journal.

At the same time, the committee believes that few opportunities exist to expose medical students to research involving patients. Unlike discrete laboratory projects, human studies are frequently multiyear studies in which a student might not be able to develop an independent portion of the project. Thus, a growing consensus of opinion postulates that the traditional medical school curriculum is not equipped to provide the necessary scientific training for clinical investigators, even for the most motivated of students. With the exception of the M.D.-Ph.D. track and a few other special programs, research experiences frequently occur during residency or following residency in a fellowship.

Training Programs for Medical Students

A few programs allow medical students to gain research experiences. These programs are funded by the federal government, the private sector, and institutions themselves. For example, NIH sponsors a short-term training grant program (referred to as a T35 training grant) to medical schools to support brief training experiences for medical students (predoctoral professional students are not generally appointed on institutional National Research Service Award training grants [T32]). The T35 program generally pays a small stipend (for example, $1,000) for 8 to 10 weeks of research experience, generally during the summer. The 1989 NIH review of the training programs indicated that between 1,000 and 1,400 short-term appointments were supported annually by NIH throughout the 1980s (National Institutes of Health, 1989a). The review panel examined the research interests of medical school graduates who were supported on T35 training grants and concluded that program participants were twice as likely to indicate an interest in a research career as were their fellow graduates.

Because of a lack of programs or deficiencies in existing programs, Duke University, Johns Hopkins University, University of Pennsylvania, and Washington University initiated The Four Schools Physician Scientist Program in Internal Medicine in 1989 (Four Schools Physician Scientist Program in Internal Medicine, 1991). In this program, two third-year medical students are selected from each institution to participate in a six-year, fully funded program of research and clinical training. The obvious advantages of this program are the total immersion into a scientific culture, exposure to other institutions, and relief of debt burden. This program is in its infancy but may provide a useful prototype for future investment in physician-scientist training. Whether these students will later participate in clinical research activities has not been determined.

In the private sector, the Howard Hughes Medical Institute (HHMI) sponsors Medical Student and Postdoctoral Training Fellowships. HHMI sponsors a national competition to encourage an interlude of basic research at NIH or elsewhere during medical school to encourage an interest in research. As of 1992, the program had placed 230 students from 73 medical schools in various NIH laboratories. Students spend 40 to 80 hours a week in the laboratory and must give a presentation of their work to their fellow students. They are also provided housing during their time at NIH. As with the previous programs and the Medical Scientist Training program discussed below, it is unclear whether these experiences enhance an individual's view of patient-oriented research.

Dual-Degree Programs

One approach to increasing the supply of physicians trained to conduct research is the development of dual-degree programs. Many medical schools offer students the opportunity to earn graduate and professional degrees in addition to the doctor of medicine degree. A combined M.D. and Ph.D. is offered at 109 schools, a combined M.D. and master's degree is available at 42 schools, a combined M.D. and doctor of jurisprudence (J.D.) degree is available in 10 schools, and a combined M.D. and master of public health degree (M.P.H.) is available in 29 schools (Jonas et al., 1991). These programs provide the student with the opportunity to undertake a unique approach to medical education. The program most touted in its record of producing physician-scientists has been the NIH-sponsored Medical Scientist Training (MST) program, which was initiated in 1962 and which is administered through the National Institute of General Medical Sciences (NIGMS) (Bickel et al., 1981).

In the MST program, students selected by admissions committees at each school pursue M.D. and Ph.D. degrees simultaneously. After spending two years in the standard medical school curriculum, students engage in a research project under the supervision of a scientist-mentor for a minimum of three years. This research project forms the basis of a thesis that is defended by the student in order to obtain the Ph.D. degree. Finally, the student completes one year of clinical rotations, after which both degrees are awarded.

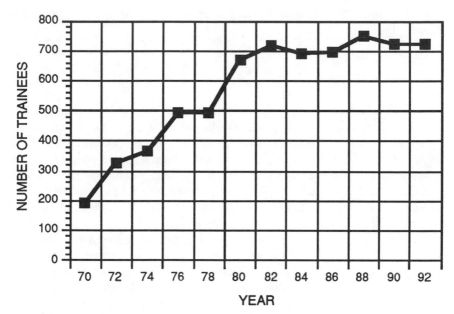

FIGURE 4-1 Total number of participants in the Medical Scientist Training program from 1970 to 1992. (Source: National Institutes of Health, National Institute of General Medical Sciences.)

The obvious advantages of the M.D.-Ph.D. program are that it requires an early commitment to science and provides continuity with the standard basic science components of the medical school curriculum, and students do not accumulate a large debt burden because the NIGMS program pays tuition costs, stipends, and some laboratory expenses for six years. Other advantages are that the student is exposed to the culture of the scientific environment and is expected to achieve scientific competency upon graduation from medical school. Nevertheless, it is not known whether these programs are effective for preparing students to undertake research involving human subjects. The disadvantage is that there often is at least a three-year hiatus between the completion of thesis work and the opportunity to return to scientific work following residency (Smith, 1989).

Data collected in 1990 on the MST program by the NIGMS revealed that of the 126 medical schools, 109 listed M.D.-Ph.D. training opportunities. Approximately 1,500 students were enrolled in these programs (Martin, 1991). NIGMS funds MST programs at only 29 of the medical schools, accounting for about 700 students annually (Figure 4-1). The 80 MST programs at the remaining medical schools are funded through institutional resources or the private sector. The NIH has invested more than $400 million through its MST program in some 2,000 double-degree graduates since its inception in the 1960s (Ahrens, 1992).

MST Program Outcomes

To date, information on the extent to which NIH's MST program has actually achieved its goal of producing independent physician-investigators, regardless of the area of research, has been sparse. One study conducted in 1981 suggested that MST program graduates outperformed their counterparts in securing faculty positions and academic promotions, obtaining NIH research grants, and publication activity (Bickel et al., 1981; Sherman et al., 1981). The extent to which these graduates were involved in basic biomedical, clinical, or patient-oriented research, however, was not examined.

Assessments of more recent graduates, although confined to individual programs and involving no comparison groups, give some sense of the research orientations of these physician-investigators. One survey of 148 MST program graduates from Washington University found 86 percent of those who completed their postgraduate training were employed in academic positions. Of this group, nearly two thirds were employed in clinical departments, 69 percent had received NIH grants, 11 percent were Howard Hughes Medical Institute investigators, and 6 percent were recipients of clinician-scientist awards from Pfizer or Squibb (Freiden and Fox, 1991).

Examinations of the outcomes for MST program graduates from other such programs reveal similar employment and research activity patterns (Bradford et al., 1986; Freiden and Fox, 1991; Martin, 1991; McClellan and Talalay, 1992). For example, a survey of M.D.-Ph.D. programs at eight medical schools revealed the following:

• Of those students who had completed their postgraduate or residency training, more than 90 percent had gone on to academic or institute research positions.

• Approximately six percent went into private practice.

• Four percent took research positions at NIH, in research institutes, and in industry.

• Of those who took faculty appointments, most were in departments of medicine.

• On average, it takes about seven years to complete the dual-degree program.

Such "snapshots" of individual programs suggest that the MST program may be instrumental in the production of patient-oriented researchers. At the same time, several important questions remain. Current data do not allow a determination of the effectiveness of the MST program in comparison with the effectiveness of other NIH mechanisms for training physician-scientists and patient-oriented researchers (for example, the Clinician-Investigator and Physician-Investigator Awards). In addition, the relative effectiveness of MST program support for training M.D.-Ph.D. researchers in comparison with the effectiveness of similar programs that do not receive such support has not been established.

This latter question is particularly important, because about half of the medical students enrolled in dual-degree programs in the 1990–1991 school year received no MST program support, and of those who received an M.D. degree in 1990, equal numbers had either graduated from dual-degree programs or had already earned their Ph.D. (Howard Hughes Medical Institute, 1992). There is some evidence suggesting that this distribution may differ across clinical specialties (Prystowsky, 1992). For example, few M.D.-Ph.D. recipients are in surgical departments, which suggests that these programs are not often designed to encompass research in the surgical disciplines. Determination of the performance of this training support, in relation to the performance of dual-degree programs or Ph.D. training prior to the receipt of the M.D. degree, would thus yield valuable data for guiding future initiatives to augment the pool of physician-investigators involved in patient-oriented research.

Whether characteristics of the training program or the preselection of the trainees is responsible for the apparent success as measured by the above indicators is not clear. There has been no study in which a control group matched for prior performance has been used to assess the outcomes of the MST program. At the very least one can assume that if intelligent, motivated people are supported financially for several years and protected from taking on responsibilities other than their research, they are likely to do research, publish papers, receive grants, and be promoted (Bland and Schmitz, 1986; Brancati, 1992; Ahrens, 1992). The success of the MST program of NIH supports this contention for a significant proportion (more than 60 percent) of MST program participants who have taken academic or institute research positions. Nevertheless, there have been no systematic analyses of the significance of research exposure in medical school in deciding on a research career, that is, how many students who were not previously so inclined turn to science as a result of such exposure. Furthermore, although the MST program is believed to be effective at training physicians to perform basic research, its effectiveness in providing training for patient-oriented research is unproven. Because many of these investigators have entered the research workforce in recent years and may not have shown their full potential as independent investigators, continued tracking and program evaluation will be useful for determining program outcomes.

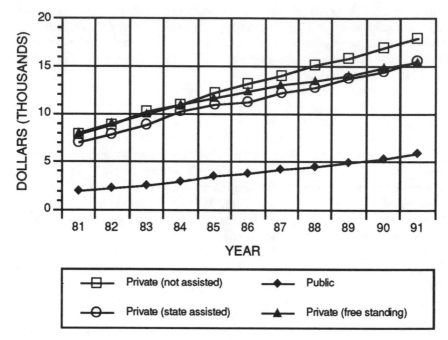

FIGURE 4-2   Average first-year, in-state medical school tuition for academic years 1981–1982 to 1990–1991.   (Source: Association of American Medical Colleges, Section for Operational Studies.)

Training in Research Ethics

Insufficient laboratory experiences and deficiencies in those experiences are not the only dilemmas experienced by physicians who choose research pathways. Scientific ethics should be introduced at some point in training for all individuals wishing to become scientists. The need for reliable instruction in scientific ethics and proper standards of behavior was evident in a survey of biomedical trainees at the University of California, San Diego. Fifty-one percent reported a first-hand observation of some kind of unethical research conduct, a personal history of unethical behavior, or a willingness to modify, perhaps even to fabricate, experimental data to get a paper accepted or, more likely, to win a research grant (Kalichman and Friedman, 1992).

Courses that formally address scientific ethics are rarely offered, much less required, in either basic science or clinical programs. Trainees from clinical departments, however, are more likely than those from basic science departments to have had a course in which scientific ethics were discussed (Kalichman and Friedman, 1992). NIH is now requiring that all institutions that receive training funds have a formal program in research ethics. Many research institutions have formulated policies for the conduct of research and scientific recordkeeping. Furthermore, all institutions that perform research involving human subjects must provide assurance to the sponsor of the ethical treatment of human subjects in their research. It is unclear, however, whether there are mechanisms to convey this information in any systematic fashion to research trainees, or whether they merely learn by trial and error in the human studies approval process.

Financing and Debt

The rapidly growing indebtedness of medical students is raising serious concerns throughout the medical education community. The committee felt strongly that the rising debt levels of medical students are deterring individuals from pursuing research careers. To further elucidate this issue, the committee commissioned a paper by Robert Beran on student indebtedness, and from which this section draws heavily (Beran, 1994).

During the 1980s, medical school tuition increased more rapidly than it had in earlier decades. Average tuition for all types of medical schools, private and public, more than doubled between 1981 and 1991 (Figure 4-2) (Association of American Medical Colleges, 1991). In the 1989–1990 academic year, tuition ranged from $8,650 to $24,300, with a median of $17,116. Student living expenses can top $10,000, and fees add several hundred dollars to the bill.

As the cost of attending medical school increases, the proportion of these costs supported by scholarships has dropped and students have been forced to make up the difference through loans (Beran, 1994; Hughes et al., 1991) (Figure 4-3). In the 1980-81 academic year, 34 percent ($137 million) of the $401.9 million in total financial assistance provided to medical students was in the form of scholarships. By the 1990–1991 academic year, the scholarship proportion had dropped to about 23 percent of the $826.5 million in student aid. This decline in the amount of aid provided through scholarship programs is largely the result of a reduction in funds available from federally sponsored scholarship programs. In 1980–1981, of the total scholarship funds ($180 million), more than 64 percent was provided through the National Health Service Corps (NHSC) ($50 million, or 36 percent) and the Armed Services Health Professional Scholarship (HPSP) program ($38 million, or 28 percent); about 17 percent was contributed from institutional funds. In the 1990–1991 academic year, however, the proportion of funds available from the NHSC program was less than 1 percent of the $186.5 million total scholarship aid, and that from the HPSP program was about 30 percent. By contrast, the proportion of scholarship funds available from the institutions rose to 41 percent.

It has long been suggested that high levels of educational debt may be a strong deterrent to interest in a career in academic research. Although the effects

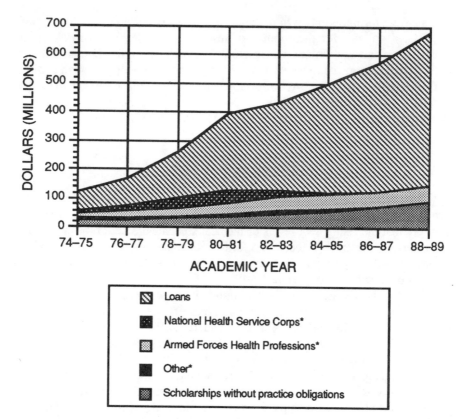

FIGURE 4-3   Loans, scholarships with practice obligations (*), and scholarships without practice obligations awarded to medical students for academic years 1974–1975 through 1988–1989. (Source: Reprinted, with permission, from Hughes et al. [1991], p. 405. Copyright 1991 by The New England Journal of Medicine.)

of debt on a career decision during residency training are largely unknown, an examination of inquiries regarding career choice and interest in research at the time of medical school graduation have not lent support to this concern. The committee reviewed the responses provided through the Association of American Medical Colleges Graduation Questionnaire. It should be noted, however, that the responses at this point of one's educational pathway may not truly reflect career choices and that querying trainees during residency or fellowship may be better indicators of career selections.

From 1980 to 1990, the average indebtedness of medical school graduates almost tripled, from about $16,500 to about $46,200 in nominal dollars (Figure 4-4) (Table 4-5). When corrected for inflation, the growth of indebtedness over the past decade was 81 percent for all schools, 65 percent for public schools, and

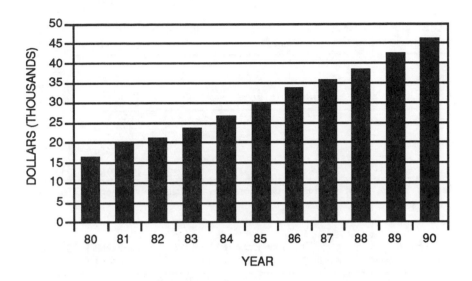

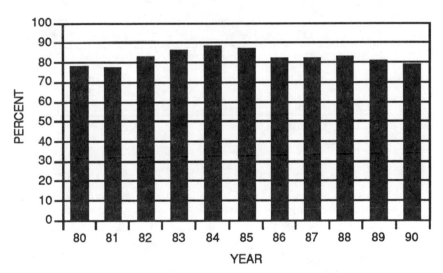

FIGURE 4-4 Average educational debt for medical students upon graduation (top panel) and percent of medical school graduates with educational debt (bottom panel), 1980–1990. (Source: Association of American Medical Colleges, Section for Operational Studies.)

105 percent for private schools (Table 4-6) (Beran, 1994). The proportion of medical students graduating with debt has hovered between 75 and 82 percent over the past decade (Figure 4-4).

TABLE 4-5 Trends in Mean Education Debt of Medical School Graduates for Selected Years from 1980 to 1990 in Current Dollars

School Type	1980	1985	1989	1990	Decade Increase (percent)
All types	$16,493	$29,943	$43,374	$46,354	181
Public school	$14,907	$25,718	$34,568	$38,189	156
Private school	$18,493	$36,417	$53,226	$58,898	218

Source: Beran, 1994; Graduation Questionnaire, Association of American Medical Colleges. Washington, D.C.

TABLE 4-6 Trends in Mean Education Debt of Medical School Graduates for Selected Years from 1980 to 1990 in Constant 1980 Dollars

School Type	1980	1985	1989	1990	Decade Increase (percent)
All types	$16,493	$22,936	$28,135	$29,907	81
Public school	$14,907	$19,700	$22,952	$24,639	65
Private school	$18,493	$27,895	$35,341	$38,000	105

Source: Beran, 1994; Graduation Questionnaire, Association of American Medical Colleges. Washington, D.C.

The mean educational debt levels for 1988, 1989, and 1990 medical school graduates who expect significant involvement in research during their medical careers is below the mean debt for all indebted medical graduates. The mean debt for the 1988 graduates anticipating research involvement was $37,821, whereas the mean debt for all indebted 1988 graduates was $38,489. Graduates expecting to pursue an exclusive career in research graduated with a mean debt of $30,015. Students graduating in 1989 who expected significant research involvement had a mean educational debt of $40,885. The mean debt for all 1989 graduates with debt was $42,374. The mean debt for the 1990 groups of graduates who expected significant involvement in research was $45,150, whereas it was $46,224 for all 1990 graduates. From these data, one could conclude that excessive debt does not appear to deter graduates' interest in research (Beran, 1994). These data, however, deal with mean debt. To gain a clearer understanding of the influence that debt has on career choice, the committee would need data on the range of debt for those choosing to pursue research careers. Furthermore, these data do not account for consumer debt, which can add additional burdens for trainees.

Although the empirical data seem to indicate that debt may not influence career choice, anecdotal reports argue otherwise. Intuitively, the pressures of an academic career and a growing likelihood that a young physician cannot service these huge debts on academic salaries leads the committee to be concerned that debt does play a key role in career choice—turning young physicians away from academic research careers. An analysis by the Association of American Medical Colleges shows that an annual income of $60,000, the starting academic salary for many internal medicine specialties and subspecialties, is insufficient for servicing debt loads of $75,000 or more (Association of American Medical Colleges, 1991).

GRADUATE MEDICAL EDUCATION

Many forces are responsible for shaping the content and structure of graduate medical education (GME). The primary goal of GME is to prepare novice medical school graduates to provide the highest quality of medical care on the basis of the vast knowledge of medical science. Confluent with that objective, the committee believes that a certain cohort must also be well prepared to pose and answer relevant scientific questions, both at the fundamental level and at the level of patients and populations. Furthermore, the scientific preparation of physicians not only should adequately prepare them for academic careers but also should be responsive to the needs of other employment sectors where clinical research talent is needed, such as government and industry. Thus, the committee explored the forces, personal as well as professional, shaping GME in an effort to find ways to overcome the barriers to investigative careers.

To probe these factors in more depth, the committee commissioned a number of papers on issues that it felt were particularly influential in developing career pathways for physician-scientists at the postdoctoral level. One paper, by Georgine Pion of Vanderbilt University, examined the training programs offered through NIH (Pion, 1994). Two other papers, one by David Atkins and colleagues at the University of Washington (Atkins et al., 1994) and one by Thomas Lee and Lee Goldman at the Brigham and Women's Hospital in Boston Lee and Goldman, 1994), dealt with models for postdoctoral training . Linda Blank of the American Board of Internal Medicine drafted a paper on the roles of the resident review committees and the certification boards on research career pathways (Blank 1994), and Judith Swazey prepared a paper on mentors and role models (Swazey, 1994). All of these papers provided valuable information to the committee in preparing this portion of the report.

How Long Should Training Be and What Should the Training Involve?

The duration of research training has long been considered a key factor in preparing for a successful research career (Levey et al., 1988; Oates, 1982). Most would agree that less than 12 months of research training is inadequate to prepare independent investigators in either the basic sciences or clinical research (National Institutes of Health, 1989a). Levey et al. (1988) have shown that at least two years of postdoctoral research training is required. Some have suggested that at least three years of training in modern biological science is necessary to prepare most individuals to perform as independent investigators (Goldstein, 1986). Similar suggestions have been made for preparing clinicians to conduct clinical effectiveness research (Goldman et al., 1990). The advantage to scientific training after the receipt of the M.D. degree is that there is temporal continuity between training and a research career. It was the model employed by many who are clinical investigators today. The drawback of this model is that by the time a student has completed training, he or she might have already decided on a clinical career without being exposed to research, and some of the flexibility in the system is thus lost.

For medical school faculty in departments of medicine, the length of postdoctoral research training was a significant predictor for subsequent involvement as an active researcher and principal investigator for a peer-reviewed research grant (Levey et al., 1988). The more that the physician is deeply immersed in the primary literature surrounding basic biology, the more likely it is research will to lead to fundamental discoveries that will further the understanding of disease processes (Martin, 1991). Along these same lines, Safran et al.(1992) has shown improved performances on various clinical knowledge measures following the implementation of a scientific curriculum in a surgical residency program. The committee believes that trainees who are exposed to clinical investigation will gain an appreciation for the results of clinical research and be prepared to pose pertinent research questions regarding humans.

Several recommendations have emerged to encourage postdoctoral research training. A 1986 survey of full-time faculty in departments of medicine advocated incorporating formal course work, particularly in the basic sciences and statistics, with less time allocated to patient care (Levey et al., 1988). In 1989, a National Research Council committee made the following recommendations (National Academy of Sciences, 1989) regarding changes that should be made in the postdoctoral institutional training programs for physician-scientists:

- a true consortium between the clinical and preclinical departments of the institution, with shared responsibilities for the design and administration of the program;
- selection of trainees on the basis of evidence of some previous experience in research and overall promise;
- formal course work in the physical and biochemical sciences sufficient to give graduates a theoretical background comparable to those of people with graduate degrees in the biological sciences;
- not less than three years of research training, primarily in direct research experience under the supervision of a mentor; and
- modules of instruction specifically tailored to the needs of the physician trainee in such areas as basic laboratory techniques, chromatography, radioimmunoassay, protein purification, advanced instrumental techniques, fundamental principles of enzymology and molecular biology, subcellular fractionation techniques, computer technology, evaluation of experimental data, epidemiology, statistics and database management, as well as grant and manuscript writing.

Although training should always be individualized, generic skills are needed. They include experimental design, biostatistics, data analysis, ethics of human experimentation and research ethics, scientific writing and presentation, general laboratory skills, including computing, and critical evaluation of scientific information (Institute of Medicine, 1988a). The investigator, for example, must understand the differences between randomized controlled trials and other experimental and nonexperimental designs. Trainees also need to be attentive to sampling methods, sample size, and analytical methods (Institute of Medicine, 1988a).

Some argue that these skills are less appreciated early in medical school and might best be taught to the beginning investigator, trainee, or fellow (Institute of Medicine, 1988a). Yet, there are dangers in waiting to introduce these concepts. Most residents elect to do research training when they are in their late twenties or thirties. Their Ph.D. counterparts might already have invested 10 years in the research laboratory. Furthermore, many clinical fellows have no coursework requirements and have no contact with basic scientists or clinical investigators. These problems point to the need for more training of physician-scientists where the research is conducted, as well as the need for formal, rigorous course work.

A few programs have attempted to provide experiences for students to conduct research during or immediately after their medical school training. The NIH Physician-Scientist Training Awards (K11 and K12) have been available since 1985. Both institutional (K12) and individual (K11) awards are made for training non-Ph.D. physicians for five years following residency. The primary intent of the awards, however, is to ensure that a period of time is spent in basic science laboratories.

Although much postgraduate training occurred at NIH in the past, most postdoctoral research training has now shifted to universities and medical centers. Furthermore, many trainees are remaining at the institutions where they completed their residencies to conduct postdoctoral research. Critics charge that this encourages institutions to select their own graduates rather than to select the best candidates in a nationally competitive manner (Martin, 1991).

The usual course for research training after receipt of the M.D. is two years of training in one of the clinical subspecialties while on a training grant. After the traineeship, individuals can apply for a two-year fellowship that allows them to pursue a research problem under the guidance of a faculty adviser or mentor. Training grants and fellowships are especially critical in enabling M.D.s to "buy out" of other administrative and clinical responsibilities that are not usually faced by Ph.D. scientists. The appropriate length of training and payback provisions have been debated frequently over the past few years (National Institutes of Health, 1989a).

Edwin Cadman, chairman of the Department of Medicine at Yale, has suggested that the best way to improve prospects for physician-scientists is to envision a future in which they spend a longer time in training, have higher salaries during training, are less dependent on the federal government for support during training, are more concentrated at research-intense medical schools, and are more concerned about population health (Cadman, 1990). Thus, postgraduate training must be streamlined to permit both adequate clinical training and the ability to continue in research.

External Factors Affecting Research Training During GME

Residency Review Committees and Certification Boards

The committee was interested to know what effect, if any, residency review committees (RRCs) and certifying boards have in promoting or hindering research careers among physicians. Both organizations have the ability to establish requirements for research training in medical subspecialties, although neither provides funding or an organizational framework to accomplish this.

Role of RRCs

The nation's 24 RRCs accredit roughly 6,900 residency training programs, which are collectively responsible for establishing the clinical training requirements of some 85,000 medical residents. (See box for list of specialties represented.) Certification boards for these 24 specialties evaluate M.D.

```
┌─────────────────────────────────────────────────────────┐
│                                                           │
│              AMERICAN BOARD OF MEDICAL                    │
│                     SPECIALTIES                           │
│                                                           │
│   American Board of Allergy and Immunology                │
│   American Board of Anesthesiology                        │
│   American Board of Colon and Rectal Surgery              │
│   American Board of Dermatology                           │
│   American Board of Emergency Medicine                    │
│   American Board of Family Practice                       │
│   American Board of Internal Medicine                     │
│   American Board of Medical Genetics                      │
│   American Board of Neurological Surgery                  │
│   American Board of Nuclear Medicine                      │
│   American Board of Obstetrics and Gynecology             │
│   American Board of Opthamology                           │
│   American Board of Orthopaedic Surgery                   │
│   American Board of Otolaryngology                        │
│   American Board of Pathology                             │
│   American Board of Pediatrics                            │
│   American Board of Physical Medicine and Rehabilitation  │
│   American Board of Plastic Surgery                       │
│   American Board of Preventive Medicine                   │
│   American Board of Psychiatry/Neurology                  │
│   American Board of Radiology                             │
│   American Board of Surgery                               │
│   American Board of Thoracic Surgery                      │
│   American Board of Urology                               │
│                                                           │
└─────────────────────────────────────────────────────────┘
```

candidates to verify that they have received adequate preparation to practice as specialists in their respective fields.

The commissioned paper by Linda Blank details the analysis she performed to assess the research requirements of the RRCs, some of which is encapsulated here. The executive secretaries of all 24 RRCs were surveyed to determine which program standards for formal training (so-called special requirements) include research experiences to obtain a description of the research criteria, to confirm the status of the research experience and documentation, and to describe any planned changes in the research experience.

Although 22 of 24 RRCs include research components in their accreditation requirements, only seven RRCs require their residents to have a research experience. Ten RRCs insist that residents should have research experience during training, and four other RRCs encourage such opportunities. The rationale for requiring or emphasizing research experiences or research training is to enhance one's clinical training to become a competent clinician.

Determination of the presence (or absence) of research in a residency program is left to RRC field surveyors, who visit residency programs as a part of the accreditation process. With the exception of information obtained from these reviews, no data are available on any programs to determine the actual levels of participation of residents in research training activities. In 1991 the RRC for internal medicine introduced a computerized system to collect and analyze accreditation data, but it is the only RRC so far to do so.

The nature and length of available research experiences are not specified in the special requirements of RRCs and are specific to the individual training program. With the exception of allergy and immunology, which requires that one quarter of the two-year residency be spent conducting research, no time commitments are specified by any of the other RRCs in their special requirements. Overall, the special requirements for research training are universally vague and difficult to interpret and measure. The committee is concerned that the RRCs do not place enough emphasis on the importance of an academic, discovery-oriented milieu for effective clinical training. The committee believes that experiences for some should go beyond exposure or superficial introduction in research methods and should have rigorous training to prepare residents in research training to undertake independent investigations with human subjects.

Role of Certification Boards

Requirements for specialty board certification generally include specified accredited training, practice experience (for some specialties), and licensure and examination. Research experience is not required for certification, although two boards—for preventive medicine and pediatrics—recognize research as an important element of clinical training. All 24 member boards of the American Board of Medical Specialties were surveyed to assess the availability of certification pathways for physicians who seek careers in clinical investigation, the number of candidates who use these pathways, examination performances, outcomes, and any expected changes in the pathways and impacts of certification and recertification for specialist who choose a career in clinical investigation (Blank, 1994).

Three of the boards—anesthesiology, dermatology, and internal medicine— offer special pathways for clinical investigators. In anesthesiology, clinical investigators are required to spend five years (rather than four, as is required for clinical-track residents) to complete the training requirement, including one and a half years conducting research.

In dermatology, research training takes place during the second or third year of residency. Residents who follow a career path in investigative dermatology usually spend more time on research during these years, although all residents are encouraged to participate in basic or clinical research at some point in their training. During an average year, between 5 and 8 percent of dermatology residents focus their training on research, and 3 of the 101 accredited training programs have 20 percent or more of their residents request additional time for basic or clinical research, according to the board.

In 1983 the American Board of Internal Medicine (ABIM) established the four-year clinical investigator pathway (CIP), which includes two years of research. From 1985 through 1990, 125 candidates completed the CIP, and 103 (82 percent) of them are now certified. Of the 80 in this group for whom career status is known, 45 (44 percent) are in private practice (including three who indicate that they remain involved in research) and 35 (34 percent) are in academic medicine (including 23 in research and 3 who combine research with teaching or consultation). From the listing in the 1991–1992 *Directory of Medical Specialties* (1991), 6,612 internists are listed as recertified by the ABIM, and 65 (or 1 percent) indicate that their major career activity is medical research. Only one of the other certifying boards—nuclear medicine—is discussing a clinical investigator pathway similar to that operated by the ABIM.

Many boards recently have initiated time-limited certification. That is, certificates have a built-in time limitation (for example, 10 years). At the end of the established period, practicing physicians will be required to take a recertification examination to continue to practice as a specialist. These programs are still too new to measure their effects on the careers of clinical researchers. The committee is very concerned that if clinical investigators, many of whom have very narrow academic interests, are required to maintain a broad-based practice to meet recertification requirements in 10-year increments, clinical research may suffer. There are no firm data to support this contention, but the committee raises it as a matter that should be watched closely.

Liaison Committee for Medical Education

Although the Liaison Committee for Medical Education (LCME) relates to medical education rather than GME, it is appropriate to consider its role here, along with the RRCs and certification boards, as an influential organization that affects the preparation of physicians. The LCME is the national authority that accredits medical education programs leading to the M.D. degree. It was formed in 1942 under the sponsorship of the Association of American Medical Colleges and the Council on Education of the American Medical Association. LCME is recognized by the Secretary of the U.S. Department of Education, the Council on Postsecondary Education, the U.S. Congress in various health-related laws, and state licensure boards (Liaison Committee for Medical Education, 1991). Thus, if changes are to be made in medical education to encourage clinical research, the committee recognizes that the LCME, its sponsors, and other parties must also be participants in these changes.

BARRIERS TO CLINICAL RESEARCH TRAINING

Physicians interested in undertaking research—particularly patient-oriented research, where the opportunities and needs seem to be greatest—during the postgraduate training period face a series of obstacles. Several of the most important are discussed below.

Inadequate Training in Research Methods

Although the conclusions of clinical studies are discussed regularly during clinical training, the methods involved in developing such studies rarely receive systematic scrutiny. Today's medical students and residents receive only desultory instruction in the basics of biostatistics, epidemiology, and health services research (Neinstein and Mackenzie, 1989). Patient-oriented researchers need expertise in study designs (such as case-control and cohort studies), and they must be familiar with the strengths and limitations of statistical techniques (such as logistic regression and Cox proportion hazards analyses). Ideally, researchers should also understand and be able to measure the costs of therapy, treatment outcomes, quality of life, and cost-effectiveness, among other variables (Atkins et al., 1994; Lee and Goldman, 1994, Roper, 1988; U.S. Government Accounting Office 1994). No single investigator is likely to master all of these skills. To be successful in a clinical research field, each investigator must be prepared to interact not just with other physicians but also with researchers in related disciplines, such as the social and quantitative sciences.

In some institutions much of the clinical research occurs in clinical research centers (CRCs), which represent a longstanding program of patient-oriented research. Funding for CRCs has declined, however, as research on the cellular and molecular bases of disease has increased. Furthermore, the model of research conducted in CRCs, which relies on detailed measurements in a small number of patients, may be too narrow for training some physicians in other important areas of clinical research, particularly studies involving the diagnosis, prognosis, and treatment of disease. Schools of public health and divisions of epidemiology and biostatistics at large medical centers offer these subjects and other relevant courses. With only 24 schools of public health and 126 medical schools in the United States, however, a minority of postdoctoral training programs have access to these resources.

Although large multicenter trials account for a substantial proportion of the clinical research conducted at many major academic centers, these sorts of studies may not provide the best training opportunities for new investigators. A junior investigator in a large randomized trial may contribute to data collection but may not be involved in the design, data analysis, or manuscript preparation. Therefore, participation in a multicenter randomized trial is unlikely to adequately prepare an independent clinical investigator unless this experience is supplemented by other training.

Inadequate Mentoring

In addition to being inadequately trained to conduct independent research through such experiences as peripheral participation in a clinical trial, research fellows pursuing clinical projects may encounter a limited supply of experienced mentors to guide them through their research endeavors. Faculty engaged in clinical research may not have been adequately trained in research methods and are even less likely to have received adequate training in clinical research methods. Many have numerous competing commitments, and they may not have the time or the resources to assist and guide the trainees' in their projects.

To further elucidate the attributes of effective mentoring, the committee commissioned Judith Swazey of the Acadia Institute to draft a paper, "Advisors, Mentors, and Role Models in Graduate Professional Education: Implications for the Recruitment, Training, and Retention of Physician-Investigators," (Swazey, 1994). In conclusion, there are few empirical data on what constitutes effective mentoring and the outcomes of mentoring. However, the committee believes that mentors who commit themselves to advising and guiding trainees through the maze of research are critical players in the research careers of young investigators. The committee also believes that some form of midcareer program to aid established investigators in becoming more effective mentors could help alleviate the shortage of clinical investigator mentors that now exists.

Timing of Training

For some specialties, the optimal timing of research training is not clear. For instance, if residents in surgery go into the laboratory for one year following the second year of clinical training, they will have to complete three clinical years after they complete their time in the laboratory. By the time they finish their residency, the data they accumulate may be too old for use as preliminary results for a grant application (see Appendix C). If instead, they go into the laboratory after the third or fourth year, many surgeons feel uncomfortable with the level of their clinical skills when they return to the senior year of residency. Furthermore,

170   CAREERS IN CLINICAL RESEARCH

brief and sporadic intervals in a laboratory are probably inadequate to prepare physicians for a research career, not to mention a clinical investigative career.

Waiting to begin research training until after the completion of clinical training has two primary drawbacks. First, many of the brightest residents will have been lost to an academic career by the passage of time. Second, if they train in research (outside the clinical setting) for two or more years after they complete their clinical training, they will feel clinically inadequate when they begin their career.

The time and expense involved in conducting clinical studies may significantly hamper research fellows who are trying to complete advanced medical training concurrently. Many patient-oriented projects take too long to complete or are too costly to attract trainees for relatively brief fellowships. In contrast, laboratory projects with established investigators can often take advantage of the existing resources of a productive laboratory, generate data more quickly, and incur more modest marginal costs. Thus, a different type of reward system may be warranted since publication may not be the currency of achievement for those clinical research trainees involved in long-term research projects.

Consistent and continuous involvement in clinical research activity throughout the training period might be one option for maintaining an interest and gaining an aptitude for clinical research—an objective that runs counter to the training requirements of residency review committees and certification boards noted earlier (Blank, 1994). This may be combined with a one-, two-, or three-year fellowship to specialize in designing and conducting clinical studies.

Competing Commitments

The average resident spends as many as 100 hours in the hospital each week delivering patient care and on clinically related issues while, at the same time, pursuing a meaningful clinical education (Safran et al., 1992). Because clinical research trainees frequently are in clinical care environments as well, the competing demands of patient care and research commitments are difficult to balance (Littlefield, 1984 and 1986). Ironically, if clinical research trainee spends time seeing patients who are not involved in a research protocol, the likelihood that the trainee will receive research support for patient-oriented studies in the future is reduced. A survey by the American Federation for Clinical Research found that every 10 hours of clinical work a week was associated with a 23 percent decrease in the odds of having federal or nonprofit foundation grant support (Lee et al., 1991). The data demonstrate an association between increased nonresearch responsibilities and decreased probability of funding, but they do not prove a cause-and-effect relationship. This does not imply that clinical research trainees should not provide patient care but, rather, that clinical research time may need to be protected from clinical training demands.

AVENUES FOR POSTDOCTORAL RESEARCH TRAINING

The vast majority of support for research training comes from the federal government—primarily NIH. Over the years, however, federal support research training has been politically charged. In 1974, the Nixon administration impounded the research training funds in an effort to phase out all research training. Congress reacted immediately by passing the National Research Service Award (NRSA) Act, which authorized training through the Public Health Service agencies, primarily NIH, ADAMHA, and the Health Resources Service Administration. Training was thus restored and funded as a separate line item in annual appropriations. Recently, however, funding has fluctuated as positions have been cut and restored and stipends have been readjusted (Institute of Medicine, 1990).

NIH currently funds training grants to support a number of trainees within an institution (T32 awards), individual research fellowships (F32 awards), and several types of career development awards (K awards). In fiscal year 1992, NIH obligated about $314 million, or about 3.5 percent of its total budget, to support research training grants (T32 awards) and fellowships (F32 awards). An additional $101.6 million was committed to career development awards (National Institutes of Health, 1993b).

A handful of private foundations and philanthropies also fund research training. In addition, a small number of programs around the country—supported by foundations and academic institutions—are taking innovative steps to improve the competence of clinical investigators. (See the section Model Programs for Research Training later in this chapter and the background papers by Atkins et al., 1994, and Lee and Goldman, 1994.) Although it is a substantial force in the area of research funding, industry is a relatively minor player when it comes to support for clinical research training.

Federal Support from NIH

Although NIH offers a variety of research training and career development opportunities, T32 training awards and F32 fellowship awards are the most common mechanisms for funding postdoctoral training of young investigators. Training grants and fellowships differ in a number of ways. For example, training grant applications are reviewed by special review panels convened by the individual institutes, and awards are made to program directors at universities or research institutes for training a certain number of individuals. The T32 awards, which may be renewed by the awardee institution every five years, provide one year or more of postdoctoral research training in a specific research area or clinical subspecialty. The actual selection of the trainees is left to the grant directors in the recipient institutions. Fellowship applications are most commonly reviewed by the initial review groups (IRGs) in the Division of Research Grants of NIH, and they are awarded to individual fellows. Fellowships are usually awarded for two years under the preceptorship of a mentor, but they may be extended for an additional year. Because of their focus, institutes are, in general, most interested in developing investigators in a particular field of research through training grants; IRG reviewers are more concerned with the substance of the research proposal presented in the fellowship application.

Financing course work in clinical research training presents a substantial problem in some training programs. Although tuition for courses is covered in predoctoral programs that support Ph.D. candidates, tuition support is not necessarily provided under the grants that support postdoctoral students—the stage when many physician-scientists require it. Although NIH institutional training grants may permit the inclusion of some tuition expenses, these must be anticipated in advance and may not be available from grants already in force. Individual NRSA fellowships (F32 awards) provide salary stipends but not tuition expenses.

Funding for training grants and fellowships grew from $180 million in 1980 to $314 million in 1992 (National Institutes of Health, 1993b). After correcting for inflation, funding actually declined from the late 1970s (Institute of Medicine, 1990). Furthermore, stipend readjustments in 1989 trimmed about 1,000 positions, which were reinstated in 1990.

Although NIH has supported about 11,000–12,000 training positions annually over the last decade, only about 5,400–5,600 of these have been postdoctoral positions (Figure 4-5). In 1992 the number of postdoctoral positions reached an estimated 5,814, surpassing the previous high of 5,690 in 1987. Of the 5,814 positions available in 1992, 2,651 (45.6 percent) were awarded to M.D.s and 3,163 (54.4 percent) were awarded to Ph.D.s. This ratio of awards to M.D.s and Ph.D.s has changed over the decade as well. Although less than 40 percent of postdoctoral awards were made to M.D.s in the early 1980s, the proportion of postdoctoral awards to M.D.s is approaching 50 percent. Of the 2,651 postdoctoral awards to M.D.s in 1992, 2,336, or 88.1 percent, were awarded through institutional training grants, and only 11.9 percent (315 awards) were individual fellowships. By contrast, 40.9 percent, or 1,293, of the 3,163 awards to Ph.D.s were individual awards (Figure 4-6).

A number of other observations can be made about fellowship and training applications and awards for M.D.s and Ph.D.s. From 1977 through 1989, the annual number of T32 training grant applications from physicians was roughly equal to the number of applications from those with a Ph.D. (Tables 4-7 and 4-8). The success rates for physicians have ranged from 44 percent in 1979 to 78

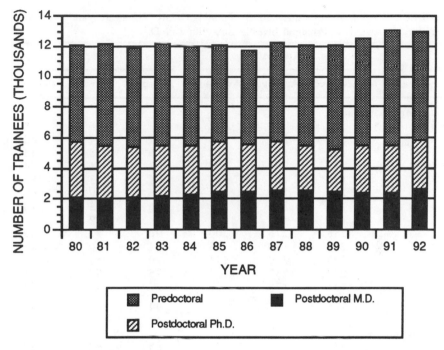

FIGURE 4-5   Number and distribution of predoctoral and postdoctoral training positions support by the NIH. (Source: National Institutes of Health, 1993b.)

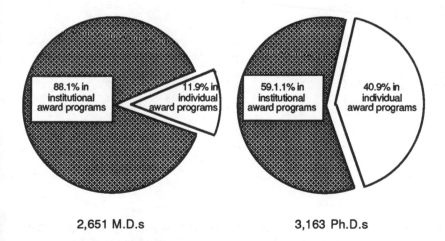

FIGURE 4-6   Distribution of NIH postdoctoral training positions between individual and institutional training grants for M.D.s and Ph.D.s in 1992. (Source: National Institutes of Health, 1993b.)

TABLE 4-7 Applications and Awards for Training Grants (T32 awards) and Individual
Fellowship Awards to Principal Investigators with a Ph.D.

Award Type and Year	Number of Applications			Rates		
	Reviewed	Approved	Awarded	Approval	Award	Success
Training grant awards						
1977	306	250	145	82	58	48
1978	277	235	173	85	74	60
1979	175	133	77	76	58	44
1980	271	248	200	92	81	74
1981	179	162	103	91	63	56
1982	197	190	131	96	69	63
1983	192	184	152	96	83	78
1984	161	146	91	91	62	57
1985	288	276	200	96	72	69
1986	211	191	96	91	50	45
1987	222	219	144	99	66	63
1988	272	257	139	95	54	51
1989	183	178	99	97	56	54
Mean	226		135	94	65	59
Fellowship awards						
1977	252	214	132	85	62	52
1978	334	279	168	84	60	50
1979	311	264	164	85	62	53
1980	310	269	137	87	51	44
1981	324	267	122	82	46	38
1982	290	253	137	87	54	47
1983	297	270	147	91	54	50
1984	362	326	151	90	46	42
1985	428	384	198	90	52	46
1986	436	401	147	92	37	34
1987	364	345	163	95	47	44
1988	396	376	166	95	44	42
1989	489	472	144	97	30	29
Mean	353		152	90	51	45

Source: Reprinted, with permission, from Ahrens (1992). Copyright 1992 by the
Oxford University Press, Inc.

percent in 1983, and is currently hovering around 50 percent. Over this same
period the success rate for Ph.D.s has been slightly lower (Ahrens, 1992).

Over the same period, the number of F32 fellowship applications by Ph.D.s
(range 1,332 to 1,648) greatly exceeded those by M.D.s (range, 252 to 489).

TABLE 4-8 Applications and Awards for Training Grants (T32 awards) and Individual Fellowship Awards (F32 awards) to Principal Investigators with an M.D.

Award Type and Year	Number of Applications			Rates		
	Reviewed	Approved	Awarded	Approval	Award	Success
Training grant awards						
1977	352	246	130	70	53	37
1978	289	232	150	80	65	49
1979	255	186	96	73	52	37
1980	298	273	176	92	65	57
1981	135	122	62	90	51	43
1982	181	168	94	93	56	51
1983	210	192	131	91	68	60
1984	171	158	87	92	55	50
1985	261	253	164	97	65	62
1986	160	149	61	93	41	38
1987	180	176	114	98	65	60
1988	235	225	133	96	59	56
1989	244	242	112	99	46	45
Mean	229		116	94	57	50
Fellowship awards						
1977	1,332	1,165	747	87	64	56
1978	1,463	1,290	876	88	68	60
1979	1,667	1,502	945	90	63	56
1980	1,421	1,277	649	90	51	45
1981	1,474	1,292	485	88	38	33
1982	1,500	1,339	619	89	46	41
1983	1,439	1,296	628	90	49	44
1984	1,452	1,324	543	91	41	37
1985	1,602	1,512	709	94	47	44
1986	1,575	1,478	415	94	28	26
1987	1,468	1,444	700	98	49	47
1988	1,430	1,384	600	97	43	42
1989	1,648	1,588	468	96	30	28
Mean	1,498		645	92	49	44

Source: Reprinted, with permission, from Ahrens (1992), p. 161. Copyright 1992 by the Oxford University Press, Inc.

Over those 13 years, however, the number of fellowship applications by M.D.s nearly doubled, while those by Ph.D.s increased by less than 20 percent. The success rates for F32 applications between the two groups were nearly identical during the 1980s, although like other NIH awards, the rates fell over the period. More important, the actual number of awards for Ph.D.s has declined from a high

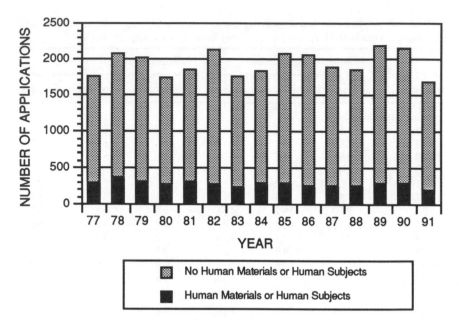

FIGURE 4-7 Number of NIH individual fellowship (F32 award) applications for studies involving the use of human subjects or human materials and those not involving human materials by all applicants. (Source: National Institutes of Health, Division of Research Grants.)

of 945 in 1979 to 468 in 1989. The number of awards to M.D.s fluctuated somewhat during the period but, for the most part, hovered between 135 and 165. There were more than twice as many F32 fellowship applications as awards for both M.D.s and Ph.D.s, which suggests that the scientific merits of the two groups' applications were judged to be nearly identical (Ahrens, 1992).

The emphasis on clinical research through these training mechanisms is difficult to discern. Because the training grants are awarded to institutions and managed locally, it is not possible to determine the nature of the training. The fellowship applications, however, must pass through the same institutional review board process as regular grant applications, and they are so identified on the cover sheet of the application. Of the 1,600 to 2,000 F32 fellowship applications submitted annually by both M.D.s and Ph.D.s, between 18 and 20 percent indicate that they intend to use human subjects or materials (Figures 4-7 and 4-8). Of the 300 to 400 applications from M.D.s, about 100 to 150 (30-40 percent) indicate the intent to use of human subjects or human materials (Figures 4-9 and 4-10). The success rates of applications not indicating the use of human subjects or human materials parallels the success rate of those applications that so indicate (Figure 4-11). The number of studies not involving humans or human

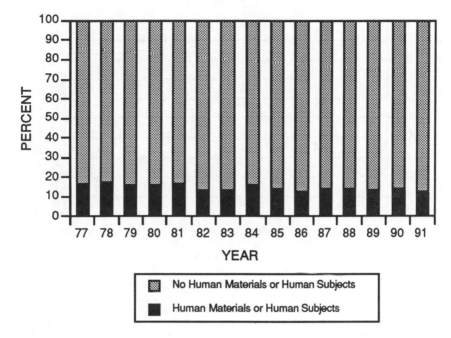

FIGURE 4-8 Proportion of NIH individual fellowship (F32 award) applications by all applicants for studies involving the use of human subjects or human materials and those not using human subjects or materials. (Source: National Institutes of Health, Office of Extramural Research.)

materials far exceeds the number of studies involving humans. If the fellowship awards for studies indicating the use of humans or human materials show the same pattern as the committee's analysis of R01 grants, which found that only about one-third of the awards indicating the use of human subjects or human materials would be for patient-oriented research, then less than 50 of the more than 300 F32 awards made annually to M.D.s are likely to be for research involving patient contact.

Although NIH has tracked the number of M.D. and Ph.D. recipients of fellowship awards and appointments on training grants, very little is known about the demographics of the trainees. For example, no data have been collected on the gender and race compositions of the trainees in the T32 training program and the F32 fellowship program. Although some data are available for those programs that encourage minority participation in research, the involvement of these awardees in clinical research is not easily determined.

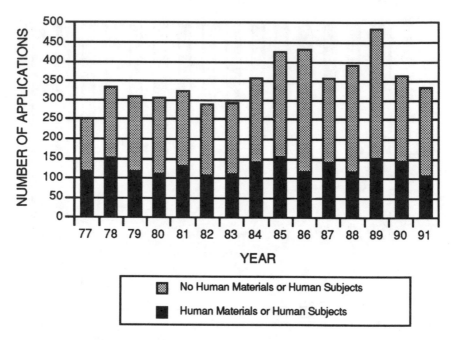

FIGURE 4-9 Number of NIH individual fellowship (F32 award) applications by all applicants for studies involving the use of human subjects or human materials and those not using human subjects or materials. (Source: National Institutes of Health, Office of Extramural Research.)

ASSESSING THE OUTCOMES OF TRAINING PROGRAMS

Since the inception of the NRSA program in the early 1970s, considerable time, money, and intellectual capital have been invested in reviewing, monitoring, and modifying the mechanisms for NIH research training. In the process, many data describing various trainee characteristics and possible relationships to subsequent outcomes have accumulated. The most recent internal evaluation was completed in 1989 and was reported in *Review of the National Institutes of Health Biomedical Research Training Programs* (National Institutes of Health, 1989a). That report devoted much attention to the recruitment and research training of professional doctorates. Recommendations focused on several issues, including early recruitment of talented individuals into biomedical research careers; the optimal structure of research training, such as length of time for training, modification of the payback provision for NRSA training, combining M.D.s and Ph.D.s in the same programs, and performance reviews; integrating research training with clinical certification requirements; trainee stipends and

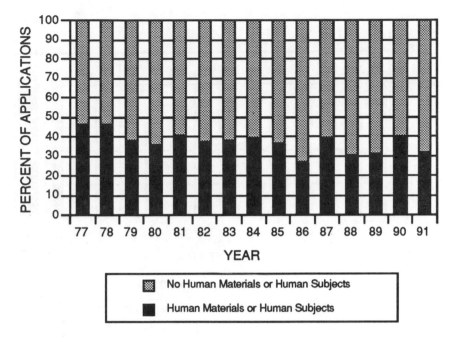

FIGURE 4-10 Proportion of NIH individual fellowship (F32 award) applications by M.D. applicants for studies involving the use of human subjects or human materials and those not using human subjects or materials. (Source: National Institutes of Health, Office of Extramural Research.)

education costs; K-series awards; and data collection and monitoring. Although the report addresses research training, the implication is that the recommendations should enhance research training for performing laboratory-based research. The panel stresses at the outset of the report's executive summary that the report should address "areas of research training not currently addressed adequately or systematically, e.g., clinical trial design and methodology, biostatistics, epidemiology, and population demography" (National Institutes of Health, 1989a, p. 1). To redress these deficiencies, the panel recommended programs at the master's degree level in epidemiology, biostatistics, or related topics and nondegree, certificate programs with emphases on epidemiology and biostatistics (National Institutes of Health, 1989a).

Despite repeated analyses over two decades, the causal linkages between research training and outcomes have yet to be identified. It appears, however, that the training grant mechanism is less successful in inducing such trainees to apply for NIH grants than is the fellowship program (Figure 4-12) (Institute of Medicine, 1989d; Quantum Research Corporation, 1991). Less than 20 percent physicians trained on T32 training grants eventually succeed in obtaining funding

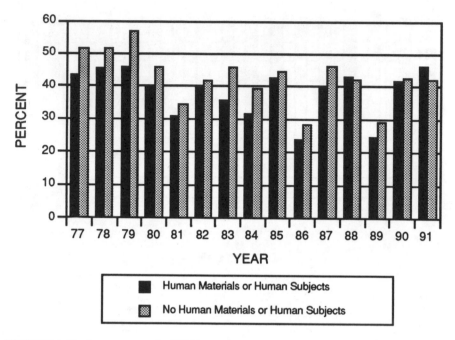

FIGURE 4-11 Success rates for NIH individual fellowship (F32 award) applications by M.D. applicants for studies involving the use of human subjects or human materials and those not using human subjects or materials. (Source: National Institutes of Health, Office of Extramural Research.)

as principal investigators on NIH grants. By contrast, those who have received F32 fellowship awards have a higher success rate than the trainees receiving support from T32 awards (Quantum Research Corporation, 1991). Moreover, success in competing for grants seems to correlate with more than two years of training (Institute of Medicine, 1989d). Since it has been shown that fellowship awardees are more successful than those trained on training grants in obtaining subsequent NIH funding and the ratio of traineeships to fellowships is higher for M.D.s (Figure 4-6), it could be inferred that Ph.D.'s might have a competitive advantage over M.D.s in obtaining NIH research grant awards.

This is not to suggest that these training mechanisms are ineffective. The available information suggests that individuals supported by NIH generally outperform other groups in research-related outcomes. The measures of success, however, are generally limited to participation rates in the NIH grant system. Whether these outcomes can be confidently attributed to the reciept of funds from NIH for training remains unclear, and any effect is likely to be small. As funds for NIH become increasingly constrained, the use of data showing the ability of

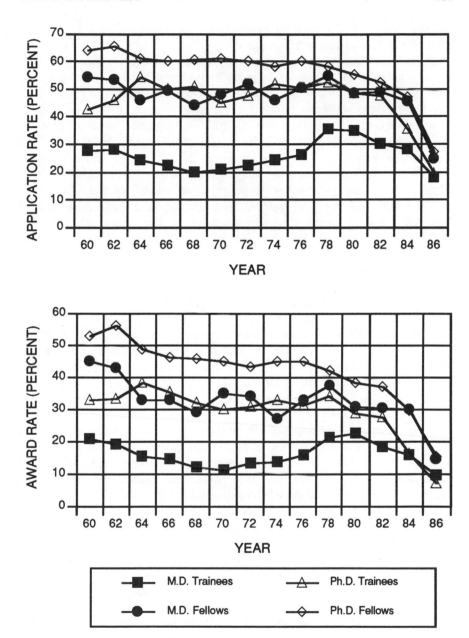

FIGURE 4-12 Application (top) and award (bottom) rates by NIH-supported M.D. and Ph.D. trainees and fellows for NIH research grants. Data for years 1982–1986 may not reflect all applicants since many may not yet have applied when the tabulations were made in 1991. (Source: National Institutes of Health, Office of Extramural Research.)

trainees to garner NIH research grants as a measurable outcome of effective training may become less and less reliable.

The time, duration, and quality of early research experiences appear to have a positive influence on the outcome of postdoctoral research training. For example, successful investigators have had longer research experiences at each stage of their careers than those who have received training but have not chosen investigative careers (Lee et al., 1991; Levey et al., 1988). Similarly, medical school research experience was strongly associated with postgraduate research involvement (Segal et al., 1990).

What is not known is how the proportion of NIH-trained individuals who go on to pursue careers in research might be increased, whether there are differences among various subgroups of trainees, and how to make fair comparisons of outcomes across the variety of training mechanisms. Furthermore, there are few data on how many training programs and fellowships might include some aspect of patient-oriented research.

Postdoctoral Ph.D. Training

The outcomes for individuals who received NIH postdoctoral traineeships and fellowships, primarily in the biomedical sciences, have been examined in relation to an assortment of post hoc-constructed comparison groups. In general, these studies have found that postdoctoral recipients, regardless of the sponsor, perform better on all research-related measures than those who did not choose to pursue postdoctoral study.

For example, NIH postdoctoral recipients were three times as likely as Ph.D. recipients with no postdoctoral plans to have applied for research support from the Public Health Service (56.9 percent of NIH-supported postdoctoral researchers did so compared with 19.6 percent of postdoctoral investigators without such training). Of those who applied, NIH-supported Ph.D. applicants were almost twice as successful in obtaining later grant support (Garrison and Brown, 1985). If the duration of training is viewed as a critical dimension of intensity, these findings suggest that a more intense "dose" of training may contribute to the production of more active researchers.

NIH-trained postdoctoral researchers were also more likely to apply for Public Health Service grants than were Ph.D.s whose training was supported by other sources (56.9 percent with training supported by NIH applied for grants compared with 34.5 percent of postdoctoral recipients trained through other means) (Garrison and Brown, 1985). More recent tabulations on the rate of application for grant awards from NIH from NIH-supported trainees by Quantum Research Corporation (1991) verify the same pattern correlating NIH-supported training with higher application and success rates in garnering research funding from NIH (Table 4-9).

TABLE 4-9 Percentage of First-Time Ph.D. Grant Applicants and Recipients with Prior NIH-Supported Training, 1964–1989

Fiscal Year of First Application for Award	All Applicants	All Recipients	Applicants with Training	Recipients with Training	Trainee Application Rate	Trainee Award Rate
1964	1,267	867	434	345	34.3	39.8
1965	1,221	688	480	321	39.3	46.7
1966	1,254	660	547	328	43.6	49.7
1967	1,247	728	572	379	45.9	52.1
1968	1,176	527	617	321	52.5	60.9
1969	1,204	625	657	394	54.6	63.0
1970	1,369	483	832	337	60.8	69.8
1971	1,339	581	804	406	60.0	69.9
1972	1,458	803	824	552	56.5	68.7
1973	1,559	601	889	406	57.0	67.6
1974	1,692	1,087	980	725	57.9	66.7
1975	1,782	1,181	1,110	835	62.3	70.7
1976	1,975	917	1,193	629	60.4	68.6
1977	2,219	918	1,331	647	60.0	70.5
1978	2,222	1,247	1,377	852	62.0	68.3
1979	2,245	1,516	1,360	1,037	56.1	68.4
1980	2,370	1,169	1,427	801	60.2	68.5
1981	2,247	1,121	1,361	765	60.6	68.2
1982	2,396	1,109	1,500	804	62.6	72.5
1983	2,376	1,283	1,351	891	56.9	69.4
1984	2,321	1,264	1,327	854	57.2	67.6
1985	2,597	1,385	1,467	922	56.5	66.6
1986	2,651	1,467	1,377	892	51.9	60.8
1987	2,488	1,388	1,286	842	51.7	60.7
1988	2,763	1,453	1,322	862	47.8	59.3
1989	2,863	1,251	1,302	689	45.6	55.1

Source: Quantum Research Corporation, 1991.

Multivariate analyses of outcomes data (such as success in obtaining grants and academic employment) that controlled for such things as the effect of selectivity of the baccalaureate institution and the prestige of the doctoral institution on training outcomes of produced small multiple R^2 values, ranging from 0.06 to 0.14 (Garrison and Brown, 1985). This indicates that several other factors foster successful career paths—factors that have not been tapped by existing databases.

Postdoctoral M.D. Training

Three studies have attempted to tease out the role of postdoctoral training for M.D.s (Garrison and Brown, 1985; National Institutes of Health, 1986; National Research Council, 1976). The findings have been fairly inconclusive because of the difficulties associated with retrospectively devising appropriate comparison groups with existing data. Physicians who have been recipients of National Research Service Award traineeships and fellowships have been contrasted with M.D.s without postdoctoral training and M.D.s who reported their primary activities to be research or teaching, but who had not pursued formal postdoctoral study. Among other findings, previously reported differences in research-related outcomes between M.D.s with postdoctoral NIH-supported appointments and M.D.s without them were significantly reduced in more recent analyses, which included those in research and teaching positions as the group of comparison. Recent tabulations by Quantum Research Corporation (1991) indicate that NIH-supported M.D. trainees were more successful in obtaining NIH research grants than were those who were not supported by NIH during training (Table 4-10).

Several studies have examined the performance of physician-investigators, relating outcomes to gross measures of length and type of training (Levey et al., 1988; Sherman, 1983, 1989). A strong relationship between the existence and length of *formal* research training and outcomes has emerged. For instance, in terms of academic employment, grant application and award rates, and average time spent in research, the performance of M.D.-Ph.D.s, a group that has undergone a formal sequence of research training, regardless of whether they had pursued postdoctoral study, outstripped that of M.D.s who did not have a Ph.D. Furthermore, if one accepts the notion that recipients of NIH postdoctoral fellowships also possess appropriate research training credentials (because their selection is based on the decisions of NIH peer review study sections), it is not surprising that NIH fellows consistently outperformed their postdoctoral trainee counterparts (National Institutes of Health, 1989a).

Although most of these retrospective analyses indicate that previous NIH support is correlated somewhat with obtaining later grant funding, the changes in the support of research may affect this measure as an outcome. As competition for NIH research funds increases, trainees may have less chance of acquiring NIH funds. Even good training and preparation may not be sufficient to garner funding, and the use of NIH funding as the yardstick of success may skew the outcomes of these programs. Thus, the committee acknowledges that outcomes must take into account other measures of research involvement.

TABLE 4-10 Percentage of First-Time M.D. Grant Applicants and Recipients with Prior NIH-Supported Training, 1964–1989

Fiscal Year of First Application for Award	All Applicants	All Recipients	Applicants with Training	Recipients with Training	Trainee Application Rate	Trainee Award Rate
1964	1,108	652	394	265	35.6	40.6
1965	999	582	395	279	39.5	47.9
1966	1,026	616	480	328	46.8	53.2
1967	930	542	444	296	47.7	54.6
1968	765	363	394	224	51.5	61.7
1969	663	376	389	258	58.7	68.6
1970	590	266	363	188	61.5	70.7
1971	597	310	369	215	61.8	69.4
1972	722	432	447	303	61.9	70.1
1973	697	314	417	186	59.8	59.2
1974	722	460	416	294	57.6	63.9
1975	804	444	496	294	61.7	66.2
1976	927	406	533	251	57.5	61.8
1977	1,019	419	616	279	60.5	66.6
1978	1,036	481	632	332	61.0	69.0
1979	973	556	581	401	59.7	72.1
1980	1,074	469	661	336	61.5	71.6
1981	983	464	584	317	59.4	68.3
1982	935	409	544	287	58.2	70.2
1983	1,000	494	550	303	55.0	61.3
1984	1,028	546	560	343	54.5	62.8
1985	1,150	592	586	363	51.0	61.3
1986	1,159	521	548	289	47.3	55.5
1987	1,029	577	485	317	47.1	54.9
1988	1,070	561	480	322	44.9	57.4
1989	1,145	512	516	269	45.1	52.5

Source: Quantum Research Corporation, 1991.

Research Career Development Awards

NIH sponsors a series of career development awards including the Physician-Scientist Award (K11 award), for M.D.s without prior research experience; a modified form of the Research Career Development Award (K04 award), which requires a minimum of three years of previous research experience; and the Clinical Investigator Award (K08 award), which requires five years of prior research training and is intended primarily for physician-investigators. In addition to the individual K11 awards, NIH supports an Institutional Physician-Scientist Award, the K12 award.

The K awards are heterogeneous in many respects, including the amount of research training expected. To date there has been very little evaluation of these transitional training-research mechanisms, particularly with regard to patient-oriented research (Biddle et al., 1988; Carter et al., 1987). NIH has plans to collect systematic information about program similarities and differences as a precursor to developing more comprehensive evaluation efforts.

In 1991, $99 million was allocated for all individual career development awards (CDAs). Of this, about $4.3 million supported 66 M.D. recipients of K04 awards, $38.7 million supported 499 M.D. recipients of K08 awards, and $24.4 million supported 306 Physician-Scientist Awards (K11 awards). An additional $4.9 million was awarded for Institutional Physician-Scientist Awards (K12 awards). Some trends for the K awards are noteworthy. On the one hand, the K04 awards, which required previous research experiences, have declined by more than half over the past 10 years, from 787 in 1982 to 313 in 1992. On the other hand, the number of Clinical Investigator Awards (K08 awards) grew from 160 to 527 over the same period, and the number of K11 awards, initiated in 1984, grew to 321.

As with all of the preceding grant and training program data, accurate data on the amount of patient-oriented studies supported through K awards are difficult to uncover. About 40 to 45 percent of K award applications indicate the intent to use human materials or human subjects; this percentage is consistently a few percentage points higher than that for the application pool for regular research grants (R01 awards). Ahrens has performed analyses on a sample of 243 abstracts from Physician-Scientist Awards to determine the fraction that are patient oriented. He concluded that about 30 percent included some research involving humans (Ahrens, 1992).

Clinical Associate Physician Program

Although any of above training programs could be used by trainees pursuing a career in patient-oriented research, the only awards specifically designed to foster this type of investigation are those supported through the Clinical Associate Physician (CAP) program. CAP awards are funded by the General Clinical Research Center branch of the National Center for Research Resources (see Chapter 3 for a description of the General Clinical Research Center program). Each center is allowed a maximum of two CAPs. Recently, the training period has been extended from two to three years. Since the program's inception in 1974, more than 260 clinical investigators have been trained through the CAP program. About 40 new CAP awards are made each year (Figure 4-13).

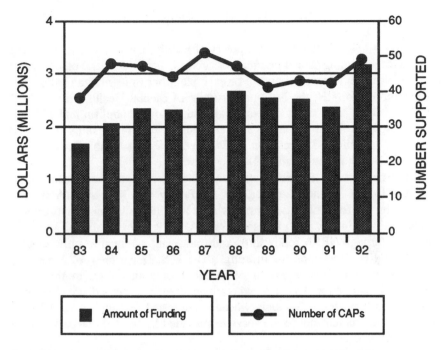

FIGURE 4-13   Number of clinical associate physician (CAP) fellows supported annually by the General Clinical Research Center program and the amount of funding, 1983–1992. (Source: National Center for Research Resources.)

Preliminary results from an ongoing analysis of the CAP program demonstrate that the CAP alumni are successful in obtaining subsequent funding from NIH. More than 40 percent of the physicians in the CAP program have received NIH funding as principal investigators. Similar numbers of K08 award recipients are successful in obtaining funding. An unknown number are probably involved in research as coinvestigators, but that number has not been determined. A survey of the clinical associate physicians is under way and should reveal how many are actually involved in NIH-sponsored research and receive funding from other sources. Given the nature of the program, it is likely that a high percentage of those funded are actively involved in patient-related clinical research. These results indicate that the CAP program and the K08 award program are effective in training competitive clinical investigators.

Non-NIH Federal Support

Although NIH is the major supporter of health-related training, including that targeted at training patient-oriented researchers, there are several other federal sponsors of health related training. For example, prior to its reorganization and incorporation into NIH, the National Institute of Mental Health, the National Institute of Drug Abuse, and the National Institute of Alcoholism and Alcohol Abuse supported about 1,500 NRSA fellowships and traineeships (pre- and postdoctoral) totaling $32.9 million in fiscal year 1990 (Alcohol, Drug Abuse, and Mental Health Administration, 1991).

Specific research training opportunities in health services research are supported by the Agency for Health Care Policy and Research (AHCPR), primarily in the form of dissertation awards and individual and institutional postdoctoral training awards. In fiscal 1992, AHCPR invested about $3 million in training through NRSA fellowships and traineeships—equal to only about 1 percent of NIH allocations for training. The U.S. Department of Veteran's Affairs also has a small program of research training efforts in this area. Postdoctoral training for physicians who are pursuing a master's degree in public health is available for individuals who are interested in health care delivery research questions relevant to the services provided by the U.S. Department of Veteran's Affairs.

Since 1951, the Centers for Disease Control and Prevention has sponsored a combined training and service epidemiology training program for postdoctoral training, the Epidemic Intelligence Service. Working under the supervision of practicing epidemiologists at the various Centers for Disease Control and Prevention sites, trainees develop their epidemiologic skills during a two-year fellowship. Although the program focuses on preparing trainees with epidemiologic skills to work in public health, it also encourages active participation in population research. More than 1,700 professionals have served in the Epidemic Intelligence Service. About 80 percent of the participants are physicians; other health professionals such as nurses and dentists with master's degrees in public health are also accepted into the program. One interesting aspect of the program is that the American Board of Preventive Medicine recognizes the training program fulfills the certification requirements of one year of supervised training and field experience. Many of the alumni are employed in public health agencies, including the Centers for Disease Control and Prevention; about 12 percent are on university faculty (Thacker et al., 1990). Whereas the program may be effective in training public health epidemiologists, it might serve as a model for patient-oriented clinical research.

The Food and Drug Administration also has developed an extensive intramural program for training Food and Drug Administration staff. For example, the Center for Drug Evaluation and Research operates a staff college that helps to train its medical reviewers. Enrollees can take courses in drug law and regulatory procedures, basic and applied statistical methods, chemistry and biotechnology, immunology, pharmacology, and clinical trials (U.S. Department of Health and Human Services, Food and Drug Administration, 1992; Peck 1988). Effectiveness of these types of programs in preparing clinical investigators, rather than train individuals to assess regulatory requirements for new drugs and devices, is not known.

Private Support

There is no current, comprehensive source of information about private sources of funding for clinical research training. A 1983 report by the Rand Corporation listed 75 foundations that provided some support for training physicians and as well as those with Ph.D.s (Carter, 1983). In 1981, according to the report, foundations funded some 400 individual junior faculty and postdoctoral awards for M.D.s. These numbers are certainly out of date, although it is not known whether they under- or overestimate the present level of funding. Non-federally supported M.D.-Ph.D. programs may be supporting as many as 700 double-degree candidates, although this number also cannot be verified (Ahrens, 1992).

Informal contacts with several voluntary health agencies and foundations by Institute of Medicine staff revealed that many support training, particularly of M.D.s. When queried whether their training programs specifically support patient-oriented clinical research trainees, most responded that they did not. Exceptions to this are the American Cancer Society, which recently started a junior faculty program for human investigation training, and the American Heart Association, which has an equally broad set of training programs. More frequently, these organizations and foundations support fundamental research training pertaining to their specific missions.

Some medical specialty groups have taken research training into their own hands. The Orthopaedic Research and Education Foundation (supported by individual contributions of members of the American Academy of Orthopaedic Surgeons and the Orthopaedic Research Society), for example, raised $3.8 million in 1991, nearly all of which went to fund peer-reviewed research and research training activities (Orthopaedic Research and Education Foundation, 1991). Again, it is not clear how much of these training funds is used to support patient-oriented clinical research training.

Health policy and health services research training are promoted by several private foundations. For example, the Robert Wood Johnson Foundation funds a Clinical Scholars Program, which has trained postdoctoral physicians in health services research since 1969 (Piccirillo, 1992; Shuster et al., 1983). Predoctoral and postdoctoral training are also supported by the Pew Charitable Trusts and Harvard Medical School's Clinical Effectiveness Program, the latter funded by the

Kellogg Foundation, the Klingenstein Fund, NIH, and the Health Resources and Services Administration (Goldman et al., 1990).

Payback of Debt

As mentioned previously, many medical residents accrue a large amount of education-related debt from undergraduate and medical schools. Under the current rules, payback must begin in the third year of postgraduate training. To accommodate this financial burden, research training often is either omitted to facilitate earlier entry into practice or is used as a time to moonlight to earn money for debt repayment. Neither scenario is likely to permit adequate or high-quality training for research on human subjects.

Other than established training programs that pay stipends during research training, some novel programs are focusing on mechanisms to repay educational debt and retain trainees. One notable example is the NIH program for AIDS researchers begun in 1989. In this program, physician research trainees are recruited to NIH to engage in AIDS research. Trainees are encouraged by the opportunity to relieve their educational debt load. NIH allows $20,000 in debt relief for each year served to a maximum of $40,000. In addition, the trainees are paid a stipend for living costs. In the first three years this program was under way, 19 trainees were accepted into the program each year. Although this is a promising avenue for encouraging ongoing participation in research, it is not evident how many of these trainees are actually engaging in patient-oriented research. Moreover, this is a small program in an area of great need. It is too early for the program to have any measurable outcomes for continued participation rates in research.

Federal programs such as those described above require authorization through public law. The NIH Revitalization Act of 1993 expanded this opportunity to other areas at the discretion of the NIH director (U.S. Congress, 1993).

MODEL PROGRAMS FOR RESEARCH TRAINING

Although many of the methodologic advances in patient-oriented research have been developed in graduate schools of public health and divisions of general medicine, investigators in subspecialties of medicine and other departments are increasingly recognizing the need for training in these techniques (Goldman, 1991; Goldman et al., 1986). This trend is the reflection of a paradigm shift in which new "horizontal" relationships are formed within a medical center, crossing the "vertical" divisions defined by preclinical sciences and clinical specialties and subspecialties (Kelley, 1992). These horizontal relationships may be defined by diseases, such as cancer, or by research methodologies. At many universities molecular biologists have developed informal or formal research interactions that play more active day-to-day roles in their lives than interactions with their subspecialties do. The same kind of cross-disciplinary associations are developing among investigators interested in advanced patient-oriented research methodologies.

A number of programs have been initiated around the country to provide investigators with the skills needed to perform patient-oriented research. A selection of these is described below; this is followed by a discussion of some of the characteristics common to most such initiatives.

Overview of Selected Programs

Robert Wood Johnson Clinical Scholars Program

One of the oldest, largest, and most successful of the existing research training programs is the Clinical Scholars Program (CSP) (Shuster et al., 1983), which was started in 1969 by the Commonwealth Fund and Carnegie Corporation. Since 1973, CSP has been funded by the Robert Wood Johnson Foundation. Each year some 25 new fellows are enrolled in six programs at seven universities and their affiliated Veterans Affairs Hospitals. The foundation does not encourage the pursuit of advanced degrees.

From 1971 through 1992 there were 600 graduates of CSP, of whom 363 (61 percent) are currently in academic medicine and another 31 (5 percent) are in government. Slightly more than half of the graduates were from internal medicine. Many have assumed leadership roles at their institutions and at various federal agencies, including AHCPR.

University of Michigan School of Public Health

The University of Michigan School of Public Health supports a program in clinical research design and statistical analyses that can lead to a master's of science degree (Penchanksy et al., 1988). The program's required core courses are taught during 18 sessions, each of which is held about once a month and lasts for four days. Student participants include physicians at various levels of training and other health care personnel.

Harvard Clinical Effectiveness Program

The Harvard Clinical Effectiveness Program provides methodologic training to postdoctoral trainees during an intensive two-month summer session administered by the Harvard School of Public Health (Goldman et al., 1990). The program was initiated in 1986 in response to interest generated among medical subspecialty fellows supported by NIH training grants.

The curriculum provides 15 credits (of the 40 needed for a master's of science or master's of public health degree) at the Harvard School of Public Health. During this period, fellows are required to be completely free of clinical responsibilities. A prerequisite for all applicants for the program is a commitment to an academic career that will utilize the methodologic skills taught in the program. All applicants must be sponsored by the chief of their clinical subspeciality division or department, who must pay the trainee's tuition (currently about $6,000) with individual or institutional training grants or other institutional funds.

Of the 80 physicians who have enrolled in the summer curriculum and who have finished their clinical training, 68 (85 percent) hold full-time academic positions and another 4 (5 percent) are in government or nonprofit research positions.

Other Programs

Among other academic centers that sponsor patient-oriented research training programs are those at Johns Hopkins University, the Mayo Clinic, Stanford University, the University of California at San Francisco, and McMaster University in Canada (Neufield, 1989).

Common Characteristics

In most instances, the programs are coadministered by schools of public health and departments of medicine. Several programs are affiliated with degree-granting schools of public health; others actively involve divisions of epidemiology and biostatistics within the medical school.

Strong emphasis is placed on issues of study design such as formulation of the research question, types of study design, subject selection, randomization, measurement, sample size, bias, pretests, quality control, compliance, discontinuing criteria, closing a trial, alternative designs, including observational studies, cohort studies, cross-sectional studies, case-control studies, and hybrid designs and multicenter trials.

All curricula stress in-depth training in statistics and epidemiology. Among the topics often covered are discrete and continuous probability theories, linear and logistic regression techniques, analysis of variance and covariance, nonparametric testing, graphical displays, data transformation, contingency-table analysis, life-table and survival-analysis techniques, mathematical modeling, meta-analysis, cost-effectiveness and cost-utility analysis, measurement error, global and specific health and functional status instruments, and questionnaire and interview design.

All programs offer training in the use of computer software and data management, as well as in the ethics of clinical research (for example, conflicts of interest, authorship, misconduct, subject selection, informed consent, institutional review boards, confidentiality, financial issues, and replication). Specific training in research management (such as resource estimation and personnel management) is included in a few of the programs. All programs include some information on how to pursue funding, and most instruct participants on how to prepare a grant proposal. Communications skills, however, are infrequently addressed.

All programs combine a basic instructional curriculum with research activities under a faculty mentor. The total duration of training ranges from 18 months to three years, with most lasting two years. The first year in most programs consists of an introductory curriculum in research methods, with the remainder of the time devoted to elective course work and a mentored research project.

The least uniform aspect of the programs reviewed by the committee is the funding mechanism. Although a large number of options were mentioned, only the few programs with department of medicine or hospital support seemed to have resources dedicated to administering their respective programs. At least one program was assisted by substantial foundation support, and others were pursuing similar funding from outside organizations. Tuition costs varied substantially, from $23,000 per year for a two-year program to $5,000 for an eight-week summer course. Finally, these programs tend to be oriented more toward population-based research or clinical trials rather than toward human pathophysiology or biology.

Remaining Obstacles

The difficulty of obtaining stable sources of funding has been the major obstacle for newly created fellowships in clinical research and may prevent other institutions from developing similar programs. Salary support for fellows can be provided through customary subspecialty training grants, but support of faculty time is often problematic. Developing and sustaining these programs require a substantial commitment of faculty and administrative time. Established programs offer from 130 to 250 classroom hours over periods of 4 to 24 months for classes of 10 to 50 fellows each. Although some of this time is accounted for by existing courses offered through other schools or departments, much of it involves new courses and seminars designed specifically to meet the needs and abilities of clinically trained physicians.

Foundation and departmental funding has been obtained to support faculty in individual programs, but this is often directed to program development, not the continuing obligations of faculty involved in teaching courses or acting as mentors to fellow-initiated projects. The ability and willingness of departments of medicine to support these activities through clinically generated revenues vary from center to center.

Ensuring program support is complicated by the variety of medical specialties and subspecialties served in such programs. No umbrella organization exists at NIH to fund comprehensive training for a variety of fellows, whose stipends are supported by separate NIH institutes. Reliance on tuition support from a collection of training grants and individual sponsors with varying budget regulations makes program planning more precarious and less efficient than if centralized support was available from a single entity at NIH or some other major sponsor.

Finally, tuition alone may not address the need to support faculty involvement as mentors. Faculty whose research activities are well-funded may not need additional support to supervise fellows who participate in their research activities. Because funding for patient-oriented research is modest, however, prospective mentors are likely to have limited extramural support to help fellows' projects. Furthermore, a substantial time commitment is required from faculty to be effective mentors, especially when fellow-initiated projects involve topics and methods outside their current research activities. Unless specific support for this time is available, mentorship is likely to be unsatisfactory for fellows and faculty alike.

CONCLUSIONS

In conclusion, the committee found that data do not exist to make an accurate assessment of the number of patient-oriented clinical investigators or the number who are being trained. Whereas career pathways for those choosing to pursue basic science investigation are clearly delineated, with established rewards and measures of productivity, comparable training pathways for patient-oriented clinical research careers are not. Given the current economic and social climate, identification of the best and most efficient ways to produce patient-oriented researchers has assumed additional importance. The escalation of health care costs, the increasing failure of the "safety net" to guarantee adequate health care for all citizens, and the emergence of AIDS and other still incurable diseases have strongly accentuated the critical need for research on the prevention, diagnosis, management, and treatment of disease. Current advances in molecular biology hold significant promise, but those advances can be fully exploited only by well-trained and committed investigators.

The responsibilities and expectations of faculty who engage in basic research are straightforward, with agreed upon standards for judging success and rewarding achievement. The same is not true for individuals choosing to become clinical investigators or faculty members who participate in clinical research. Few programs rigorously train clinical scientists to provide them with a substantive foundation in clinical research methods. The responsibilities and expectations of the clinical research faculty are ambiguous and there are no agreed upon standards for measuring success. Furthermore, there appears to be few rewards even when consensus agrees that success has been achieved. Given this scenario, it is clear that medical students and other health professionals do not perceive clinical research pathways as viable options for academically based careers or careers in other employment sectors as well.

The prospect of a significant infusion of funds for postdoctoral research training may be low, given such problems as the federal budget deficit and other economic woes. What is more likely is a scenario in which resources for research training remain constant or increase only minimally. Thus, future policy and program decisions will most likely involve such issues as identifying which training mechanisms work best, what is needed for their implementation in other settings, and how such programs could be fine-tuned to increase their efficiency. In addition, situations of constant or reduced funding will require policymakers to decide which mechanisms should be eliminated or scaled back to permit the expansion of other programs or experiments with promising new strategies.

The committee concluded that some means must be developed for determining what programs are, in fact, training patient-oriented clinical investigators. Only then can the scientific community be confident that an appropriate number are being trained. Once those programs are identified and suitable outcomes measures are determined, the programs that are effective in training patient-oriented clinical investigators should be expanded. Some programs, such as the Clinical Associate Physician program, train this type of investigator by design. Since the General Clinical Research Center infrastructure is already in place around the country, these centers seem to be an appropriate place to begin developing programs that involve medical students and residents in human research.

Finally, the desire for change will have to come from all sectors with an interest in clinical research and professional education. The federal government will have to assume the leadership role in effecting change, but it will need the full cooperation of the academic medical centers, the pharmaceutical biotechnology and medical device industries, medical and life insurance companies, professional societies, and organizations with a stake in professional education and certification for all groups of clinical investigators. All of those listed above as well as other groups need to work together progressively to improve the training of patient-oriented clinical investigators and create rewarding career paths to encourage clinicians to pursue careers in clinical research. The committee fears that failing to be proactive and addressing training pathways at this critical juncture in science and its relationship to medical care could jeopardize future progress in biomedicine.

5

Academic-Industry Relationships

There is a long tradition of industry support for biomedical research, and there have been numerous types of academic-industry relationships. As noted in Chapter 3, industry funded more than half of all health sciences research in the United States before World War II, largely in the area of pharmaceutical research and development (R&D). Following the war, however, federal support for health research, primarily from the National Institutes of Health (NIH), grew at very rapid pace and soon eclipsed the investment by industry. Through the 1960s and early 1970s, industry support for research, in-house as well as sponsored research in academic institutions, slowed. The reasons for this waning of research investment have never been confirmed, but possibly include disappointing returns on overly optimistic expectations of the role and potential returns of broadly conceived basic research by industry, cost-accounting approaches to management that tended to put lower priority on long-range activities like fundamental research, and economic recessionary periods limiting corporate investment in research (National Science Board, 1981). The decline of in-house research was paralleled by a perception of slackening industrial support for academically based research. It has even been hypothesized that the Vietnam war aggravated antibusiness ideology on college campuses, further suppressing industry investment in academic research (National Science Board, 1981). However, industrial support, when measured in constant dollars, remained steady. As a result of these many forces, the proportion of funding from industry declined, and by the end of the 1970s, industry supported only 29 percent of the total national investment in health sciences research.

The availability of rapidly increasing federal funds for academic scientists possibly contributed to a weakening of the interactions and channels of communication between academic research institutions and industry through the 1950s and 1960s (White House Science Council, 1986). Industrial support of health R&D grew from 29 percent in 1979 to 48 percent in 1992. Of the estimated $13.5 billion that industry invested in health R&D in 1992, less than $1 billion went toward research at institutions of higher education (National Institutes of Health, 1993b).

During the late 1970s and throughout the 1980s several factors led to renewed interest in partnerships between academic institutions and industry. The rapid pace of technological change and the lack of U.S. competitiveness in world markets stemming from a relative decline in productivity and quality required a greater awareness by U.S. industry of academic research developments (National Science Foundation, 1987b and 1988b; U.S. Congress, Office of Technology Assessment, 1984). There was a growing sense that the lines between basic knowledge and its application were becoming blurred in a number of areas and an awareness that fundamental research often provides solutions to industry's challenges (Low, 1983). The declining rate of increase in federal funding for research at a time of unprecedented scientific opportunities exist encouraged academic institutions to seek other sources of funding, notably from industry. Additionally, predictions of impending shortages of scientific and engineering talent in many fields led industry to reconsider their linkages with academic institutions (White House Science Council, 1986). A growing interest in the results of research by the public, particularly as it relates to their own health and welfare, also has been a driving force for innovation and more scientific investigation in the health arena. These and many other factors have influenced a renewed interest in academic-industry relationships.

Legislation that also stimulated increased interactions between academic institutions and industry was passed. The Stevenson-Wydler Technology Innovation Act of 1980 established a federal policy for increasing the pace of translation of research results from federal laboratories into commercial products and directed federal agencies with research funds to allocate 0.5 percent of the research funds for technology transfer. In 1982 the Small Business Innovation Development Act required that all federal agencies with research budgets in excess of $100 million award 1.25 percent of their research funds to small, for-profit companies to encourage innovation and stimulate economic competitiveness through the translation of fundamental research into commercial products. These goals were reinforced by the passage of the Federal Technology Transfer Act in 1986, which provided incentives for collaboration between industry and the federal agencies. It authorized government laboratories to develop Cooperative Research and Economic Development Agreements with other federal agencies, state and local governments, and nonprofit and profit-making organizations. Finally, the federal government provided tax incentives for R&D investment in the 1981 Economic Recovery Act, which provided a 20 percent tax credit for incremental increases in R&D spending. Similar research investment incentives to encourage research activity and the translation of research into products have been used since that time.

During the 1980s there was also increased interest in the commercialization of the results of academic research. The 1980 Patent & Trademarks Act stipulated that inventions made by academic scientists on federally funded research projects were subject to institutional policies and were not the property of the government. In effect, academic institutions were granted the authority and incentive to protect the intellectual property of their faculty who were supported by federal research funds, own patents resulting from federally sponsored research, and seek industrial partners to transfer technology to the marketplace (Waugaman and Porter, 1992). The U.S. General Accounting Office, an investigative arm of U.S. Congress, reports that large numbers of faculty have linkages with for-profit companies, and the control of inappropriate access to federally funded research results is causing growing uneasiness in many sectors (U.S. Government Accounting Office, 1992b). This was particularly evident in the Scripps Institute/Sandoz Company agreement announced recently in which Sandoz was to have exclusive rights to license the research results of scientists at Scripps even when the research was underwritten by U.S. taxpayers. This agreement has subsequently not materialized. In the worst light, this has been described as "science for sale" (Malone, 1992).

The increased interaction between academic institutions and industry has also stimulated an increase in technology transfer, which some would argue has reached its highest level of expression in the biotechnology industry. Biotechnology is defined as "any technique that uses living organisms [or parts of organisms] to make or modify products to improve plants or animals or to develop micro-organisms for specified uses" (U.S. Congress, Office of Technology Assessment, 1988b). These methods were revolutionized during the 1980s, and there has been a huge investment by the federal government in such research. This explosion of biological knowledge, together with the ability to apply the knowledge to increasing the understanding of disease states and the development of biotechnology products to modify diseases, led to intensive activity in the academic community to commercialize the discoveries. This activity has led to the formation of hundreds of biotechnology companies, which often represent a positive interaction between the academic community and the investment community (Blumenthal et al., 1986a and 1986b).

These dramatic changes have created unprecedented opportunities for innovative new product development to improve health care, but the new developments have also led to novel situations that must be dealt with by industry, government, and academic institutions. Clearly, innovation and the translation of fundamental research to improved health care rely on the interdependent relationships of research institutions, government, and industry.

The cultural differences and frequent misperceptions between academia and industry have clouded their complementary relationships and the opportunity for positive collaborations between them. Cooper and Novitch (1992) have described the long-range needs of industry from academic medical centers, which include the following: patients, prestige, patents, publications, and personnel.

The committee sought to explore these relationships in general terms as well as from the perspective of clinical research. In the development of these opportunities, the clinical investigator plays a key role in transferring the technology to improved patient care. The extent, consequences, and management of these new academic-industry relationships in the life sciences have been reviewed recently by Blumenthal (1992). This chapter discusses the relationships between research institutions and industry and the implications of the changing patterns of interactions.

OBJECTIVES OF ACADEMIC-INDUSTRY RELATIONSHIPS

Linkages between academic institutions and industry are often viewed with suspicion and disdain because the motivations and cultures of the two participants are quite different. Knowledge for its own sake is the accepted and desired output from academic research, and industry is motivated by the potential for the efficient production of goods and services in a competitive marketplace (Low, 1983). According to Cooper and Novitch (1992), there is nothing inherently corrupting about the presence of industrial funding in academic medical centers because all research funding has economic components and determinants. They also posit that regulatory rules and requirements to gain Food and Drug Administration (FDA) approval, not industry's profit-making orientation, are the major impediments to academic-industry collaborations. Academicians, on the other hand, perceive that research structured to gain regulatory approval removes the freedom to pursue their own research paths and is not highly regarded by promotion committees. Although academic norms are founded on the open communication and publication of research findings, industry must protect proprietary information to remain competitive. Nonetheless, there are also many common objectives and common needs by both parties. Industry needs a continuous stream of highly skilled talent to work at the cutting-edge of research and product development. Academicians may be better prepared to teach and perform cutting edge research with potential practical applications through close ties to industry (Low, 1983). Melding the unique contributions each can make to positive research collaborations can facilitate the rapid and efficient transfer of new knowledge to medical care.

TWO CULTURES

In the past the two very different cultures of industrial research and academically based research have defined the interactions between them. Some of these cultural differences have had the unfortunate effect of unnecessarily inhibiting open and full interaction between academic scientists and industry (National Academy of Sciences, 1991). The notion that each sector has its own well-delineated and isolated role in the R&D process is outmoded in today's research environment. The long-standing paradigm that new fundamental knowledge that is discovered in academic settings flows to industry, where it is transformed into useful commercial applications, is no longer entirely valid. However, too much emphasis has been placed on the dichotomy between the "pure" basic research performed in academic settings and the applied research considered the province of industry (Varrin and Kukich, 1985).

Universities are largely recognized as the marketplace of ideas where knowledge is pursued following the norms of free discussion and free access to and exchange of information in concert with the uninhibited freedom to publish scholarly works. Such an environment relies on trust and openness and a clear understanding of a set of principles governing scholarly pursuit. Simply stated, these principles include the following: the academic institution and the faculty pledge themselves to the open, unimpeded, and objective pursuit of ideas; to the exchange of ideas openly and without deceit; and to the full and wide dissemination of knowledge through teaching and written publication of the results of scholarly inquiry (Giamatti, 1983; Merton, 1942). Largely through publication in peer-reviewed journals faculty submit their research findings to the critical scrutiny of their peers to ensure that there has been completeness in investigation and citation and that rigorous and logical conclusions have been applied in the process.

Whereas industrial research may be subjected to the same rigor during the research process, the primary driving force is the commercial potential of products and processes derived from new knowledge, basic or applied. Commercial application of new knowledge typically requires substantial investment in applied R&D to bring products or processes to market. Companies will make such investments and take the associated risks only when they can expect a reasonable return on investment (Giamatti, 1983). Thus, the opportunity for generating profit provides the incentive for companies to develop socially beneficial applications of new knowledge. However, to realize profits from technological innovation and remain competitive in the marketplace, companies strive to protect their proprietary knowledge from other companies. This emphasis on protecting trade secrets, often through limiting the exchange of information, is antithetical to those investigators in academia. As a result, industry-sponsored research has often been perceived as being of lower intellectual caliber than investigator-initiated investigations of the type supported by the federal government or nonprofit organizations. Because of the close linkages between academic clinical researchers and industry in conducting clinical trials for pharmaceutical development, this type of research frequently has been regarded with disdain in the academic community.

One notable contrast between the cultures of industry and academia is the different approaches to performing research between the two. In academia, investigators are expected to conduct scholarly research in an area of investigation to gain recognition, climb the academic ladder, and, in many cases, achieve tenure. Thus, academic scientists frequently tend to work independently, or in small collaborative units, to achieve their scholarly goals. Whereas companies stifle the flow of proprietary information among competitors, research within companies frequently is undertaken by a team approach (testimony to the committee by Dr. Louis Sherwood of Merck Sharp & Dohme Laboratories, 1991). Teams involve not only a wide spectrum of scientists in various fields but also others who are actively involved in the development process, such as marketing and regulatory affairs personnel. The committee drew the corollary that clinical researchers in academia often combine the attributes of the independent scholarly achievement of the academic setting with the team approach common to corporate researchers.

TYPES OF ACADEMIC-INDUSTRY LINKAGES

Over the past decade substantial efforts have been made by federal, state, and local governments to foster greater and more effective ties between academic institutions and industry through mechanisms such as cooperative programs, research centers, and research parks (National Academy of Sciences, 1986). The globalization of research and the pressure of international competition have introduced a critical time dimension into the stream of product development (National Academy of Sciences, Government-University-Industry Roundtable, 1992; President's Council of Advisors on Science and Technology, 1992). Whereas the United States has enjoyed a competitive advantage in many high technology fields, other countries have developed effective means for the direct translation of new knowledge into commercial products. As inferred by a report by the Task Force on the Health of Research of the House Committee on Science, Space, and Technology, it is likely that federal funding for research will become increasingly tied to societal goals (U.S. House of Representatives, Committee on Science, Space, and Technology, 1992). The same emphasis has been echoed by the Carnegie Commission on Science, Technology, and Government (1992).

As a result of these legislative forces and the initiative of the academic institutions and industry, many varieties of mechanisms for industry support of academic research have evolved (National Academy of Sciences, 1986 ; Price,

1985). According to Waugaman and Porter (1992) there are five critical elements in academic-industry collaboration including: (1) contract research, (2) consultantship, (3) employment, (4) technology transfer, and (5) gifts. These elements lead to a number of relationships that satisfy industry's needs, but they also raise conflicts with the investigators and academic institutions.

Blake (1994) has outlined "a spectrum of relationships" that the academic clinical investigator can have with one or more companies, including: consultant, sponsored research basic, sponsored research clinical trials, patent licensing, and company founder. All of these relationships can provide financial gain for the investigator and each has a particular set of issues related to conflict of interest and conflict of commitment.

The type and magnitude of gain vary as do the potential conflict with obligations to the investigator's employer, the academic institution, but some distinctions should be recognized. A consulting fee or support of salary through a research grant provides concurrent reimbursement for research services rendered. In this case, no direct future financial benefit ensues to the investigator other than the potential for a continuation of the consultantship or continued research support. Although these future potential benefits are valuable, they are not unique to relationships with industry. Indeed, future continuous support from NIH for grant recipients depends largely on achieving a certain level of research productivity. In addition, if industry did not reimburse academic organizations for the effort of their faculty and staff, the academic institution in effect would be subsidizing the R&D program of a for-profit company.

Independent fee-for-service consulting and salary support under sponsored research agreements traditionally have been accepted by academic institutions, government, and public representatives, particularly in areas such as law, business, and engineering schools, long before they arose in schools of medicine. However, the concern in the health sciences arena reflects, in part, the unique element that health research sometimes involves patients whose welfare might conceivably be compromised in the service of corporate-sponsored investigations (Blumenthal, 1992). The doctor-patient relationship is built on a foundation of trust and respect, and any compromise of this relationship to further the interests of business or financial gain runs counter to medical ethics and academic principles. As recently stated by David Kessler, FDA Commissioner, FDA could not do its job without complete trust in the clinical trials of medical products performed by academic clinical investigators (St. George's Society Lecture, Johns Hopkins University, 1992). The special concern about the clinical investigator in the setting of a randomized clinical trial (RCT), the core of clinical investigation, is ironic in that this is rigorously designed research that is subjected to substantial scrutiny by committees and government agencies. The clinical investigator in a multicenter RCT, with oversight by a separate data and monitoring group, has virtually no opportunity to bias the results.

Probably the most common model in the clinical research realm is funding provided by industry as direct support to individual academic investigators to perform clinical trials on a specific drug or device under development utilizing their access to patient populations. A few industry programs support basic research without specified commercial product or process development. These fund research programs or centers that support many research projects and that are closely tied to general academic research and teaching activities. An existing model of industry involvement in academically based research is several collaborative relationships that emerged during the 1980s. For example, the Monsanto Corporation established a collaborative research effort with Washington University in St. Louis to conduct basic research into peptides and proteins. Monsanto initiated the relationship in 1982 to support research in areas in which the company lacked expertise. Although the funding allows uninhibited pursuit of fundamental knowledge, the company reserves the right to review research results 30 days prior to submission for publication in order to have adequate time to decide on exclusive licensing to develop commercial products (National Academy of Sciences, Government-University-Industry Research Roundtable, 1986). A similar collaborative arrangement was established between Hoechst AG and the Massachusetts General Hospital to fund facilities and provide research support to the hospital's Department of Molecular Biology.

Another kind of academic-industry interaction is a focus project, which involves well-defined practical objectives and intellectual goals. This arrangement often uses the research of both academic and corporate scientists. An example of this type of arrangement is Becton Dickinson Corporation support for research in the infectious diseases section of the Department of Medicine at Wake Forest University's Bowman Gray School of Medicine (Waugaman and Porter, 1992).

Various consortia of academic institutions have been formed to combine the strengths of the various institutions to focus on a specific problem or set of problems (Low, 1983). One notable example in the arena of clinical research is the Consortium of Teaching Hospitals that was recently formed to facilitate the efficient conduct of clinical trials. As numerous small clinical trials companies have begun to siphon away some multicenter clinical studies from academic institutions, this consortium provides a central access point for companies to negotiate multicenter trials through one organization. Thus, companies will be able to negotiate one agreement for many centers rather than dealing with the different rules and committees of numerous institutions to conduct their trials.

In some fields industry has also formed cooperatives when the entire industry perceives a need for more research and research personnel. Although these types of relationships may be uncommon in the medical field presently, they have been formed in other fields such as in semiconductor R&D. These cooperatives, like SEMATECH raise funds through membership fees and award research funds to academic institutions in response to specific proposals.

Many institutions have formed affiliate programs by which companies can acquire access to an institution's or a department's research results through conferences, mutual visits, and publications. Often these results are available to affiliates prior to public release, and thus may enable them to gain a competitive edge. The relationships are frequently bidirectional, in which the academic institution receives important advice on the needs of the marketplace.

Universities and state and local governments have also been creating incubators and research parks to facilitate technology transfer. In many instances, these start-up ventures are provided inexpensive space, scientific advice, and laboratory and library services. The benefits include a mutually supportive environment for industry and the academic institution, with the potential for collaboration that may spawn new ideas and the synergism for a dynamic academic-industry enterprise.

An evolving paradigm of academically based research with significant involvement of industry might be the creation of centers of excellence focusing on a specific research theme combining the support of academic institutions, industry, the federal government, and other sources. One example of a center with such a funding portfolio is the Transplantation Biology Research Center at the Massachusetts General Hospital that was formed to bring together a critical mass of basic scientists and clinical investigators to move fundamental research results more efficiently into clinical practice. As federal research support becomes ever more constrained, these collaborative efforts may become important means of leveraging scarce resources and achieving high-quality research.

Industry also may provide operating or capital funds for academic institutions in terms of gifts. Such gifts do not obligate the investigator or the academic institution to provide anything in return.

Support for training is another important contribution to the academic sector. Some companies directly sponsor fellowships for trainees both in industrial laboratories and in academic laboratories. Others may contribute to a common fund for training that is overseen by a third party such as Merck's support for clinical research fellowships offered by the American Federation for Clinical Research.

PROGRAMS TO HELP COMMERCIALIZE
FACULTY RESEARCH

Many academic institutions have developed expertise in patenting the novel findings of their scientists with the hope that the patents will yield products and return capital to the academic institution. In the past, academic institutions generally have not had the resources for or the experience of transforming novel research discoveries into marketable products. Thus, academic institutions have licensed these patents to industry to develop them into products.

Some institutions have had nonprofit affiliates for some time such as the Wisconsin Alumni Research Foundation formed at the University of Wisconsin in 1925 and the MIT Development Corporation founded by the Massachusetts Institute of Technology in 1972 to facilitate the transfer of technology. Others have created for-profit buffer corporations to develop real and intellectual property on behalf of the institution. For example, the Dome Corporation was established by the Johns Hopkins University and the Johns Hopkins Health System with a cadre of professional technology transfer managers, many of whom thrive on the compensation arrangements of the private sector, to facilitate technology transfer. The Dome Corporation, in turn, created another for-profit corporation, Triad Investors, to provide venture capital for start-up companies. Although the latter does not have more access to faculty than other venture capital firms, and is free to work with nonacademic personnel, these firms allow an avenue for commercial development by faculty (Blake, 1994).

The committee believes that patenting and licensing will continue to play an increasing role in academic institutions, and faculty need to be apprised of the process. For example, the growing area of biological therapies derived from investigator-initiated research such as genetically engineered proteins and peptides might lead to a novel therapy for a disease with a low incidence rate or may not have significant commercial interest at the outset. Not unlike the provisions for developing orphan drugs in the private sector, such findings might not capture the interest of industry if the market is small and the potential for an adequate return on investment is marginal. Thus, academic institutions may be placed in the position of working through their own buffer corporations to bring these therapies to market themselves. In fact, a new therapy developed by University of California researchers for systemic lupus erythematosus is, for various reasons, being brought to market by the institution.

PREVALENCE OF ACADEMIC-INDUSTRY RELATIONSHIPS

According to Blumenthal (1992), information on the prevalence and outcomes of academic-industry relationships in the health sciences is outdated. However, it is useful to recap results of earlier studies to gain an appreciation of the involvement of faculty and students in these relationships. In 1985 a survey by the Harvard Project on University-Industry Relationships of 800 faculty at 40 of the top 50 U.S. universities involved in biotechnology research revealed that 47 percent provided consultant services to industry, 23 percent participated as principal investigators on at least one industry-funded project, and 8 percent owned equity in a privately traded company that marketed products that were based on the faculty member's academic research (Blumenthal at al., 1986a). More recently, Krimsky et al. (1991), have shown that nearly one third of the faculty in selected life sciences departments had some link to private firms. Gluck et al. (1987) also surveyed 700 graduate students and postdoctoral fellows in the life sciences departments of six research universities and found that 19 percent received some research or educational support from industry.

The level of industry participation in academic research relationships is also worthy of mention. Although research-intensive pharmaceutical companies have had long-standing relationships with academic institutions, the relative importance of these relationships could be measured by the escalation of arrangements with biotechnology firms. A 1984 survey by Blumenthal et al. (1986b), of 106 firms conducting research in biotechnology revealed that nearly half supported research in universities. Thus, it can be inferred that there are many positive aspects of academic-industry linkages that are important to the successful translation of this new technology to commercial products and applications.

BENEFITS FOR INDUSTRY

Access to Fundamental Scientific Advances

The boundaries of the earlier paradigm of developing new knowledge and theoretical concepts in academia and the transformation of this knowledge into practical application by industry are becoming more blurred. Although the pharmaceutical and biotechnology industries conduct fundamental research in many areas, they are still highly dependent on the results of the discovery process, which is embedded in the biomedical research laboratories of academia and certain government agencies such as NIH. Development and the clinical application of new discoveries are, on the other hand, highly dependent on the interest of the pharmaceutical and biotechnology industries. This interdependence became even more relevant when universities, academic medical centers, and government agencies obtained the right to protect their intellectual property through the patent process. Nonetheless, the R&D process works best for the health of the public when there is a rapid and facile pace of discovery, disclosure, and technology transfer.

Some scientific fields have evolved in such a manner that commercial applications derive more readily and rapidly from academically based research than was previously the norm. In the health research arena, biotechnology could be cited as a prime example. Not only is industry involved in developing technology for end-use patient care, but, in cooperation with academic institutions, is also actively involved in commercializing midstage fundamental knowledge into commercial products such as recombinant DNA procedures and transgenic animals. Thus, the shrinking interval between fundamental research and industrial applications also is serving to foster linkages between academic institutions and industry.

In an earlier survey, the factors perceived to be benefits by the majority of industrial respondents from biotechnology firms included the following:

- the likelihood of the collaboration resulting in product or process licenses,
- the ability of the company to keep current with important research,
- reduction in the costs of mounting R&D programs in a new field,
- enhancement of the firms' public image, and
- training and staff development for company scientists (U.S. Congress, Office of Technology Assessment, 1987).

There are certainly many other benefits too numerous to cover in this section. However, it is evident that collaborations with academic institutions allow companies to tap into existing pools of scientific talent and resources to increase their competitive edge without having to duplicate efforts already in place. Thus, academic-industry relationships enable both parties to achieve research objectives that neither could accomplish alone.

Access to Academic Personnel

Historically, industry has needed access to scientific personnel employed in academia to conduct research, basic as well as applied, on potentially marketable products. In the clinical research arena this has involved clinicians in the design and execution of clinical studies or trials during the various phases of the drug or device approval process. The unique contributions of academic clinical investigators have been access to sufficiently large patient populations and the objective assessment of the compound or device under investigation. Although some of these studies have merely involved clinicians as data collectors, others have provided the opportunity for clinical investigators to learn methods of conducting large-scale clinical investigations while they have participated in the design, execution, and subsequent data analysis of these studies. With the growing interrelationships between industry and academia, old paradigms of collaboration are being reinforced or remodeled, and new ones are being shaped. The various types of faculty-industry relationships were discussed above in more detail in the section on types of academic-industry relationships.

Human Resources Needs

The pharmaceutical and biotechnology industries not only need highly qualified investigators in academia to catalyze the discovery process and conduct research on behalf of the corporate sector, but they also need academia as a source of corporate talent. Industry needs access to highly trained personnel who can undertake basic research and health professionals to run clinical trials, including physicians, pharmacists, nurses, and other professionals, such as biostatisticians, who are essential for the design and execution of clinical trials. For example, many biotechnology companies are just bringing their first products into the clinical trial stage; thus, a substantially greater number of personnel probably will be needed both in the companies and in academic medical centers. In addition, corporate leadership often comes from academia. Thus, industry is highly dependent on the preparation of highly skilled individuals from academia.

BENEFITS FOR ACADEMIC INSTITUTIONS, FACULTY, AND STUDENTS

With the increasing competition for and the reduced rate of growth of the available federal funds for research, academic institutions have actively sought other sources of support, particularly from industry. Universities and their faculty generally would prefer that industry provide unrestricted funds for both basic research and clinical trials. Nevertheless, industry is most likely to invest large amounts of money in work with potential for product development. The U.S. pharmaceutical industry spent over $2 billion on clinical research in 1991, making it one of the largest sources of support for patient-oriented clinical research.

Although many of these financial resources are viewed as contractual research with prescribed outcomes, participation in industry research also can spin off some investigator-initiated studies simultaneously. Thus, the exposure of faculty to these opportunities can enhance their scholarly pursuits.

Just as industry benefits from access to academic talent, academic institutions can also benefit by interaction with scientific personnel in the private sector. Exchanges of scientific talent with industry allows the infusion of new ideas into the academic realm in the same fashion as academics provide advice to industry.

Students can benefit from academic-industry relationships by participating in industry-sponsored research. Such experiences can open up new opportunities for investigation and career opportunities. However, students should not be beholden to industrial support for their thesis research and certain precautions should be taken to insulate students from any negative consequences of industrial support.

RISKS, CONCERNS, AND CONFLICTS

Increasing academic-industry relationships also raise the specter of the inherent risks involved in these collaborations. Low (1983) has summarized the principal concerns as the following:

• The possible erosion of basic academic values of the educational goals of teaching and research, of giving faculty members their choice of questions to pursue, and of maintaining the academic institution as a credible and impartial resource.

• The conflicts of interest that may arise when trade secrets interfere with the freedom to publish, or when managing one's investments interferes with one's commitment to teaching and scholarly work.

• The possible leakage of information from company to domestic or foreign competitors when research results are communicated openly in traditional academic fashion.

Concerns about the commercialization of academic biomedical research and linkages with industry have been scrutinized throughout the past decade. This was reflected by hearings convened by the U.S. House of Representatives Committee on Science and Technology in 1981 that focused on two primary issues: whether academic-industry research relationships violated scientific and academic freedom and responsibilities, and whether these relationships best served the interests of the American public. A year later, then Congressman Albert Gore, Jr., stated, "We do not view such agreements as bad per se, but rather as a development that needs to be examined in detail" (U.S. Congress, Office of Technology Assessment, 1988). To date, few empirical data from few isolated studies have been generated and little evidence exists to confirm or refute the risks to academia as a result of academic-industry relationships (Blumenthal, 1992). Nonetheless, a slate of issues has emerged, and these issues need to be considered in developing positive interrelationships between academic institutions and industry (National Academy of Sciences, 1991).

Scientific Communication and Proprietary Rights

The apparent conundrum is one of preserving basic academic values while protecting the rights of ownership of commercially valuable products or processes (Low, 1983). As mentioned above, academic principles are generally understood to be the educational goals of teaching and research, in which the faculty have the uninhibited choice to pursue questions of their own choosing, while maintaining the academic institution as a credible and impartial resource. By contrast, commercial value is inherent in the competitive advantage gained through the application of new knowledge in the application of a process or the design of a product that is uniquely available to one company and not to its competitors. To this end, commercial value relies on the control of proprietary information or control of the use of the information (Low, 1983). Thus, the academic freedom of academia and the desire to advance knowledge for its own sake conflicts with the needs of both industry and the academic institution to develop products.

Results of the survey reported by Blumenthal et al. (1986a) suggest that academic-industry relationships in the biotechnology research arena were associated with some potentially worrisome departures from the traditional Mertonian academic behaviors and norms (Merton, 1942). For example, approximately one third of faculty engaged in biotechnology research reported that their choice of research topics had been influenced by the likelihood that the research results would have commercial application, whereas less than 10 percent of those without industry support indicated that their choice had been so influenced. Moreover, biotechnology faculty with industrial support were more than four times as likely as their colleagues without such support to report that proprietary information had resulted from their investigations (Blumenthal et al., 1986a). Additionally, faculty involved in industry relationships were nearly five times as likely to report that their research results were the property of their industrial sponsors and could not be published without the sponsor's consent. These reports have raised concerns about the whether academic-industry linkages can potentially compromise the objective role of academic institutions in the development of fundamental biological knowledge (Blumenthal, 1992).

The main commodity of the biomedical academic-industrial research enterprise is unique proprietary information that can be used to develop competitive products. Many research projects arrive at a crossroads—where following one path of investigation would provide interesting information with no near-term application to product development, whereas an alternate path may lead to more immediate product development. Industry that is funding research at academic institutions would prefer the strategy that leads to near-term product development; the academic investigator may have a different objective. Industry needs to protect this information to justify a large investment, and patents provide a way to protect the information. However, academic faculty, in the spirit of open and uninhibited communication of research findings, wish to present these findings at scientific meetings and publish scholarly works in peer-reviewed journals. Prompt publication of findings or presentation of findings at a scientific meeting may conflict with the need of industry to protect information and release it at a later time to limit competitor access as long as possible. Furthermore, academic institutions have now recognized the value of patents, and the timing of release of information from academic research is an emerging issue that needs further scrutiny.

Ownership of Proprietary Rights for New Discoveries

Questions arise about the ownership of novel discoveries made at academic institutions while performing investigations that are based on proprietary information from industry. Blake (1994) has suggested that the clinical investigator who discovers a useful new effect of a drug studied under the manufacturer's sponsorship should have patent rights. Most companies believe that because they own the patent they should also own any use patents if the discovery occurred during the performance of a study. Universities could argue that the patent belongs to the inventor (or the inventor's institution) because it is a reward for the inventor's creative effort. Is the academic clinical investigator an employee of the sponsor—without intellectual property rights—or an independent scholar whose creative talents can benefit the sponsor's R&D program?

The matter of who should own the use patent if a clinical investigator discovers a new activity of the drug that the investigator is studying under manufacturer's sponsorship is a complex one. The ability of the investigator to make novel observations has been made possible by the company through its novel product and by support of the investigator's research. A company cannot be regarded in the same way as a publicly funded government agency. In drug development, investors have placed their money at risk in the hope that they will realize a return on their dollars. By the time the product is in clinical trials, tens of millions of dollars have already been invested by company shareholders. Many of these potential products fail at earlier stages, or even at the clinical trial stage. Industry will promote scholarship while commercializing products, but it is clearly in the context of shareholder risk. A company will not be willing to relinquish its rights to these discoveries. Regardless of the resolution of these issues, the public gains from the commercialization effort because it brings forth novel therapies that improve medical care.

Exclusivity of Information

Recently, growing concern has been voiced in many sectors regarding the exclusivity of scientific results stemming from federally supported research. Although academic institutions have the legal right to patent and license technologies derived from federally supported research, some of these arrangements call into question the inappropriate licensing of exclusive rights because of undisclosed conflicts of interest or other relationships (U.S. General Accounting Office, 1992). Particularly troublesome are arrangements that might stifle the release of important research results from research that has been underwritten by taxpayers for reasons of commercial or financial gain. Thus, some companies might gain an unfair advantage in commercializing the results of federally sponsored research.

Probably even more troublesome is the involvement of foreign interests in gaining exclusive rights to federally sponsored research results emanating from U.S. research institutions. In some cases, this information can be bought freely, through membership fees paid to an institution, to obtain information prior to its public release. Thus, information is available to those people, domestic or foreign, who can afford to pay. In the extreme, foreign companies can develop relationships with research institutions to effectively gain the rights of exclusive licensing for all research performed at an institution or in a particular department without regard to the public sponsor. Although the committee is not aware of any documented case of abuse in these types of relationships, the potential exists for controlling information paid for by U.S. citizens and relationships of this sort require careful monitoring in the event that public policy changes need to be made.

Conflicts of Interest

The issue of conflicts of interest is a complicated one and is the subject of a book by Porter and Malone (1992). Most reports have focused on the clinical investigator, because the relationships of clinical investigators with industry (described above) create the setting for such conflicts. From the point of view of industry, there is a desire to avoid conflicts of interest that may inject bias into research results. Talented academic investigators with relevant special expertise, especially those who provide advice as consultants, are given incentives by industry to provide their best effort through remuneration. Some firms provide a basic modest consulting fee along with equity opportunities such as stock options. However, this kind of compensation is not provided for academic investigators who perform clinical trials with company products, because it might create an investigator bias in the interpretation of results. Such conflicts, which could lead to loss of objectivity, are counterproductive for the company as well as the academic stature of the investigator.

Although investigator conflict of interest has received considerable scrutiny, institutional conflict of interest has begun to emerge, in which officers and managers of academic institutions own equity in companies whose success may be influenced by their faculty's research. The leadership of academic institutions is ultimately held responsible and accountable for the faculty's research and providing assurance of objectivity and integrity. The personal ownership or institutional ownership of equity in companies with which they have a professional research relationship raises the specter of improprieties and questions the ability of these institutions to manage their own academic-industry relationships (Blumenthal, 1992). With the relatively recent approach of patenting academic research discoveries, institutions that wish to take new discoveries from the laboratory to the clinic, such as was described above with the formation of the Dome Corporation and Triad Investors by the Johns Hopkins University, will have to take careful measures to avoid conflicts of interest. This is clearly a topic that needs careful monitoring and attention from a public policy standpoint.

Clearly, bias created through conflicts of interest by investigators undermines the academic research process and the credibility of academic research institutions. The heterogeneity of academic research institutions and their affiliates suggests that there is no universally applicable standard or formula for dealing with conflicts of interest. Furthermore, according to Shipp (1992), the goal in managing conflicts of interest should not be to eliminate all potential sources of conflicts: rather, the objective should be to control the injection of inappropriate bias into research and other professional activities.

Although investigators can be expected to exert some level of self-control over their outside interests, it is probably unreasonable and unwise to depend entirely on researchers to identify, disclose, and manage all of their own potential conflicts of interest (Shipp, 1992). Ambiguity in guidelines often makes distinguishing between acceptable and questionable practices difficult and requires oversight by institutions. Thus, institutions must have a role in aiding their researchers in identifying, monitoring, and controlling conflicts of interest. Whatever the policies of the institution, many would agree that avoiding conflicts of interest by the faculty requires full, timely, and public disclosure to avoid even the perception of impropriety (Blake, 1992).

Conflict of Commitment

With regard to academic-industry relationships, conflict of commitment is quite different from conflict of interest. Conflict of commitment pertains to whether a faculty member is fulfilling institutional obligations while subjected to competing demands for one's time (Porter, 1992). Conflicts of commitment frequently are more difficult to address and resolve than conflicts of interests, because they are often subtle and of varying degrees (Low, 1983). Resolution generally falls into one of two categories: discontinuing or reducing one's outside commitments in the commercial venture that caused the conflict or leaving the academic institution (Low, 1983). Because of the complexity of conflict of commitment, few policies exist, and those that do are generally vague and ambiguous. However, the Association of American Medical Colleges has suggested the following guidelines to obviate conflict of commitment:

• Ensure that research, teaching, and public service obligations to the academic institution are met.

• Abide by restrictions on the type and amount of outside activity, as determined by the academic institution or by subsequent agreements between faculty and the academic institution or hospital administration.

• Abide by commitments of effort as specified in the contractural research and grant applications.

MANAGING ACADEMIC-INDUSTRY RELATIONSHIPS

The management of academic-industry relationships poses challenges to both academic institutions and industry. It is imperative that these relationships not threaten the fabric of academic principles or freedoms nor compromise the proprietary information of industry. Varrin and Kukich (1985) have proposed a partial list of management guidelines for academic institutions to consider in these relationships that include the following: retain publication rights, retain ownership of all patents, minimize the use of proprietary information in research and do not require graduate students to sign confidentiality agreements, create research units with faculty, and hire full-time researchers to staff such units if necessary, do not permit faculty to consult with sponsors in the area of the sponsored research, do not permit a faculty entrepreneur's company to sponsor his or her research on campus, share personnel and resources with industry, which is beneficial for both parties, and prepare model research agreements for potential industrial sponsors. The preceding list is not exhaustive nor is it totally inclusive; it is merely intended to raise consciousness about several potential pitfalls in striving to develop fruitful academic-industry collaborations.

To prevent improprieties, academic institutions could require full disclosure of the commercial interests of faculty, academic officers, and senior management in their institutions on a regular basis. Academic institutions could develop criteria or standards of what is and what is not acceptable in the various types of academic-industry relationships. This is particularly applicable in clinical research, in which the financial interests of the faculty or administration could cause bias to be injected into a study (Blumenthal, 1992).

Academic institutions also need to be concerned about the balance of interdepartmental and intradepartmental resources. Whereas some departments may engender the interest of industry, financially as well as scientifically, other departments fear that they will be starved of resources (U.S. Congress, Office of Technology Assessment, 1987). Thus, institutions should take care to provide balance in the allocation of resources in light of some lucrative academic-industry collaborations.

SUMMARY AND CONCLUSIONS

In summary, academic-industry relationships are growing in number and frequency (Blumenthal, 1992). The real benefit from academic-industry research relationships is the potential to achieve results that neither partner could achieve alone (U.S. Congress, Office of Technology Assessment, 1987). The respect and objectivity inherent in academic research must not be compromised by academic-industry relationships. A clearer understanding of each others' motivations, responsibilities, and mechanisms to facilitate constructive relationships will undoubtedly allow each to contribute to research in mutually beneficial relationships. These collaborative arrangements should not be so rigidly uniform as to squelch creativity. Rather, each should be tailored individually to achieve objectivity, valid clinical ends, mutually agreeable financial results, and legally acceptable consequences. As the pattern of academic-industry research collaboration strengthens in the future, sound policies and respect for each others' interests will be major factors in determining the extent and fruitfulness of such relationships (Cooper and Novitch, 1992).

Examining the overall picture of academic-industry interactions, many important advantages can be seen. The major winners are the American people, who benefit from the increasing pace of development of new products to improve health care. The relationships should provide more revenues to academic institutions and improved product development and profits for industry. Individual clinical investigators who have made important contributions can benefit financially from the evolution of their discoveries into products that improve health care. One of the most important contributions that a biomedical scientist can make is to improve the health care of millions of people.

At the same time, the pitfalls of this new process are clear. Academic freedom and pursuit of knowledge for its own sake require protection at academic institutions. Academic faculty must continue to perform their faculty duties, despite the financial incentive of interacting with industry. Continued federal support of research is needed, because NIH-supported research has been an important incubator of new ideas and novel discoveries.

A cohort of clinical investigators must also be trained to transfer technology between the laboratory bench and the bedside. They will oversee the transmission of new products and interventions to the clinic and, conversely, the transfer of clinical aberrancies to the laboratory for explanation. Highly trained individuals who can accomplish this in an efficient and cost-effective manner are needed. Incentives must be created to attract physicians and other health professionals to clinical investigations to ensure that new technology will generate new medical therapy.

There continues to be debate about whether the current supply of individuals appropriately trained as clinical investigators is seriously deficient. There is nearly unanimous agreement that the explosion of new knowledge in molecular biology, medicine, and medical informatics will create a need in the future for substantially more expertise (Kelley, 1988). Fully trained physicians and other health professionals in academia, government service, and industry will be particularly crucial in the transformation of these discoveries into cost-effective treatments for human disease. Thus, clinical investigators trained in academia will also be needed in industry to help in the translation of advances in biomedical research to the development and application of new products. Given the monumental opportunities that will soon be available and the current nature of the enterprise, the critical human resource pool will be seriously deficient. The pharmaceutical and biotechnology industries have a special interest in facilitating training and in the initial discovery process, which often occurs in academia.

The translation and application of advances in research to patient care require a strong partnership between the academic institutions and industry. Facilitation of technology transfer by both parties is important and deserves special support. The relationship among faculty, the academic institution, and industry is changing dramatically and represents a new paradigm. This will require new standards in the definition and resolution of conflicts of interest at all levels in support of this change. Issues related to conflicts of interest must be explicitly defined, and for the alleviation of both individual and institutional conflict of interest must be implemented at the local level.

References

Abrahamson, S. 1991. The dominance of research in staffing of medical schools: Time for a change? Lancet 337:1586–1588.

Agency for Health Care Policy and Research (AHCPR). 1992. Program, Evaluation, and Legislation Plan, FY 1994–1998. OPD 2/92. Rockville, Md.

Ahrens, E.H. 1992. The Crisis in Clinical Research: Overcoming Institutional Obstacles. New York: Oxford University Press.

Alcohol, Drug Abuse, and Mental Health Administration. 1991. ADAMHA Extramural Activities. ADAMHA Program Analysis Report No. 91-23. Rockville, Maryland.

American Federation for Clinical Research. 1992. Draft recommendations on policy issues to be considered in the NIH strategic plan. Clin. Res. 40:189–196.

American Medical Association (AMA). 1991. Women in Medicine in America: In the mainstream. Chicago.

American Medical Association (AMA). 1992. Physician Characteristics and Distribution in the U.S. G. Roback, L. Randolph, and B. Seidman, eds. Chicago.

Antman K., L. Schnipper, and E. Frei III. 1988. The crisis in clinical cancer research: Third-party insurance and investigational therapy. N. Engl. J. Med. 319:46–48.

Antman, K., L.M. Aledort, J. Yarbro, et al. 1989. Cost-effectiveness and reimbursement in patient care. Semin. Hematol. 26:32–45.

Applegate, W.B. 1990. Career development in academic medicine. Am. J. Med. 88:263–267.

Arias, I.M. 1989. Training basic scientists to bridge the gap between basic science and its application to human disease. N. Engl. J. Med. 321:972–974.

Association of American Medical Colleges (AAMC). 1984. Physicians for the twenty-first century. Report of the Project Panel on the General Profesional Education of the Physician and College Preparation for Medicine (GPEP). Part II. J. Med. Educ. 59(suppl.)

219

Association of American Medical Colleges (AAMC). 1987. Research Activity of Full-Time Faculty in Departments of Medicine. Washington, D.C.

Association of American Medical Colleges (AAMC). 1991. Financing a Medical Education in the '90s: Collective Concerns—Paying the Bills and Preventing Defaults. Washington, D.C.

Association of American Medical Colleges (AAMC). 1992a. AAMC Data Book: Statistical Information Related to Medical Education. P. Jolly and D.M. Hudley, eds. Washington, D.C.

Association of American Medical Colleges (AAMC). 1992b. Educating Medical Students. Washington, D.C.

Association of American Medical Colleges (AAMC). 1993. U.S. Medical School Faculty 1993. Washington, D.C.

Atkins, D., R.A. Deyo, R.K. Albert, D.J. D.J. Sherrard, and T.S. Inui. 1994. Models of postdoctoral training for clinical research. Background paper for the Institute of Medicine Committee on Career Paths for Clinical Research. Washington, D.C.

Austrian, R, G.S. Mirick, D.E. Rogers, et al. 1951. The efficacy of modified oral penicillin therapy of pneumococcal lobar pneumonia. Bull. Johns Hopkins Hosp. 88:264–269.

Batshaw, M.L., L.P. Plotnick, B.G. Petty, et al. 1988. Academic promotion at a medical school: Experience at Johns Hopkins University School of Medicine. N. Engl. J. Med. 318:741–747.

Battelle. 1991. The Value of Pharmaceuticals: An Assessment of Future Costs for Selected Conditions. Washington, D.C.: Battelle Human Affairs Research Centers.

Beaty, H.N., D. Babbott, E.J. Higgins, P. Jolly, and G.S. Levey. 1986. Research activities of faculty in academic departments of medicine. Ann. Intern. Med. 104:90–97.

Beran, R.L. 1994. Considerations of educational debt and the selection of clinical research careers. Background paper for the Institute of Medicine Committee on Career Paths for Clinical Research. Washington, D.C.

Bickel, J. 1988. Women in medical education. N. Engl. J. Med. 319:1579–1584.

Bickel, J. 1991. The changing faces of promotion and tenure at U.S. medical schools. Acad. Med. 66:249–256.

Bickel, J., and B.E. Whiting. 1991. AAMC data report: Comparing the representation and promotion of men and women faculty at U.S. medical schools. Acad. Med. 268:173.

Bickel, J.W., C.R. Sherman, J. Ferguson, et al. 1981. The role of MD-PhD training in increasing the supply of physician-scientists. N. Engl. J. Med. 304:1265–1268.

Biddle, A.K., G.M. Carter, J.S. Uebersax, and J.D. Winkler. 1988. Research Careers of Recipients of the Research Scientist and Research Scientist Development Awards. Publication No. R-3688-NIMH. Bethesda, Md.: National Institute of Mental Health.

Bishop, M.J. 1984. Infuriating tensions: Science and the medical student. J. Med. Educ. 59:91–102.

Blackburn, R.T. 1979. Academic careers: Patterns and possibilities. Curr. Issues Higher Educ. 2:25–27.

Blake, D.A. 1992. The opportunities and problems of commercial ventures: The university view. Pp. 88–92 in Biomedical Research: Collaboration and Conflict of Interest. R. Porter and T.E. Malone, eds. Baltimore: Johns Hopkins University Press.

Blake, D.A. 1994. University-industry relationships in clinical research: University perspective. Background paper for the Institute of Medicine Committee on Career Paths for Clinical Research. Washington, D.C.

Bland, C.J., and C.C. Schmitz. 1986. Characteristics of the successful researcher and implications for faculty development. J. Med. Educ. 61:22–33.

Blank, L. 1993. Roles and responsibilities of resident review committees and certification boards in promoting research careers. Background paper for the Institute of Medicine Committee on Career Paths for Clinical Research. Washington, D.C.

Blumenthal, D. 1992. Academic-industry relationships in the life sciences: Extent, consequences, and management. J. Am. Med. Assoc., 268:3344–3349.

Blumenthal, D., M. Gluck, K.S. Louis, and D.Wise. 1986a. Industrial support of university research in biotechnology. Science 231:242–246.

Blumenthal, D., M. Gluck, K.S. Louis, M.A. Stoto, and D.Wise. 1986b. University-industry relationships in biotechnology: Implications for the university. Science 232:1361–1366.

Boniface, Z.E., and R.W. Rimel. 1987. U.S. Funding of Biomedical Research. Philadelphia: The Pew Charitable Trusts.

Boyer, E.L. 1990. Scholarship reconsidered: Priorities of the professoriate. Princeton, N.J.: The Carnegie Foundation for the Advancement of Teaching.

Bradford, W.D., S. Pizzo, and A.C. Christakos. 1986. Careers and professional activities of graduates of a medical scientist training program. J. Med. Educ. 61:915–918.

Brancati, F.L., L.A. Mead, D.M. Levine, et al. 1992. Early predictors of career achievement in academic medicine. J. Am. Med. Assoc. 267:1372–1376.

Bryan, G.T. 1991. Physicians and medical education. J. Am. Med. Assoc., 266:1407–1408.

Burke, D.L. 1992. Physicians in the academic marketplace. Westport, Conn.: Greenwood.

Burke, J.D., H.A. Pincus, and H. Pardes. 1986. The clinician researcher in psychiatry. Am. J. Psychiatry 143:968–974.

Bush, V. 1945. Science—The Endless Frontier, A Report to the President on a Program for Postwar Scientific Research. Washington, D.C.: Office of Scientific Research and Development. (Reprinted by the National Science Foundation, Washington, D.C., May 1980.)

Cameron, S.W. 1981. Sponsorship and academic career success. J. Higher Educ. 52:369–377.

Cadman, E.C. 1990. The new physician-scientist: A guide for the 1990s. Clin. Res. 38:191–198.

Cadman, E.C. 1994. The image of the clinical investigator. Background paper for the Institute of Medicine Committee on Career Paths for Clinical Research. Washington, D.C.

California Institute of Technology (CIT). 1991. Summer Undergraduate Research Fellowships, 1991 Annual Report. Pasadena, Calif.

Calkins, E.V., and R. Wakeford. 1982. Perceptions of instructors and students of instructors' roles. J. Med. Educ. 58:967–969.

Cantor, J.C., A.B. Cohen, D.C. Barker, et al. 1991. Medical educators' views on medical education reform. J. Am. Med. Assoc. 265:1002–1006.

Carnegie Commission on Science, Technology, and Government. 1992. Enabling the Future: Linking Science and Technology to Societal Goals. Washington, D.C.

Carter, G.M., A. Robyn, and A.M. Singer. 1983. The Supply of Physician Researchers and Support for Research Training. Part I. Evaluation of the Hartford Fellowship Program. Santa Monica, Calif.: The RAND Corporation.

Carter, G.M., J.D. Winkler, and A.K. Bibble. 1987. An Evaluation of the NIH Research Career Development Award. Publication No. R-3568-NIH. Santa Monica, Calif.: The RAND Corporation.

Chin, D., D. Hopkins, K. Melmon, and H. Holman. 1985. The relation of faculty academic activity to financing sources in a department of medicine. N. Engl. J. Med., 312:1029–1034.

Choppin, P.W. 1989. Howard Hughes Medical Institute: Training the next generation of medical scientists. Acad. Med. 64:382–383.

Cohen, R.A. 1991. New foundations for young investigators. Clin. Res. 39:505–513.

Cole, J.R., and H. Zuckerman. 1987. Marriage, motherhood, and research performance in science. Sci. Am. 256:119–125.

Commonwealth Fund. 1985. The future financing of teaching hospitals. In Prescription for Change: Report of the Task Force on Academic Health Centers. New York: Harkness.

Cooper T. and M. Novitch. 1992. The research needs of industry working with academia and with the federal government. Pp.187–198 in Biomedical Research: Collaboration and Conflict of Interest. R. Porter and T.E. Malone, eds. Baltimore: Johns Hopkins University Press.

Cooperative Institutional Reseach Program. 1982

Cotton, P. 1992. Harassment hinders women's care and careers. J. Am. Med. Assoc., 267:778–783.

Cotton, P. 1992. Women scientists explore more ways to smash through the "glass ceiling." J. Am. Med. Assoc. 268:173.

Cuca, J. 1983. NIH grant applications for clinical research: Reasons for poor ratings or disapproval. Clin. Res. 31:453–461.

Cuca, J., and W.J. McLoughlin. 1987. Why clinical research grant applications fare poorly in review and how to recover. Cancer Invest. 5:55–58.

Davis, W.K., and W.N. Kelley. 1982. Factors influencing decisions to enter careers in clinical investigation. J. Med. Educ. 57:275-281.

Detsky, A.S. 1989. Are clinical trials a cost-effective investment? J. Am. Med. Assoc., 262:1795–1800.

DiBona, G.F. 1979. Whence cometh tomorrow's clinical investigator's? Clin. Res. 27:253–256.

DiMasi, J.A., R.W. Hansen, H. G. Grabowski, and L. Lasagna. 1991. Cost of innovation in the pharmaceutical industry. J. Health Econ. 10:107–142.

Directory of Medical Specialists. 1991. Marquis Who's Who, 25th Edition. Willmette, Illinois: Macmillan Directory Division.

Dwyer, M.M., A.A. Flynn, and P.S. Inman. 1991. Differential progress of women faculty: Status 1980–1990. In J.C. Smart, ed. Higher Education: Handbook on Theory and Research, Volume 3. New York: Agathon Press.

Eddy, D.M. 1984. Variations in physician practice: The role of uncertainty. Health Affairs 4:74–89.

Educational Testing Service. 1988. National Assessment of Educational Progress: The Science Report Card: Elements of Risk and Recovery. Princeton, N.J.

Eisenberg, D. 1989. Medicine is no longer a man's profession. Or when the men's club goes coed, it's time to change the regs. N. Engl. J. Med. 321:1542–1544.

Eisenberg, J.M. Cultivating a new field: Development of a research program in general internal medicine. J. Gen. Intern. Med. 1(Suppl.):S8–S18.

Farrell, K., M. Witte, M. Holguin, and S. Lopez. 1985. Women physicians in medical academia: A national survey. J. Am. Med. Assoc. 254:781–787.

Federal Coordinating Committee for Science, Engineering, and Technology (FCCSET), Committee on Education and Human Resources. 1991. By the Year 2000, First in the World. Washington, D.C.: White House Office of Science and Technology Policy.

Feinstein, A.R. 1985. Additional basic approaches in clinical research. Clin. Res. 33:111–114.

Feinstein, A.R. 1985. Clinical epidemiology: The architecture of clinical research. Philadelphia: W.B. Saunders.

Fletcher, R.H. 1989. The costs of clinical trials. J. Am. Med. Assoc. 262:1842.

Fletcher, R.H., S.W. Fletcher, and E.H. Wagner. 1982. Clinical Epidemiology: The Essentials. Baltimore: Williams & Wilkins.

Flexner, A. 1910. Medical education in the United States and Canada. Bulletin No. 4. New York: Carnegie Foundation for the Advancement of Teaching.

Forrest, J.N., Jr. 1980. The decline in the training of clinical investigators: Data and proposals from the 1970's. Clin. Res. 28:246–247.

Four Schools Physician Scientist Program in Internal Medicine. 1991. Information booklet. Baltimore.

Fox, R.C., J.P. Swazey, and J.C. Watkins eds. 1992. The Study of the Sick. Proceedings of an Oral History Conference on the Development of Clinical Research. Philadelphia: The Medical College of Pennsylvania.

Freireich, E.J. 1990. A study of the status of clinical cancer research in the United States. J. Natl. Cancer Inst. 83:829–837.

Frieden, C., and B.J. Fox. 1991. Career choices of graduates from Washington University's medical scientist training program. Acad. Med. 66:162–164.

Friedman. M.A. 1987. Patient accrual to clinical trials. Cancer Treatment Rep. 71:557–558.

Friedman, M.A., D.F. Cain, D. Bronzert, and R.S. Wu. 1991. Poor funding rates of cancer clinical research: Intractable problem or solvable challenge. J. Natl. Cancer Inst. 83:838–841.

Fye, W.B. 1991. The origin of the full-time faculty system. Implications for clinical research. J. Am. Med. Assoc. 265:1555–1561.

Garrison, H.H., and P.W. Brown. 1985. Minority Access to Research Careers: An Evaluation of the Honors Undergraduate Research Training Program. Institute of Medicine. Washington, D.C.: National Academy Press.

Garrison, H.H., and P.W. Brown. 1986. The Career Achievements of NIH Postdoctoral Trainees and Fellows. Washington, D.C.: National Academy Press.

George, Y.S. 1991. Investing in the Human Potential: Science and Engineering at the Crossroads. M.L. Matyas and S.M. Malcom, eds. Washington, D.C.: American Association for the Advancement of Science.

George, Y.S., B. Chu-Clewell, and N. Watkins. 1987. Lessons for HBCUs from Precollege Science and Mathematics Programs. Washington, D.C.: White House Initiative on Historically Black Colleges and Universities.

Giamatti, A.B. 1983. Free market and free inquiry: The university, industry, and cooperative research. Pp. 3–9 in Partners in the Research Enterprise: University-Corporate Relations in Science and Technology. T.W. Langfitt, S. Hackney, A.P. Fishman, and A.V. Glowasky, eds. Philadelphia: University of Pennsylvania Press.

Gill, G. 1984. The end of the physician-scientist? Am. Scholar 53:353–368.

Ginzberg, E., and A.B. Dutka. 1989. The Financing of Biomedical Research. Baltimore: The Johns Hopkins University Press.

Glickman, R.M. 1985. The future of the physician scientist. J. Clin. Invest. 76:1293–1296.

Gluck, M., D. Blumenthal, and M. Stoto. 1987. University-industry realtionships in the life sciences: Implications for students and postdoctral fellows. Res. Policy 16:327–336.

Goldman, L. 1991. Blueprint for a career in general internal medicine. J. Gen. Intern. Med. 6:331–334.

Goldman, L., E.F. Cooke, J. Orav, A.M. Epstein, A.L Komaroff, T.L. Delbanco, A.G. Mulley, and H.H. Hiatt. 1990. Research training in clinical effectiveness: Replacing "In my experience. . . . with rigorous clinical investigation. Clin. Res. 38:686–693.

Goldman, L., S. Shea, M. Wolf, and E. Braunwald. 1986. Clinical research training in parallel: The internal medicine research residency track at the Brigham and Women's Hospital. Clin. Res. 34:1–5.

Goldstein, J.L. 1986. On the Origin and Prevention of PAIDS (Paralyzed Academic Investigator's Disease Syndrome). Presidential address delivered before the 78th Annual Meeting of the American Society for Clinical Investigation, Washington, D.C., May 3, 1986. J. Clin. Invest 78:848–854.

Goodman, L.J., E.E. Brueschke, R.C. Bone, et al. 1991. An experiment in medical education: A critical analysis using traditional criteria. J. Am. Med. Assoc. 265:2373–2376.

Grant, L. 1988. The gender climate of medical school. J. Am. Med. Women's Assoc. 43:109–119.

Graves, P., and C. Thomas. 1985. Correlates of midlife career achievement among women physicians. J. Am. Med. Assoc. 254:781–787.

Green, K.C. 1989. A profile of undergraduates in the sciences. Am. Sci. Sept/Oct:475–480.

Greenlick, M.R. 1992. Educating physicians for population-based clinical practice. J. Am. Med. Assoc. 267:1645.

Healy, B. 1988. Innovators for the 21st century: will we face a crisis in biomedical research brainpower. N. Engl. J. Med. 319:1058–1064.

Herman, S.S., and A.M. Singer. 1986. Basic Scientists in Clinical Departments of Medical Schools. Clin. Res. 34:149–158.

Hewitt, N.M., and E. Seymour. 1991. Factors contributing to high attrition rates among science, mathematics, and engineering undergraduate majors. Report to the Alfred P. Sloan Foundation. Boulder: University of Colorado.

Holmes, B.L. 1992. Current strategies for the development of medical devices. In Medical Innovation at the Crossroads, Volume 3, Technology and Health Care in an Era of Limits. A.C. Geligns, ed. Washington, D.C.: National Academy Press.

Howard Hughes Medical Institute. 1992. Attracting Students to Science, Undergraduate and Precollege Programs. Bethesda, Maryland.

Hughes, R.G., D.C. Barker, and R.C. Reynolds. 1991. Are we mortgaging the medical profession? N. Engl. J. Med. 325:404–407.

Hunter, C.P., F.W. Frelick, A.R. Feldman, et al. 1987. Selection factors in clinical trials: Results from the community clinical oncology program physician's patient log. Cancer Treatment Rep. 71:559–565.

Institute of Medicine. 1979. DHEW's Research Planning Principles: A Review. Washington, D.C.: National Academy of Sciences.

Institute of Medicine. 1980. DHEW Health Research Planning, Phase II: A Review. Washington, D.C.: National Academy of Sciences.

Institute of Medicine. 1985. Personnel Needs and Training for Biomedical and Behavioral Research. Washington, D.C.: National Academy Press.

Insitute of Medicine. 1987. Organization of NIH. Washington, D.C.: National Academy Press.

Institute of Medicine. 1988a. Resources for Clinical Investigation. Washington, D.C.: National Academy Press.

Institute of Medicine. 1988b. A Healthy NIH Intramural Program, Structural Change or Administrative Remedies? Washington, D.C.: National Academy Press.

Institute of Medicine. 1989a. A Stronger Cancer Centers Program. Washington, D.C.: National Academy Press.

Institute of Medicine. 1989b. Government and Industry Collaboration in Biomedical Research and Education. Washington, D.C.: National Academy Press.

Institute of Medicine. 1989c. Physician Staffing for the VA, Volume 1. Washington, D.C.: National Academy Press.

Institute of Medicine. 1989d. Biomedical and Behavioral Research Scientists: Their Training and Supply. Washington, D.C.: National Academy Press.

Institute of Medicine. 1990. Funding Health Sciences Research: A Strategy to Restore Balance. Washington, D.C.: National Academy Press.

Institute of Medicine. 1992. Strengthening Research in Academic OB/GYN Departments. Washington, D.C.: National Academy Press.

Janowsky, D.S., I.D. Glick, L. Lash, et al. 1986. Psychobiology and psychopharmacology: Issues in clinical research training. J. Clin. Psychopharmacol. 6:1–7.

Jennett, P. 1988. Medical school M.D. graduates' activities in research and teaching. In Research in Medical Education, 1988: Proceedings of the Twenty-Seventh Annual Conference, D.S. Dabney, compiler. Washington, D.C.: Association of American Medical Colleges.

Jolin, L.D., P. Jolly, J.Y. Krakower, and R. Beran. 1992. US medical school finances. J. Am. Med. Assoc. 268:1149–1155.

Jonas, H.S., S.I. Etzel, and B. Barzansky. 1991. Educational programs in U.S. medical schools. J. Am. Med. Assoc. 266:913–920.

Jonas, H.S., S.I. Etzel, and B. Barzansky. 1992. Educational programs in U.S. medical schools. J. Am. Med. Assoc. 268:1083–1090.

Jones, R.F., M.F. Mirsky, and J.A. Keyes, Jr. 1985. Clinical practice of medical school faculties: An AAMC survey of problems and issues. J. Med. Educ. 60:897–910.

Kalichman, M.W., and P.J. Freidman. 1992. A pilot study of biomedical trainees' perceptions concerning research ethics. Acad. Med. 67:769–775.

Kelley, W.N. 1980. A positive approach: Things could be even better. Clin. Res. 28:267–270.

Kelley, W.N. 1985. Personnel needs for clinical research: role of the clinical investigator. Clin. Res. 33:100–104.

Kelley, W.N. 1988. Are we about to enter the golden era of clinical investigation? J. Lab. Clin. Med. 111:365–370.

Kelley, W.N. 1992. Primary care and subspecially medicine. Fostering a unified internal medicine. J. Gen. Intern. Med. 7:221–224.

Kelley, W.N. and J.K. Stross. 1992. Faculty tracks and academic success. Ann. Intern. Med. 116:645–659.

Kennedy, T.J. 1990. The rising cost of NIH-funded biomedical research. Acad. Med. 65:63–73.

Kimes, B.W., V. Cairoli, E.J. Freireich, J. Carp, and S.S. Yang. 1991. Training in clinical research in oncology. Cancer Res. 51:753–756.

Krimsky, S., J.G. Ennis, and R. Weissman. 1991. Academic-corporate ties in biotechnology: A quantitative study. Sci. Tech. Hum. Values 16:275–287.

Kyle, W.C. 1984. What became of the curriculum development projects of the 1960s? How effective were they? What did we learn from them that will help teachers in today's classrooms? In Research Within Reach: Science Education. D. Holdzkiom and P.B. Lutz, eds. Charlestown, W.V.: Appalachia Educational Laboratory.

Laetz, T., and G. Silverman. 1991. Reimbursement policies constrain the practice of oncology. J. Am. Med. Assoc. 266:2996–2999.

Lapoint, A.E., N.A. Mead, and G.W. Phillips. 1989. A World of Differences: An International Assessment of Mathematics and Science. Princeton, N.J.: Educational Testing Service.

Leaf, A. 1989. Cost-effectiveness as a criterion for Medicare coverage. N. Engl. J. Med. 321:898–900.

Lederman, L.M. 1991. Science: The end of the frontier. Science 251(Suppl.)

Ledley, F.D. 1991. The physician scientist's role in medical research and the mythology of intellectual tradition. Perspect. Biol. Med. 34:410–420.

Lee, T., and L. Goldman. 1994. Models of postdoctoral training for clinical research. Background paper for the Institute of Medicine Committee on Career Paths for Clinical Research. Washington, D.C.

Lee, T.H., F.P. Ognibene, and J.S. Schwartz. 1991. Correlates of external research support among respondents to the 1990 American Federation for Clinical Research survey. Clin. Res. 39:135–144.

Levey, B.A., N.O. Gentile, P. Jolly, H.N. Beaty, and G.S. Levey. 1990. Comparing research activities of women and men faculty in departments of internal medicine. Acad. Med. 65:102–106.

Levey, G.S., C.R. Sherman, N.O. Gentile, and L.J. Hough. 1988. Postdoctoral research training of full-time faculty in academic departments of medicine. Ann. Intern. Med. 109:414–418.

Levinson, W., S. Tolle, and C. Lewis. 1989. Women in medicine: Combining career and family. N. Engl. J. Med. 321:1511–1517.

Levinson, W., and J. Weiner. 1991. Promotion and tenure of women and minorities on medical school faculties. Ann. Intern. Med. 114:63–67.

Liaison Committee on Medical Education (LCME). 1991. Functions and Structure of a Medical School. Washington, D.C.: Association of American Medical Colleges and American Medical Association.

Littlefield, J.W. 1984. On the difficulty of combining basic research with patient care. Am. J. Hum. Genet. 36:731–735.

Littlefield, J.W. 1986. The need to promote careers that combine research and clinical care. J. Med.Educ. 61:785–789.

Lockheed, M.E., M. Thorpe, J. Brooks-Gunn, P. Casserly, and A. McAloon. 1985. Understanding sex/ethnic related differences in mathematics, science and computer science for students in grades four to eight. Princeton, N.J.: Educational Testing Service.

Low, G.M. 1983. The organization of industrial relationships with universities. Pp. 68–80 in Partners in the Research Enterprise: University-Corporate Relations in Science and Technology. T.W. Langfitt, S. Hackney, A.P. Fishman, and A.V. Glowasky, eds. Philadelphia: University of Pennsylvania Press.

Malcom, S.M. 1983. Equity and excellence: Compatible goals. Washington, D.C.: American Association for the Advancement of Science.

Malone, T.E. 1992. The moral imperative for biomedical research. Pp 3–32 in Biomedical Research: Collaboration and Conflict of Interest. R.J. Porter and T.E. Malone, eds. Baltimore: Johns Hopkins University Press.

Marshall, E. 1994. Strong medicine for NIH. Science 264:896–898.

Martin, J.B. 1991. Training physician-scientists for the 1990s. Acad. Med. 66:123–129.

Martin, J.F., W.G. Henderson, F.R. Rickles, et al. 1984. Accrual of patients into a multihospital cancer clinical trial and its implications on planning future studies. Am. J. Clin. Oncol. 7:173–182.

Massachusetts Institute of Technology (MIT). 1990. Education that works: An action plan for the education of minorities. Cambridge, Mass.: MIT Press

Matyas, M.L. 1994. Early Exposure to Research: Opportunities and Effects. Background paper for the Institute of Medicine Committee on Career Paths for Clinical Research. Washington, D.C.

Matyas, M.L., and S.M. Malcom, eds. 1991. Investing in the Human Potential: Science and Engineering at the Crossroads. Washington, D.C.: American Association for the Advancement of Science.

McClellan, D.A., and P. Talalay. 1992. M.D.-Ph.D. training at The Johns Hopkins University School of Medicine, 1962–1991. Acad. Med. 67:36–41.

McManus, I.C. 1991. How Will Medical Education Change? Lancet 337:1519–1521.

Medical Research Council. 1948. Streptomycin treatment of pulmonary tuberculosis. Br. Med. J. 2:769–783.

Menkes, J.H. 1981. The physician-scientist: Past, present and future. Johns Hopkins Med. J. 148:175–178.

Merton, R.K. 1942. Science and technology in a democratic order. J. Leg. Polit. Sci. 1:15–26.

Meyer, C.T., and A. Price. 1992. The crisis in osteopathic medicine. Acad. Med. 67:810–816.

Moertel, C.G. 1991. Off-label drug use for cancer therapy and national health care priorities. J. Am. Med. Assoc. 266:3031–3032.

Moody, F.G. 1992. The changing health care economy: Impact on surgical techniques. In Medical Innovation at the Crossroads, volume 2. Technology and Health Care in an Era of Limits. A.C. Geligns, ed. Washington, D.C.: National Academy Press.

Movsesian, M.A. 1990. Effect on physician-scientists of the low funding rate of NIH grant applications. N. Engl. J. Med. 322:1602–1604.

Nathan, D.G. 1987. Sounding Board: Funding subspecialty training for clinical investigators. N. Engl. J. Med. 316:1020–1022.

Nathan, D.G. 1988. Training in Clinical Investigation. In Resources for Clinical Investigation. Institute of Medicine. Washington, D.C.: National Academy Press.

National Academy of Sciences (NAS), Government-University-Industry Research Roundtable. 1986. New Alliances and Partnerships in American Science and Engineering. Washington, D.C.: National Academy Press.

National Academy of Sciences (NAS), Government-University-Industry Research Roundtable. 1987. Nurturing Science and Engineering Talent: A Discussion Paper. Washington, D.C.: National Academy Press.

National Academy of Sciences (NAS), Government-University-Industry Research Roundtable. 1991. Industrial Perspectives on Innovation and Interactions with Universities. Washington, D.C.: National Academy Press.

National Academy of Sciences (NAS), Government-University-Industry Research Roundtable. 1992. Fateful Choices: The Future of the U.S. Academic Research Enterprise. Washington, D.C.: National Academy Press.

National Institutes of Health (NIH). 1986. Review of the Mission of the Clinical Center. D.W. Seldin, panel chair. Bethesda, Md.

National Institutes of Health (NIH). 1989a. Review of the National Institutes of Health Biomedical Research Training Programs. Bethesda, Md.

National Institutes of Health (NIH). 1989b. Biomedical Research: The Next Generation of Scientists. Proceedings of the 59th Meeting of the Advisory Committee to the Director, National Institutes of Health. Bethesda, Md.

National Institutes of Health (NIH). 1992a. Clinical Trials Report: FY 1988–FY 1989. Office of Medical Application of Research. Bethesda, Md.

National Institutes of Health (NIH). 1992b. DRG Peer Review Trends; Member Characteristics: DGR Study Sections, Institute Review Groups, Advisory Councils and Boards, 1981–1991. Bethesda, Md.: National Institutes of Health.

National Institutes of Health (NIH). 1992c. NIH Data Book 1992. Bethesda, Md.

National Institutes of Health (NIH). 1992d. Summary report of meeting of Dr. Bernadine Healy, Director, National Institutes of Health, with Chairpersons of NIH Initial Review Groups. Bethesda, Md.

National Research Council (NRC). 1987a. Minorities: Their Underrepresentation and Career Differentials in Science and Engineering. Proceedings of a Workshop. Washington, D.C.: National Academy Press.

National Research Council (NRC). 1987b. Women: Their Underrepresentation and Career Differentials in Science and Engineering (Proceedings of a Workshop). Washington, D.C.: National Academy Press.

National Research Council (NRC). 1989a. Biomedical and Behavioral Research Scientists: Their Training and Supply, Volume 1, Findings. Washington, D.C.: National Academy Press.

National Research Council (NRC). 1989b. Everybody Counts: A Report to the Nation on the Future of Mathematics Education. Washington, D.C.: National Academy Press.

National Research Council (NRC). 1990. Fullfilling the Promise: Biology in the Nation's Schools. Committee on High School Biology. Washington, D.C.: National Academy Press.

National Research Council (NRC). 1991. Women in Science and Engineering: Increasing Their Numbers in the 1990s. Washington, D.C.: National Academy Press.

National Science Board (NSB). 1981. University-Industry Research Relationships: Myths, Realities and Potentials. Fourteenth Annual Report of the National Science Board. Washington, D.C.: National Science Foundation.

National Science Board (NSB). 1991. Science and Engineering Indicators. NSB 91-1. Washington, D.C.: National Science Foundation.

National Science Foundation (NSF). 1987a. Report on Funding Trends and Balance of Acitivities: National Science Foundation 1951–1988. NSF 88-3. Washington, D.C.

National Science Foundation (NSF). 1987b. Biotechnology Research and Development Activities in Industry: 1984 and 1985. NSF 87-311. Washington, D.C.

National Science Foundation (NSF). 1988a. The Science and Technology Resources of Japan: A Comparison with the United States. NSF 88-318. Washington, D.C.

National Science Foundation (NSF). 1988b. Science Resource Highlights: Industrial Biotechnology R&D Increased an Estimated 12 Percent in 1987 to $1.4 Billion. NSF 88-306. Washington, D.C.

National Science Foundation (NSF). 1989. Science and Technology Resources: Funding and Personnel. NSF 89-300. Washington, D.C.

National Science Foundation (NSF). 1990. Women and Minorities in Science and Engineering. NSF 90-301. Washington, D.C.

National Science Foundation (NSF). 1992. America's Academic Future: A Report of the Presidential Young Investigator Colloquium on U.S. Engineering, Mathematics, and Science Education for the Year 2010 and Beyond. NSF 91-150. Washington, D.C.

Neinstein, L.S., and R.G. Mackenzie. 1989. Prior training and recommendations for future training of clinical research faculty members. Acad. Med. 64:32–35.

Neufeld, V.R., C.A. Woodward, and S.M. MacLoed. 1989. The McMaster M.D. program: A case study of renewal in medical education. Acad. Med. 64:423–432.

Newcomer, L.N. 1990. Defining experimental therapy—a third-party payer's dilemma. N. Engl. J. Med. 323:1702–1704.

Nickerson, K.G., N.M. Bennett, D. Estes, and S. Shea. 1992. The status of women at one academic medical center: Breaking through the glass ceiling. J. Am. Med. Assoc. 264:1813–1817.

Oates, J.A. 1982. Presidential Address: Clinical investigation: A pathway to discovery. Trans. Assoc. Am. Physicians 95:1xxviii–xc.

Orthopaedic Research and Education Foundation. 1991. Defining the Current Status of Orthopaedic Research: Scope, Funding, Personnel, Facilities and Areas of Study. Chicago, Il.: Council on Research, American Academy of Orthopaedic Surgeons.

Osborne, E.H.S., V.L. Ernster, and J.B. Martin. 1992. Women's attitudes toward careers in academic medicine at the University of California, San Francisco. Acad. Med. 67:59–62.

Paiva, R.E., C. Donnelly, H.B. Haley, et al. 1975. Factors Related to Medical Students' Research Activities. J. Med. Educ. 50:339–345.

Pak, C. 1994. Role of the GCRC in Establishing Career Paths in Clinical Research. Background paper for the Institute of Medicine Committee on Career Paths for Clinical Research. Washington, D.C.

Parris, M., and E.J. Stemmler. 1984. Development of clinician-educator faculty track at the University of Pennsylvania. J. Med. Educ. 59:465–470.

Peck, C. 1988. Training of Clinical Investigators. In Resources for Clinical Investigation. Institute of Medicine. Washington, D.C.: National Academy Press.

Penchansky, R., J.R. Landis, and M.B. Brown. 1988. Education for clinical research: An experiment at the University of Michigan. Clin. Res. 36:21–32.

Pharmaceutical Manufacturers Association. 1989. Annual Survey Report of the U.S. Pharmaceutical Industry, 1987–1989. Washington, D.C.

Piccirillo, J.F. 1992. The Robert Wood Johnson Scholars Program: A research training plan. Otolaryngol. Head Neck Surg. 106:25–26.

Pion, G. 1994. The effectiveness of federally supported research training in preparing clinical investigators: Important questions but few answers. Background paper for the Institute of Medicine Committee on Career Paths for Clinical Research. Washington, D.C.

Pool, R. 1991. The social return of academic research. Nature, 352:661.

Porter, R.J. 1992. Conflicts of interest in research: The fundamentals. Pp. 121–134 in Biomedical Research: Collaboration and Conflict of Interest. R.J. Porter, and T.E. Malone, eds. Baltimore, Md: Johns Hopkins University Press.

President's Council of Advisors on Science and Technology. 1992. Renewing the Promise: Research-Intensive Universities and the Nation. Washington, D.C.: White House Office of Science and Technology Policy.

Price, F.D. 1985. Industry and academia in collaboration: The Pfizer experience. Circulation 72(Suppl. I):13–17.

Prystowsky, J.H. 1992. Factors influencing the pursuit of careers in academic medicine: A survey of M.D.-Ph.D. residents in dermatology programs in the United States. J. Invest. Dermatol. 98:125–127.

Quantum Research Corporation. 1991. Prospective and retrospective trainee analysis. Developed for the Planning and Policy Research Branch, Office of Science Policy and Legisation, National Institutes of Health. Bethesda, Md.

Rahimtoola, S.H. 1990. The sad plight of the clinician-clinical investigator: "Don't boil the frog in the pot." Circulation 81:1702–1706.

Raskin, I. 1992. Research Funding at the Agency for Health Care Policy and Research. Presentation at the IOM workshop on Clinical Research and Training: Spotlight on Funding. Washington, D.C.

Reigelman, R.K, G.J. Povar, and J.E. Ott. 1983. Medical student's skills, attitudes, and behavior needed for literature reading. J. Med. Educ. 58:411–417.

Robert Wood Johnson Foundation. 1987. Special Report: The Foundation's Minority Medical Training Programs. Number 1. Princeton, N.J.

Roper, W.L., W. Winkenwerder, G.M. Hackbarth, and H. Krakauer. 1988. Effectiveness in health care: An initiative to evaluate and improve medical practice. N. Engl. J. Med. 319:1197–1202.

Ross, R.S. 1985. Boundaries of the General Clinical Research Center in an academic medical center. Clin. Res. 33:105–110.

Sackett, D.L., R.B. Haynes, and P. Tugwell. 1985. Clinical Epidemiology: A Basic Science for clinical Medicine. Boston: Little Brown.

Sadeghi-Nejad, A.B., and M.M. Marquardt. 1991. Academic physicians: Today's dinosaurs? Am. J. Med. 90:371–373.

Safran, D.B., H.D. Crombie, L. Allen, et al. 1992. Preliminary assessment of a scientific curriculum in a surgical residency program. Arch. Surg. 127:529–535.

Schaller, J.G. 1990. The advancement of women in academic medicine. J. Am. Med. Assoc. 264:1854–1855.

Science Services, Inc. 1991. 1992 Directory of Student Science Training Programs for Precollege Students. Washington, D.C.

Segal, S., T. Lloyd, P.S Houts, et al. 1990. The association between students' research involvement in medical school and their postgraduate medical activities. Acad. Med. 65:530–533.

Seggel, R.L. 1985. Stabilizing the Funding of NIH and ADAMHA Research Project Grants. Washington, D.C.: National Academy Press.

Selker, L. 1994. Clinical Research in Allied Health. In Career Paths for Clinical Research, Volume 2. Institute of Medicine. Washington, D.C.: National Academy Press.

Shapley, W.H. 1992. The Budget Process and R&D. New York: Carnegie Commission on Science, Technology, and Government.

Shaw, L. 1992. A misunderstood specialty: A survey of physicians in the pharmaceutical industry. J. Clin. Pharmacol. 31:419–422.

Sherman, C.R. 1983. Notes on the NIH Role in Support of Postdoctoral Research Training of Two Groups of Physicians. Bethesda, Md.: National Institutes of Health.

Sherman, C.R. 1989. The NIH Role in the Training of Individual Physician Faculty: A Supplementary Analysis. Bethesda, Md.: National Institutes of Health.

Sherman, C.R., H.P. Jolly, T.E. Morgan, et al. 1981. On the Status of Medical School Faculty and Clinical Research Manpower, 1986–1990. Bethesda, Md.: National Institues of Health.

Shipp, A. 1992. How to control conflict of interest. Pp. 163-184 in Biomedical Research: Collaboration and Conflict of Interest. R. Porter and T.E. Malone, eds. Baltimore, Md.: Johns Hopkins University Press.

Shulkin, D.J., J.J. Escarci, C. Enarson, and J.M. Eisenberg. 1991. Impact of the Medicare fee schedule on an academic department of medicine. J. Am. Med. Assoc. 266:3000–3003.

Shuster, A.L., L.E. Cluff, M.A. Haynes, et al. 1983. An innovation in physician training: The Clinical Scholars Program. J. Med. Educ. 58:101–111.

Smith, D.B. 1992. The future of research at the Department of Veterans Affairs. Acad. Med. 67:836-837.

Smith, D.B. 1992b. Research Funding in the Department of Veterans Affairs. Presentation at the IOM Workshop on Clinical Research and Training: Spotlight on Funding. Washington, D.C.

Smith, L.H. 1989. Training of physician/scientists in biomedical and behavioral research: Their training and supply. In Biomedical and Behavioral Scientists: Their Training and Supply. National Research Council. Washington, D.C.: National Academy Press.

Smith, R. 1988. Medical researchers: Training and straining. Br. Med. J. 296:920–924.

Smith, W.C.J. 1992. Report on medical school faculty salaries 1991–1992. Washington, D.C.: Association of American Medical Colleges.

Spilker, B. 1992. Career opportunities for physicians in the pharmaceutical industry. J. Clin. Pharmacol. 29:1069–1076.

Stolley, P. 1988. The training of clinical investigators. In Resources for Clinical Investigation. Institute of Medicine. Washington, D.C.: National Academy Press.

Stossel, T.P., and S.C. Stossel. 1990. Declining American representation in leading clinical research journals. N. Engl. J. Med. 322:739–742.

Strickland, S.P. 1972. Politics, Science, and Dread Disease: A Short History of United States Medical Research Policy. Cambridge, Mass.: Harvard University Press.

Swazey, J.P. 1994. Advisers, mentors, and role models in graduate and professional education: Implications for the recruitment, training, and retention of physician-investigators. Background paper for the Institute of Medicine Committee on Career Paths for Clinical Research. Washington, D.C.

Telling, F.W. 1992. Managed care and pharmaceutical innovation. In Medical Innovation at the Crossroads, Volume 3. Technology and Health Care in an Era of Limits. A.C. Geligns, ed. Washington, D.C.: National Academy Press.

Thacker, S.B., R.A. Goodman, and R.C. Dicker. 1990. Training and service in public health practice, 1951–90—CDC's Epidemic Intelligence Service. Public Health Rep. 106:599–604.

Thier, S.O. 1980. Clinical investigation in the 1980s: Perspective of the medical schools. Clin. Res. 28:248–251.

Thier, S.O., D.R. Challoner, J. Cockerham, et al. 1980. Proposals addressing the decline in the training of physician investigators: report of the ad hoc committee of the AAMC. Clin. Res. 28:85–93.

Tobias, S. They're Not Dumb, They're Different: Stalking the Second Tier. Tuscon, Ariz.: Research Corporation.

Tudor, C.G., and D.W. Lindley, eds. 1988. Trends in Medical School Applicants and Matriculants—1978–1987. Washington, D.C.: Association of American Medical Colleges.

U.S. Congress. 1993. National Institutes of Health Revitalization Act of 1993. Public Law 103–43. Washington, D.C.: U.S. Government Printing Office.

U.S. Congress, Office of Technology Assessment. 1984. Commercial Biotechnology: An International Analysis. OTA-BA-218. Washington, D.C.: U.S. Government Printing Office.

U.S. Congress, Office of Technology Assessment. 1985. Demographic Trends and the Scientific and Engineering Workforce. OTA-TM-SET-35. Washington, D.C.: U.S. Government Printing Office.

U.S. Congress, Office of Technology Assessment. 1988a. Educating Scientists and Engineers: Grade School to Grad School. OTA-SET-377. Washington, D.C.: U.S. Government Printing Office.

U.S. Congress, Office of Technology Assessment. 1988b. New Developments in Biotechnology: U.S. Investment in Biotechnology—Special Report. OTA-BA-360. Washington, D.C.: U.S. Government Printing Office.

U.S. Congress, Office of Technology Assessment. 1990. Proposal Pressure in the 1980s: An Indicator of Stress on the Federal Research System. A staff paper. Washington, D.C.: OTA.

U.S. Congress, Office of Technology Assessment. 1991. Federally Funded Research: Decisions for a Decade. OTA-SET-490. Washington, D.C.: U.S. Government Printing Office.

U.S. Department of Commerce, Bureau of the Census. 1983. Projections of the Population of the United States by Age, Sex, and Race, 1983 to 2080. Current Population Reports Series P-25, No. 925. Washington, D.C.

U.S. Department of Education, Office of Educational Research and Improvement. 1991. The Condition of Education, 1991: Postsecondary Education, Volume 2. NCES 91-637. Washington, D.C.: National Center for Education Statistics.

U.S. Department of Education, Office of Special Education and Rehabilitative Services. 1991. NIDRR Program Directory: Fiscal Year 1991. Silver Spring, Md: National Rehabilitation Information Center.

U.S. Department of Health, Education, and Welfare. 1958. Secretary's Consultants Report: Advancement of Medical Research and Education. Washington, D.C.:

U.S. Department of Health, Education, and Welfare, Public Health Service. 1976. Report of the President's Biomedical Research Panel. DHEW Publication No. (OS)76-500. Washington, D.C.

U.S. Department of Health and Human Services, Food and Drug Administration; Center for Drug Evaluation and Research. 1992. Office of Professional Development and Staff College Catalog. Publication No. HFD-3. Rockville, Md.

U.S. Department of Health and Human Services, Public Health Service. 1985. DRG Peer Review Trends, Workload and Actions of DRG Study Sections, 1975–1985. Bethesda, Md.: National Institutes of Health.

U.S. Department of Health and Human Services, Public Health Service. 1989. ADAMHA Data Source Book FY 1988. ADAMHA Program Analysis Report No. 89-18. Rockville, Md.: Alcohol, Drug Abuse, and Mental Health Administration.

U.S. Department of Health and Human Services, Public Health Service. 1991a. General Clinical Research Centers. Publication No. 91-1433. Bethesda, Md.: National Institutes of Health.

U.S. Department of Health and Human Services, Public Health Service. 1991b. Report to Congress: Progress of Research on Outcomes of Health Care Services and Procedures. Publication No. 91-0004. Bethesda, Md.: Agency for Health Care Policy and Research.

U.S. Department of Health and Human Services, Public Health Service. 1991c. A Research Agenda for Primary Care: Summary of a Conference. Publication No. AHCPR 91-08. Bethesda, Md: Agency for Health Care Policy and Research.

U.S. Department of Health and Human Services, Public Health Service. 1991d. Primary Care Research: Theory and Methods: AHCPR Conference Proceedings. Publication No. AHCPR 91-0011. Bethesda, MD: Agency for Health Care Policy and Research.

U.S. Department of Health and Human Services, Public Health Service. 1991e. NIH Almanac. Publication No. 91-5. Bethesda, Md.: National Institutes of Health.

U.S. Department of Health and Human Services, Public Health Service. 1992a. Extramural Trends, FY 1982–91. Bethesda, Md.: National Institutes of Health, Division of Research Grants.

U.S. Department of Health and Human Services, Public Health Service. 1992b. NIH Advisory Committees: Authority, Structure, Function, Members. Publication No. 92-11. Bethesda, Md.: National Institutes of Health.

U.S. Department of Health and Human Services, Public Health Service. 1992c. NIH Data Book 1992. National Institutes of Health Publication No. 92-1261. Bethesda, Md.

U.S. Department of Health and Human Services, Public Health Service. 1992d. National Institutes of Health Loan Repayment Program for AIDS Researchers, Applicant Information Bulletin, 1992 Fiscal Year. Bethesda, Md.: National Institutes of Health.

U.S. Department of Veterans Affairs. 1991. Final Report of the Department of Veterans Affairs Advisory Committee for Health Research Policy: January 1990–January 1991. Washington, D.C.

U.S. General Accounting Office. 1988. Biomedical Research: Issues Related to Increasing Size of NIH Grant Awards. Report No. GAO/HRD-88-90BR.

U.S. General Accounting Office. 1991. Off-Label Drugs: Reimbursement Policies Constrain Physicians in their Choice of Cancer Therapies. No. GAO/PEMD-91-14. Washington, D.C.

U.S. General Accounting Office. 1992a. Cross-Design Synthesis—A New Strategy for Medical Effectiveness Research. No. GAO/PEMD-92-18. Washington, D.C.

U.S. General Accounting Office. 1992b. Controlling Inappropriate Access to Federally Funded Research Results. Publication No. RCED-92-104. Washington, D.C.

U.S. House of Representatives, Committee on Science, Space, and Technology. 1992. Report of the Task Force on the Health of Research. Washington, D.C.: U.S. Government Printing Office.

Vaitukaitis, J.L. 1991. The future of clinical research. Clin. Res. 39:145–156.

Vance, C. 1982. The mentor connection. J. Nurs. Admin. 38:7–13.

Varrin, R.D., and D.S. Kukich. 1985. Guidelines for industry-sponsored research at universities. Science 227:385–388.

Waugaman, P.G., and R.J. Porter. 1992. Mechanisms of interaction between industry and the academic medical center. Pp. 93–118 in Biomedical Research: Collaboration and Conflict of Interest. R.J. Porter and T.E. Malone, eds. Baltimore, Md.: Johns Hopkins University Press.

Weiss, I.R. 1987. Report of the National Survey of Science and Mathematical Education. Research Triangle Park, N.C.: Research Triangle Institute.

Weiss, I.R., B.H. Nelson, S.E. Boyd, and S.B. Hudson. 1989. Science and Mathematics Education Briefing Book. Washington, D.C.: National Science Teachers Association.

Wennberg, J.E. 1990. What is outcomes research? In Medical Innovation at the Crossroads, Volume 1. Modern Methods of Clinical Investigation. A.C. Gelings, ed. Washington, D.C.: National Academy Press.

Wennberg, J.E., K. McPhearson, and P. Caper. 1984. Will payment based on diagnosis-related groups control hospital costs? N. Engl. J. Med. 311:295-300.

Wennberg, J.E., A.G. Mulley, Jr., D. Hanley, R.P. Timothy, F.J. Fowler, Jr., N.P. Roos, M.J. Barry, K. McPherson, E.R. Greenberg, D. Soule, et al. 1988. An assessment of prostatectomy for benign urinary tract obstruction. Geographic variations and the evaluation of medical care outcomes. J. Am. Med. Assoc. 259:3027–30.

White House Science Council. 1986. A Renewed Partnership. Washington, D.C.: White House Office of Science and Technology Policy.

Whybrow, P.C. 1988. Clinical research training in psychopharmacology—context and climate: Notes from the chairman's perspective. Psychopharmacol. Bull. 24:285–287.

Witt, M.D., ed. 1991. Industry/University/Government Biomedical Research Alliances in the Public Interest: Models for the Future. Adapted from a Symposium at the Forsythe Dental Center, Boston, MA. Washington, D.C.: The Journal of NIH Research.

Wittes, R.E. 1987a. Antineoplastic agents and FDA regulations: Square pegs for round holes? Cancer Treatment Rep. 71:795–806.

Wittes, R.E. 1987b. Paying for patient care in treatment research—who is responsible? Cancer Treatment Rep. 71:107–113.

Wittes, R.E. 1988. From research to approved treatment: Overcoming the obstacles. Semin. Oncol. 25:38–42.

Woods, D. 1979. Can students and practicing doctors be encouraged to do medical research, and should they? Can. Med. Assoc. J. 121:352–355.

Wyngaarden, J.B. 1979. The clinical investigator as an endangered species. N. Engl. J. Med. 301:1254–1259.

Wyngaarden, J.B. 1983. Encouraging young physicians to pursue a career in clinical research. Clin. Res. 31:115–118.

Wyngaarden, J.B. 1986. The priority of patient-oriented research. Clin. Res. 33:95–104.

Appendix A

Report of the Task Force on Clinical Research in Dentistry

EXECUTIVE SUMMARY

Energized by the highly successful national investment in biomedical and behavioral research, the discipline of clinical research has undergone a remarkable evolution in the scope, sophistication, and power of its methodologies. Development of clinical research is expected to accelerate in the future, driven by the explosion of science in biotechnology, molecular biology, computer technology, diagnostic systems, decision analysis, and clinical measurements technology. The task force supports the conclusion that there is an overall need to expand the pool of biomedical clinical investigators and the monies available for clinical research. Its specific charge was to focus on the unique barriers and, particularly, the unique opportunities in oral health research that warrant specific attention and remedies.

Past successes of clinical research in dentistry underscore the need for continued clinical dental research to take full advantage of opportunities for transfer of fundamental information to patients. No example is more dramatic than the significant reduction in dental caries and corresponding improvements in the oral health of school-age children and young adults that is estimated to have saved over $39 billion, in 1990 dollars, from 1979 through 1989. The application of basic science research findings to dental practice as a result of clinical research has also saved the American public from much suffering and lost productive time.

This change in the oral disease pattern has triggered a marked change in the dental profession, with a shift of focus to diseases that were formerly ignored.

237

Most notable of these are the periodontal diseases, affecting some 7 out of 10 adults, which are responsible for much of the tooth loss in adults, and are now replacing caries as the most prevalent infection in humans. Other oral diseases include oral cancer; salivary dysfunction; oral mucous membrane lesions such as aphthous ulcers; oral herpes; oral diseases in patients with systemic diseases, such as periodontal disease in diabetics; and oral candidiasis and necrotic periodontal lesions in AIDS patients. There are many opportunities for improving the general health of humankind from expanded clinical research in oral health. In view of the opportunities for application of knowledge and technologies to manage and prevent oral diseases and their sequelae, specific barriers and opportunities for clinical research were examined.

The product of the task force's assessment was a series of recommendations that can be summarized as follows:

• Increase the funding for population-based clinical studies and technology transfer.

• Educate dental scientists to existing resources that can be used in clinical dental research.

• Improve the peer review structure for clinical dental research proposals.

• Address the shortage in human resources needed to accomplish dental clinical research objectives by developing an essentially new type of investigator, the *senior dental clinical scientist*; improving the clinical research competencies of both seasoned and young dentist-scientists with basic science training; and capitalizing on the capabilities of existing dental clinical faculty through the implementation of an innovative short-term training program for dental clinical research associates.

• Address important structural barriers existing in many dental schools that limit their clinical research capabilities and facilitate the transition of these institutions into viable and productive members of the academic health centers.

To accomplish many of these recommendations, the task force would ideally prefer the provision of new or augmented resources. At the same time, cognizant of not only the financial constraints presently faced by government, industry, and the educational sectors but also the oral health benefits that would follow an expansion of dental clinical research, the task force endorses the refocusing of existing resources to significantly expand national dental clinical research capabilities. The critical issue(s) or problem(s) in each area was identified, together with specific recommendations. These recommendations have a reasonable chance of success—most can be carried out almost immediately—and they have measurable endpoints.

CLINICAL RESEARCH IN DENTISTRY

There is an acute need for focused, high-quality clinical dental research. A relatively small investment in clinical dental research can have a large impact, improving both oral and general health.

Over the past several decades there have been remarkable improvements in the oral health of the U.S. population that have been made possible, to a great extent, by clinical research advances in dentistry. Among these advances are such notable examples as the fluoridation of public water supplies, which has resulted in a marked decrease in the incidence of dental caries, and the development of improved dental materials such as composite resins and dental sealants. There are a number of additional areas in which there is a sufficient base of laboratory investigation for the initiation of clinical trials. The main barrier to this transfer of technology is the lack of resources for clinical investigation in dentistry.

Background

Clinical research in dentistry encompasses a number of different areas focusing on the human oral cavity. Epidemiologic studies determine oral health care needs in the United States regarding dental caries and periodontal disease, which are the traditional foci of dental clinical investigations. Other areas that could benefit from clinical research include salivary function, oral cancer, taste and smell, craniofacial anomalies and acquired defects (for example, trauma), temporomandibular joint disorders, nutritional deficiencies affecting the oral cavity, and the oral sequelae of systemic diseases such as diabetes mellitus and human immunodeficiency virus (HIV) infection. On the basis of the perceived oral health care needs of the U.S. population, clinical studies in dentistry examine the etiologies of these oral diseases and encompass such basic science disciplines as microbiology, immunology, and biochemistry, and clinical sciences including radiology. Determination of the etiology of the various oral diseases consequently leads to a major focus on research in clinical intervention. This research includes clinical trials comparing treatment regimens; product testing, such as that required for dental materials; local antimicrobial and antiplaque agents; and studies of health care delivery. Behavioral science studies in clinical dental research examine issues such as patient compliance, utilization of specific self-care or provider-based prevention or treatment intervention, and health promotion. Furthermore, utilizing the oral cavity as a "window to the body," clinical dental research offers a model with broad applicability to biomedical research in such areas as pain control, mucosal immunity, and the pathobiology of secretions and secretory glands.

Although clinical dental research activities encompass a relatively broad spectrum of areas currently being examined by a small number of appropriately trained clinical investigators, the explosion of basic research applicable to clinical dentistry sets the stage for unprecedented opportunities for the clinical research needed to accelerate appropriate technology transfer. This is likely to have a major impact on oral health in the United States and throughout the world. Advances in anti-infective therapy for periodontitis; in the clinical, radiographic, and laboratory diagnoses of oral disease; in the remineralization of carious lesions; and in the regeneration of oral tissues destroyed as a result of chronic infection are but a few of the areas ripe for clinical application. Furthermore, there have been major advances in the science of clinical dental research itself, with significant improvements in data collection instruments and statistical analysis of hypothesis-oriented clinical problems. Future advances in areas such as molecular epidemiology will find ready application in clinical dental studies.

In addition to a backlog of basic science developments that need immediate clinical testing, a number of other conditions or factors will require increased clinical dental research efforts. Prime among these, as for biomedical science in general, is the desire for increased knowledge in order to diagnose and treat oral diseases. The growing regulatory requirements from the Food and Drug Administration (FDA) and other agencies that must be fulfilled prior to the marketing of dental products also will increase the need for clinical research.

The primary source of support for oral health research is the National Institute of Dental Research (NIDR). For this reason, the task force was particularly interested in assessing the current NIDR funding for dental clinical research. Preliminary results from a recent general assessment indicate that approximately one-fifth of the NIDR extramural budget and one-fifth of the number of research grants supported by the NIDR in fiscal year 1991 involved clinical investigators to at least some extent. The task force and the NIDR leadership recognize that this may be an overestimate.

In addition to the support from the National Institutes of Health (NIH), an unknown amount of support for clinical dental research is provided by industrial sources. With few exceptions, however, this research is restricted to narrow, product-oriented studies including randomized clinical trials and studies required by the FDA or other regulatory agencies and as defined by the sponsoring organizations. There is, however, anecdotal evidence of increasing industrial support from traditional industries and from new biotechnology companies for exploratory projects, some of which may lead to potentially commercial findings.

Recommendations

In order to expand clinical dental research, the task force recommends an increase in funding for population-based clinical studies and technology transfer. Clinical dental research often can be accomplished through NIDR-directed reallocation of existing resources through the request for application (RFA) mechanism. In addition, by allocating increases in the NIDR budget to clinical research and by better using existing resources—such as integrating clinical oral health studies with clinical general health studies and using clinical center grant mechanisms—clinical studies can be funded. For example, studies of the oral manifestations of systemic diseases such as diabetes mellitus and HIV infection can often be combined with a parent medical study, thus avoiding redundancy and affording better utilization of the general health database.

The task force recommends that it will be necessary to educate clinical dental scientists about resources that can be used in clinical dental research. NIH supports a number of core facilities and repositories that are designed to serve as resources for clinical investigators. Prominent among these are the Clinical Research Centers, which can assist the clinical investigator in study design, data and material collection, and data analysis. In addition, private industry has made a large investment in science and technology. Methods and results from these activities have great relevance to clinical dental researchers. Information regarding the availability of these resources should be disseminated to clinical dental scientists.

The task force recommends that improvements are needed in the structure and organization of peer review for clinical dental research proposals. Clinical dental research has emerged as a highly sophisticated and specialized field addressing major public health problems. The level of education and expertise necessary both to formulate and to review clinical dental research proposals is akin to that required in other highly specialized biomedical fields, such as molecular biology. Accordingly, the success of clinical dental research proposals may be enhanced by improving the quality of the research proposals. Modification of the structure or organization of peer review of population-based clinical research proposals by NIH—with the inclusion of more seasoned clinical investigators—would likely lead to more responsive and informed decisions. This may be accomplished by one or more of the following:

- the establishment of a separate study section dealing exclusively with clinical dental research proposals for investigator-initiated support,
- greater use of teleconferencing and site visits for the evaluation of clinical dental research proposals,

• greater attention to the selection of highly qualified and experienced clinical researchers to serve on study sections and more willingness on the part of clinical scientists to agree to participate on chartered study sections, and

• utilizing the RFA mechanism of NIDR to encourage high-quality, hypothesis-oriented, population-based research in oral conditions and diseases.

HUMAN RESOURCES

More well-trained, clinical investigators are needed in dental research.

Background

The task force defines a senior dental clinical scientist as one who plans, develops, coordinates, directs, and analyzes "patient-oriented or patient-related" clinical dental research. This scientist should ideally be a dentist or dental scientist with a full-time effort and a long-term commitment in clinical investigation. This individual should have training in a specific clinical specialty; a Ph.D. or comparable training in an area required for directing clinical investigations, such as epidemiology, biostatistics, or behavioral or social science, with additional training in clinical research methodology; and knowledge, either through training or experience, of cutting-edge laboratory methods from such fields as molecular and cellular biology, immunology, genetics, microbiology, and radiography that is sufficiently developed for application in patient-related research. These scientists should be able to answer fundamental questions in the clinical sciences through clinical trials, clinical studies of small populations, and epidemiologic investigations of small and large populations. In addition, they should be able to collaborate with practitioners in the transfer of relevant basic and clinical research to the patient care setting.

There are few senior dental clinical scientists in dentistry today. The task force is convinced that special effort is warranted to train a cadre of such investigators to bring the energy, direction, and unique competency needed to move dental clinical research into the large, well-coordinated, multicenter research arena.

Another group of scientists who can participate in clinical research are the dentist-scientists. Dentist-scientists presently exist in dental research, although in inadequate numbers. The preparation of dentist-scientists includes both a clinical specialty and extensive postdoctoral research training and, in most cases, a Ph.D. in a relevant basic science discipline. Such individuals usually begin their research careers in basic science. As their careers progress, some recognize the need or potential to expand their research into clinical settings. The dentist-scientists who make this transition most often have become self-educated in clinical research study design and methodology. Those fortunate enough to be located in research-intensive academic health centers frequently have developed productive alliances with epidemiologists, biostatisticians, and other clinical researchers who have helped them in the design and conduct of their clinical investigations.

The increasing backlog of needed clinical studies mandates that such individuals should either have enhanced opportunities during their initial research training to develop clinical research competencies or should be able to take advantage of specially designed senior clinical research career development opportunities.

The third category of clinical researcher the task force feels is needed is the dental clinical research associate. Within academic dentistry there is a large pool of dental clinical faculty who, although very limited in formal research training or experience, have superior clinical capabilities. Encouraged by the increasing pressure of the university for all faculty to be engaged in scholarly activity, many of these faculty would welcome the opportunity to actively assist in the conduct of clinical studies and trials.

The availability of specially designed and highly focused short-term training would quickly build a cadre of clinicians capable of executing rigorous clinical research protocols. Such research plans would typically be developed by the senior dental clinical scientists or a dentist-scientist with special clinical research training. The ability of the dental research community to carry out the needed dental clinical research agenda is dependent on a cadre of such dental clinical research associates who would function as examiners, operators, or in other roles to assist in clinical research.

To prepare for future clinical research activities in dentistry, the availability of human resources must be assured. Most urgently needed are appropriate expertise and skills to meet the expected need and demand for senior dental clinical scientists, dentist-scientists, and dental clinical research associates. This need exists in dental institutions, health science centers, private industry, and government facilities, including the FDA. A projection of the potential future need and demand for clinical researchers is provided in the section entitled Projecting the Potential Need for Clinical Researchers at the end of this appendix. A conservative estimate is that 42 senior dental clinicians and dentist scientists and 84 dental clinical research associates are needed now, assuming the present level of funding for clinical research from NIDR. If federal funding levels and industrial support are increased for clinical research, these estimates may be very low.

Recommendation

The task force recommends the establishment of a well-defined clinical research training track to develop a cadre of

senior dental clinical scientists. It is not sufficient to say that more clinical investigators are needed. What is needed is something that does not exist, or exists only in a few institutions, and that is a well-defined track, possibly leading to a graduate degree, that will train clinical investigators in all of the skills and concepts needed to carry out the full spectrum of clinical studies. Senior dental clinical scientists should be trained in (1) the ability to recognize significant clinical problems, for example, based on prevalence or impact of condition; (2) protocol design including the use of statistics for the appropriate application of such functions as power calculations and randomization and stratification methodologies; (3) implementation of the studies with detailed information on pretesting and pilot testing methodologies and assessment techniques; (4) monitoring the quality of the studies; (5) data collection, recording, management, and editing; (6) analysis of the data, including assessment of methodologic errors; and (7) data and report preparation and publication. They should also be able to design new experiments based on data interpretation and subsequent hypothesis generation.

Current federally funded options for supporting the training of dental researchers include the Dentist-Scientist Award, Physician-Scientist Award, and the National Research Service Award. Although the development of clinical research skills is provided in some programs, none of these award mechanisms emphasizes the training of clinical investigators. For this reason, NIDR should be encouraged to develop a special research training program or to modify one of the existing training or career development programs to prepare senior dental clinical scientists. Industrial and foundation support for such training is limited but could be expanded to develop sufficient numbers of well-trained clinical researchers.

The elements of training senior dental clinical scientists include academic and clinical epidemiology, research design and methods, biostatistics, clinical measurements, and clinical laboratory methodologies. Training in a clinical specialty or subspecialty may also be necessary for a fully trained, independent clinical investigator. Secondary elements in their training include ethics, conflict of interest, FDA regulatory issues, industrial issues, and commercialization such as patenting and licensing. Original thesis research involving a major representative clinical investigation would also be of importance. It is envisioned that this clinical investigator track would require full-time effort and a long-term commitment of possibly five to seven years, and that it would be comparable to a Ph.D. in basic science.

It is likely that dental schools on health sciences campuses that also have a school of public health or strong departments of public health, preventive medicine, or comparable fields with Ph.D. programs in epidemiology and biostatistics can offer the opportunity for high-quality training in clinical research.

The task force suggests the following strategies to increase the number of dentist-scientists with clinical research competencies:

• Require that essential clinical and epidemiologic research components be included in current Dentist-Scientist Awards or National Research Service Award postdoctoral research training and fellowship programs. Requests for applications for these training programs should request inclusion of specific training programs and experience in clinical research.

• Modify current or develop new clinical research career training opportunities for existing dentist-researchers who desire to move their research into clinical application.

• Provide short-term training opportunities for biostatisticians, epidemiologists, and scientists in other areas related to clinical research to facilitate the formation of dental clinical research teams.

The following strategies would increase the number of dental clinical research associates.

• Establish short-term (two to four week), highly structured training in the execution of population-based clinical studies under the terms of a clinical protocol. Such training would include not only the technical aspects of a study but, more important, an understanding of the rigors of a clinical study and the requirements for strict adherence to protocol and proper data management and data analysis procedures.

• Work with the American Dental Association, FDA, and other regulatory agencies to develop guidelines for every large clinical studies and, most important, multicenter clinical trials to ensure the training, calibration, and continued quality control of dental clinical research associates who function as examiners or operators.

BARRIERS TO THE DEVELOPMENT AND SUPPORT OF CLINICAL INVESTIGATORS IN DENTISTRY

The conduct of high-quality clinical research is hampered by several barriers to the development, support, and long-term retention of qualified and motivated clinical scientists. These barriers include inadequate fiscal resources, lack of adequately trained dental school faculty, constraints in the dental curriculum, and the culture of the dental school environment.

Background

The financial positions of most dental schools present special problems in the generation of discretionary funds that could be used to train fellows in clinical research, as frequently occurs in the hospital/medical school setting. Unlike medical education, which relies upon university or university-affiliated hospitals for clinical training, the dental school staffs, finances, and operates its own dental hospital. The cost of clinic operations, which are fundamental to the teaching program, are often borne entirely by the dental school. Unlike the teaching hospital, dental school clinics must offer care at 50 to 75 percent less than the customary fee as a patient incentive. Furthermore, dental schools frequently provide care without charge to the indigent and the uninsured. As a result, dental school clinics often operate at a financial loss.

Some 150 million people in the United States do not have dental insurance. Furthermore, unlike the universal federal medical coverage of older Americans under Medicare, dental care is not covered. Indeed, there is limited and clearly inadequate coverage of dental treatment under the federal Medicaid program. In this regard, dentistry stands outside the broader health care system. This has resulted in dental schools, hospital-based graduate dental schools, and hospital-based graduate specialty programs that lack access to significant federal clinical service funding. These constraints significantly limit the ability of dental schools to support clinical research.

There are few faculty members in dental schools adequately trained in the science of clinical research. As a result of the small number of qualified clinical researchers, few dental schools have active, state-of-the-art clinical research programs. The lack of role models may result in negative feedback that results in few faculty and students becoming committed to this career path. The availability of senior investigators who have made significant contributions through clinical research to serve as mentors may be required for the long-term development of a faculty oriented toward clinical research.

In contrast to medicine, advanced dental education is generally not based on stipends, and many programs require tuition. On the basis of 1991 estimates, the average student leaves dental school with an indebtedness of $52,130, thereby limiting the possibilities of financing further training through personal resources. The NIDR training programs provide a mechanism to overcome this problem for a limited number of trainees.

The often lockstep, four-year dental curriculum demands a major commitment of time from clinical faculty to train independent dental practitioners. Because dental schools must graduate competent clinicians, dental students cannot be mere observers but must be the active providers of care. Therefore, in addition to providing didactic education in the basic and clinical sciences, the dental school provides hands-on training in all aspects of clinical dentistry. With dental students performing mainly irreversible procedures on patients, the need for intensive, direct, and constant supervision by clinical faculty is clear. As a result, clinical researchers are not always recognized or compensated for participating in clinical research. One recognition would be commensurate release from clinical teaching responsibilities. Such release time is critical both to the successful conduct of the individual study and for maintaining an environment that rewards success in scholarly endeavors.

The culture of U.S. dental schools also presents special problems in the development of an environment conducive to successful clinical research. Most of the mature dental faculty have the formal qualifications to practice general dentistry or a dental specialty; few, however, have training or experience in scholarly activity. Faculty background, training, and interest, coupled with the need to prepare students to be independent practitioners in a technically demanding discipline, have resulted in an understandable emphasis on clinical training and technique in four short years. Unfortunately, emphasis on the clinician as a scholar has suffered.

Perhaps the most critical barrier to the development of mature, independent scientists in dentistry is that few dental schools provide an environment in which this development can easily occur. For example, there is often a lack of critical mass of scientists, mentors are not available, and resources needed in the early years of a scientist's career are often not allocated. Although more schools provide such an environment than was the case just 10 or 20 years ago, it still is difficult for the Ph.D. or D.D.S.-Ph.D. to succeed as a competitive, productive scientist without postdoctoral training and extended association with more mature scientists in the field. The clinical investigator is no exception. There are few schools where the environment is supportive of the young clinical investigator. The task force strongly believes that it is at this step in the training and maturation of a clinician-scientist (including the clinical scientist) that the dental academic system is most apt to fail.

Recommendations

The task force recommends that tenure-track appointments be reserved for faculty who participate fully in teaching, research, and service. Faculty devoted only to teaching or only to research may be placed on a fixed contract. Dental faculties and dental schools are in a time of transition from being institutions focused on technical training to becoming institutions that are true members of the university academic community.

It is also recommended that institutions with minimal ongoing research recruit as department chairs successful midcareer clinical scholars who will be capable of building a research program and serving as role models and mentors. It is recognized that many dental schools want to increase their research enterprises. Newly trained individuals need the support of such an environment to be successful over the long term. New clinical scientists (immediately after training) should not be appointed to positions where they do not have the time or the environment to be mentored and developed into independent investigators.

The task force recommends that time and other resources such as space and start-up funds need to be made available to faculty undertaking clinical research. When research projects are extramurally supported, the salary released should be used to free investigators from their teaching load in keeping with the scope of the projects. These funds can then be used to expand the number of faculty and the research base of the department and institution. Over the long term, means of restructuring the financing of preventive and therapeutic dental care and the financial struture of the dental education system should be explored.

The task force recommends that mechanisms need to be established at each dental school to ensure that discretionary funded release time, overhead recovery, and salary release are used to provide support for innovative high-risk, start-up, or carry-over research activities.

Measurement of Outcomes

Long-term measures of the success of implementation of the task force recommendations include an estimate of the number of drugs, devices, and technologies that are made available to clinicians resulting in better treatment and more effective prevention of oral diseases in the years after implementation of the recommendations. More specific and near-term measures of success include more research funds devoted to clinical dental research by government and private industry, more clinical researchers engaged in population-based studies of oral disease, and more frequent and higher-quality publication of the results of clinical research projects.

Projecting the Potential Need for Clinical Researchers

It is difficult to project the potential need and demand for clinical researchers among private industry, the federal government, health science centers, and other such institutions. One can try to project possible needs, however, at least among U.S. dental institutions, which will be the most likely future employers of most of these individuals.

The methodologic approach used to project personnel needs in the near future is based on approximations of the number of clinical research grants that could be funded through NIDR support and the number of clinical researchers (that is, senior dental clinical scientists, dentist-scientists, and dental clinical research associates) needed to direct and conduct these investigations. A conservative approach is based on a situation of no growth in the percentage of grant dollars awarded for clinical research by NIDR. The assumptions include the following:

- In fiscal year 1991, between 20 and 25 percent of NIDR extramural research support went to clinical research studies, and approximately 20 percent of NIDR extramural research funds for new and competing renewal applications supported clinical research projects. In the immediate future, it is assumed that the distribution of NIDR extramural support for clinical research will be about 20 percent. This does not imply, however, that this ratio should be perpetuated.
- The average cost of a clinical research grant may remain approximately $160,000. This is based on data for fiscal year 1991. (It is highly probable, however, that the average cost of these grants will increase substantially in the future.)
- Each senior dental clinical scientist and dentist-scientist could be involved, as a principal investigator, in no more than two active grants. (This is based on NIDR data which showed that, in fiscal year 1990, 80 principal investigators had two active NIDR research grants and 16 had three or more active awards.)
- One full-time dental clinical research associate is needed for each grant as a coprincipal investigator.
- Existing clinical researchers are working at maximum capacity. Therefore, the projected number of clinical researchers needed is assumed to be in addition to those already holding positions at dental institutions. (The actual number of the latter is unknown.)

The projected number of research personnel needed by U.S. dental institutions—on the basis of current level of NIDR funding for clinical research and the assumptions listed above—are 42 well-trained senior dental clinical scientists and dentist-scientists and 84 dental clinical research associates. Changes in funding levels or in the set of assumptions will necessitate a revised estimate for needed clinical investigators. It should also be noted that these individuals would be *in addition to* those more oriented to the basic laboratory sciences who are already being trained through the dentist-scientist and physician-scientist award programs of NIDR. Further, and perhaps most important, this does not account for the clinical research personnel needs of private industry and nondental institutions in health science centers, hospitals, and the other employees of clinical dental researchers, which are not easily estimated but may be large and growing.

TASK FORCE MEMBERS

ROBERT J. GENCO, Chair, Associate Dean for Graduate Studies,
Distinguished Professor and Chairman, Department of Oral Biology,
School of Dental Medicine, State University of New York at Buffalo,
Buffalo, New York

JAMES W. BAWDEN, Alumni Distinguished Professor, Department of
Pediatric Dentistry, School of Dentistry, University of North Carolina,
Chapel Hill, North Carolina

MARJORIE K. JEFFCOAT, Rosen Professor and Chairman, Department of
Periodontics, School of Dentistry, University of Alabama,
Birmingham, Alabama

JAMES A. LIPTON, Special Assistant for Scientific Development,
Epidemiology and Oral Disease Prevention Program, National Institute
of Dental Research, National Institutes of Health, Bethesda, Maryland

PRESTON A. LITTLETON, JR., Executive Director, American Association of
Dental Schools, Washington, D.C.

JOSEPH J. ZAMBON, Professor, Department of Oral Biology and Department
of Periodontology, State University of New York at Buffalo, Buffalo,
New York

Appendix B

Report of the Task Force on Clinical Research in Nursing and Clinical Psychology

CLINICAL RESEARCH IN NURSING

Nurses who conduct clinical research share commonalities and differences with professionals in other health-related disciplines who are engaged in research. Advances in science, health crises such as AIDS, changes in health care delivery, and population changes over the past few decades have yielded opportunities for clinical research that nurses need to improve health care delivery and the health of the American public. Nevertheless, the limited number of nurses with the doctoral training needed to conduct clinical research and oversee research training, the erosion of federal funding for research and research training, and the frequent lack of administrative and financial incentives to pursue research rather than more financially rewarding administrative or other positions in the clinical and private sector mitigate against the pursuit of careers in clinical research.

Although the focus of nursing research has shifted over more than a century, its roots were formed in clinical practice and remain in clinical practice. Nursing research dates to the mid-1800s and the work of Florence Nightingale on the impact of nursing care on morbidity and mortality of soldiers during the Crimean War. From the turn of the century through the 1940s, nursing research focused on nursing education. Much of the preparation of nurses during that period was oriented toward providing an apprentice service rather than what most would consider an education. With World War II, the unprecedented demand for nurses shifted the focus of research to the supply and demand for nurses, the hospital environment, and the status of staff nurses. A variety of converging forces resulted in an escalation in nursing research in the 1950s. This included an increase in the number of nurses with advanced educational degrees and the availability of many master's programs that required a thesis, the establishment of the nursing research grants and fellowship programs of the Division of Nursing of the Public Health Service, establishment of the American Nurses' Foundation to foster research, and the establishment of the professional journal *Nursing Research* (Polit and Hungler, 1978; Wilson, 1985). In the 1960s the focus was on theoretical bases for nursing practice, along with a continuing attention to students and nursing education. From the 1970s to the present the focus of research in nursing has been on the improvement of patient care. Establishment of the National Center for Nursing Research at the National Institutes of Health (NIH) in 1985 not only fostered these efforts but also, by establishing a national nursing research agenda, served to draw the research efforts of nurses into priority areas.

In nursing research, training is well developed from the undergraduate level, through the postdoctoral level, and through midcareer development. Nurses currently holding doctorates may have been prepared for clinical research through a nursing doctoral program or a doctoral program in a related discipline such as one in the biological, social, or behavioral sciences. The pool of doctorate-prepared nurses capable of pursuing careers in clinical research is on the increase. The number of such individuals, however, is insufficient to meet the current demand in academic and clinical settings where research and research training are conducted. In addition, the frequent lack of administrative and undervaluing of support of clinical research, combined with the availability of lucrative administrative, clinical, and consultative positions, reduces the number of individuals drawn to and retained in clinical research.

Research Opportunities

There are numerous opportunities for clinical research in nursing. Nursing research focuses on major public health issues with the purpose of providing accurate and reliable information that will improve nursing practice. The ultimate goal is to promote health and ameliorate disease for the American public. The critical issue is the need to accelerate the conduct and support of nursing research and research training to more effectively attack public health concerns.

Nursing research involves the study of the human biological and psychological responses to health and illness across the life span. Nursing research does not focus on disease or the treatment of disease but rather on individuals' and families' responses to the disease and subsequent treatments. There is a strong orientation toward health promotion and disease prevention and enhancing individuals' and families' independence in health and illness. Taking a holistic perspective, nursing research generates knowledge about:

- health promotion and disease prevention across the life span,
- therapeutic actions to mitigate the effects of illness and treatment,
- optimal functioning in chronic illness,
- special and physical environments that influence health and illness,
- innovative and efficient systems for enhancing quality care and desired individual and family outcomes,
- maximal independence in health and disease, and
- emphasis on vulnerable populations.

A strong interdisciplinary focus is evident and encouraged for nursing research and research training. Given the complexity of clinical nursing research concerns and questions, synthesis of knowledge from across many disciplines is required in the quest to generate new information for nursing practice.

The scope of nursing research opportunities is broad. To focus resources in several critical public health areas, the nursing research community as well as the Advisory Council and staff of the National Center for Nursing Research have identified a National Nursing Research Agenda consisting of seven priorities. These are staged in a three-step framework that allows for refinement of the priorities and implementation with targeted resources. The priorities include:

- Stage I
  — Low birthweight: mothers and infants
  — HIV infection: prevention and care
- Stage II
  — Long-term care for older adults
  — Symptom assessment and management of acute pain in adults
  — Nursing information: support for patient care
- Stage III
  — Health promotion for children and adolescents
  — Technology dependency across the life span

In addition to the identified priorities, much research has arisen from the science evolving from the current nursing research base. These include:

- symptom management of clinical conditions secondary to illness and treatment,
- women's midlife health issues,
- health promotion and disease prevention (community and environmental issues),
- biobehavioral interface issues with increased biological studies,

- clinical bioethics concerns,
- health promotion within chronic illnesses for vulnerable populations (older persons, individuals at high risk for a specific illness, children, and so forth),
    - rural health problems,
- innovative practice systems to enhance desired individual and family outcomes,
    - nurse-sensitive patient outcomes and cost factors, and
    - culturally sensitive interventions.

These are only samples of the current opportunities for nursing research; many others could be cited or will evolve over time.

Barriers

Several barriers inhibit the growth of nursing research and impede the ability of nurses to take full advantage of the numerous research opportunities. These include the following:

- In several of the areas of research opportunities, there are a limited number of individuals with the clinical and research training required to investigate crucial areas, for example, biobehavioral interface, clinical bioethical issues, and symptom management with biologically based problems.
- The opportunities and the need to attack critical public health problems are growing more rapidly than the resources available for clinical nursing research and research training. Although this reflects a "fighting success" phenomenon, the lack of resources limits the profession's ability to respond fully to important health problems.
- Well-established research programs that can provide a strong base for clinical knowledge and for research training are limited. These programs and the accompanying cadre of nurse-scientists need to be enhanced.
- The number of research-intensive environments that can respond quickly to health crises is limited but developing rapidly. The growth of such institutional environments needs to be facilitated to support research and research training.
- Access to clinical settings and to consenting human subjects needs to be enhanced. Both institutional and professional barriers are evident in clinical nursing research. Access for independent nurse-investigators is critical to the quality of the research conducted and the science developed for nursing practices.

Recommendations

The task force recommends the promotion of the development of mechanisms, long-term plans, and strategies to focus research efforts; the enhancement of the development of research-intensive environments for clinical nursing research and research training and career development; and increased funding and resources to support the rapid growth of clinical nursing and its focus on critical public health issues.

Human Resources

There are approximately 9,000 doctorate-prepared nurses in this country; about 20 to 25 percent of this group is conducting research. Approximately 80 percent of doctorate-prepared nurses hold educator or administrative positions in academic and service settings where there is little expectation for research. Only in the late 1970s could one note an expectation of nursing research by the faculty in schools with master's degree programs and developing doctoral programs. Even into the 1980s, however, only 15–20 schools of nursing had achieved a sufficient research base each year to qualify for Biomedical Research Support Grants, which require only that the institution have federal grant awards totaling $200,000 from at least three separate grant awards.

There is a need to encourage the development of nursing doctoral programs in research-intensive institutions and to develop cadres of nurse researchers in schools that prepare nurse researchers. Although nurses had received limited federal funding for research in the mid-1980s with the establishment of the National Center for Nursing Research at NIH, increased resources became available for nurse-researchers to engage actively in federally funded research. Additionally, nurse researchers are encouraged to seek funding from other federal sources and from private funding sources.

In addition to the group of doctorate-prepared nurses conducting clinical research, there are tens of thousands of nurses trained at the master's level who are involved in clinical research. This involvement includes serving as research nurses in clinical centers, working as research project managers, serving as data collectors, or conducting small-scale, limited clinical practice studies.

Because doctoral programs in nursing are relatively new, many nurses who hold doctorates received them in related disciplines such as psychology, education, sociology, physiology, and the like. In 1963 there were 4 doctoral programs, whereas there were 52 in 1988. Doctoral programs in nursing currently are producing approximately 330 new graduates annually (Bednash et al., 1992).

An examination of the human resource profile of clinical researchers in nursing reveals two clear needs. First, although the number of nurses with doctorates has increased rapidly over the past 20 years, more are needed. Second, there is an equal need to maintain the productivity of those already engaged in research and research training. Because of the limited pool of nurses with doctorates prepared for and engaged in research, this small group bears the heavy burden of conducting clinical research studies to develop the underpinnings of clinical practice to improve care and of conducting research training at all levels. One mechanism that has been effective in developing nursing research has been to involve nurses in interdisciplinary clinical research centers and programs. Such participation by nurses has served both to provide nurses with valuable research experience and to add a nursing perspective to the study of patient problems.

The numbers of doctorate-prepared faculty are insufficient to fill positions in graduate programs, and heavy faculty workloads further compromise research activities. Of the full-time faculty teaching in graduate programs, 78 percent hold a doctorate (approximately 31 percent in nursing), and only 45 percent of the part-time faculty hold a doctorate (11 percent in nursing) (National League for Nursing, 1989). The lack of adequate numbers of nurses with doctorates to serve as faculty exercises a qualitative as well as a quantitative constraint on the continued growth in the numbers of doctorally prepared nurses and hampers research training at all levels. Heavy faculty work-loads are also problematic. Data from the National League for Nursing (NLN) indicate that only faculty teaching at the graduate level report any time devoted to research.

This same limited pool of doctorate-prepared nurses is also actively involved in clinical research. In funding year 1988, 91 percent of the research applications from schools, colleges, or departments of nursing were headed by doctorate-prepared investigators, compared with 76 percent in 1984 (U.S. Department of Health and Human Services, Public Health Service, National Institutes of Health, 1989).

Barriers

The barriers to increasing the numbers of doctorate-prepared nurses capable of conducting independent clinical research studies and research training include a lack of money for research training and the conduct of research, the lack of competitive salaries in academic settings to promote research and training, too few mechanisms to promote career development in clinical research, and a need to enhance the research intensity in some of the environments preparing doctoral students in the discipline.

Although increased numbers of doctorate-prepared nurses are needed, there is an equal need to maintain the productivity of those already engaged in the conduct of research and research training. Salaries for doctorate-prepared nurse faculty are not competitive with those for nurses in the practice setting. In some areas of the country, the annual salaries of doctorate-prepared nurses working in academic settings are approximately equal to those of a newly graduated staff nurse with an undergraduate preparation. This disparity draws some doctorate-prepared nurses out of the academic setting and into more financially rewarding roles in the service and private sectors.

There is a need to enhance the research intensity at some research training sites to ensure the rigor of clinical research training. The current need for this enhancement has arisen, in part, from the rapid growth of doctoral programs in nursing, which draw from the limited pool of doctorate-prepared individuals in the discipline.

Recommendations

The task force recommends that the development of more Ph.D. programs in nursing at research-intensive institutions be encouraged. In addition, it urges the promotion of the development of more targeted research centers in schools of nursing that prepare nurse-researchers and the involvement of nurse faculty in strong interdisciplinary clinical research centers and programs. Organizational mechanisms that reward nursing faculty economically for conducting research should also be encouraged.

Clinical Research Training

Formal research training in nursing is well developed. It begins at the undergraduate level and proceeds through the postdoctoral level and midcareer development. The NLN, the profession's educational accrediting body for the undergraduate and master's programs, emphasizes and requires instruction in research methods in the curriculum. In 1981 the American Nurses' Association Commission on Nursing Research outlined the investigative functions for nurses at the baccalaureate, master's, and doctoral levels on the basis of the research training provided to nurses.

At the baccalaureate level, the focus of training is to prepare a knowledgeable research consumer. All baccalaureate nursing programs have an identifiable research content, which may be taught in separate courses or integrated into several courses. Such courses often focus on the critique and basic design of research as a problem-solving process. Basic statistics may be required as a separate course or integrated into nursing research courses. The basic baccalaureate prepared nurse should be prepared to do the following:

   • read, interpret, and evaluate research for applicability to nursing practice,

   • identify nursing problems that need to be investigated and participate in the implementation of scientific studies,

   • use nursing practice as a means of gathering data for refining and extending practice,

   • apply established research findings of nursing and other health-related research to nursing practice, and

   • share research findings with colleagues (American Nurses Association, Commission on Nursing Research, 1981).

     At the master's level, the nurse is prepared to be an active collaborator in research. The focus of the research component of the master's curriculum in nursing is on a more in-depth critique of research, deriving testable hypotheses or research questions from theory or practice, and application or utilization of research in clinical settings. Applications may be focused in a clinical specialty area and functional area (practitioner, teaching, or management role). Most programs have at least one formal research course, statistics content, and basic computer science content that builds upon baccalaureate research instruction. A thesis is often required; some programs, however, require research-focused clinical projects that involve literature review and critique in a topical area, written research reports, case studies, or research-oriented clinical assignments.

     The American Nurses' Association (ANA) Commission on Nursing Research's (1981) guidelines for the investigative functions for the master's prepared nurse are as follows:

   • analyze and reformulate nursing practice problems so that scientific knowledge methods can be used to find solutions,

   • enhance the quality and clinical relevance of nursing research by providing expertise in clinical problems and by providing knowledge about the way in which these clinical services are delivered,

   • facilitate investigations of problems in clinical settings through such activities as contributing to a climate supportive of investigative activities, collaborating with others in investigations, and enhancing nursing's access to clients and data,

   • conduct investigations for the purpose of monitoring the quality of the practice of nursing in a clinical setting, and

   • assist others in applying scientific knowledge in nursing practice.

     At the doctoral level, nurses may be prepared for clinical research through a nursing doctoral program or through a doctoral program in a related discipline, such as in the biological, social, or behavioral sciences.

There are three kinds of doctoral nursing programs: doctor of philosophy (Ph.D.), doctor of nursing science (D.N.S., D.S.N., D.N.S.C.), and the doctor of education (Ed.D.). The Ph.D. focuses primarily on research and builds upon the clinical specialty training most nurses obtain at the master's level. The doctor of nursing science generally focuses on high-level preparation for nursing practice, with additional research training above the master's degree level. The Ed.D. in nursing emphasizes teaching of nursing and conducting research on nursing education problems. The standard doctoral program in nursing requires 60 semester credits above the master's degree, with about 75 percent of required credits in nursing and 25 percent in related cognate areas or electives. Approximately 50 percent of total required credits focus on research (Ziemer et al., 1992). The environments and actual mentorship experiences in research in doctoral programs in nursing, however, are uneven.

The ANA Commission on Nursing Research (1981) specified guidelines for the research functions of nurses from both practice-oriented and research-oriented programs. The graduate of a practice-oriented nursing doctoral program:

- provides leadership for the integration of scientific knowledge with other sources of knowledge for the advancement of practice,
- conducts investigations to evaluate the contributions of nursing activities to the well-being of clients, and
- develops methods to monitor the quality of the practice of nursing in a clinical setting and to evaluate contributions of nursing activities to the well-being of clients (American Nurese Association, 1981).

The graduate of a research-oriented program:

- develops theoretical explanations of phenomena relevant to nursing by empirical research and analytical processes,
- uses analytical empirical methods to discover ways to modify or extend existing scientific knowledge so that it is relevant to nursing, and
- develops methods for scientific inquiry of phenomena relevant to nursing (American Nurses' Association, Commission on Nursing Research, 1981).

Postdoctoral research training in nursing provides intensive research mentorship with a productive and established investigator in the area of specific research interest to the trainee. A nursing postdoctoral trainee may be mentored by a nurse-investigator, an investigator in a related discipline, or a nurse-investigator in collaboration with an investigator from another discipline. A nurse may receive National Research Service Award support for full-time postdoctoral study if approved for funding within the first five years after graduation from a doctoral program. Nurses who choose to engage in their own postdoctoral research with the support of a mentor for 50 percent of their time while also working may obtain a FIRST award (R29). Approval for a FIRST award, however, must also be obtained within the first five years after graduating from a doctoral program. Academic Career Awards (K series awards) may be obtained by nurse-investigators who have been out of their doctoral program for more than five years and who wish to initiate a postdoctoral midcareer mentorship by becoming a coprincipal investigator or research associate on the R01 grant of a senior investigator. In addition to federal awards, some private foundations support nurses for postdoctoral training.

Nursing has relatively little difficulty attracting nurses into doctoral education or research-oriented programs. A major challenge, however, is developing nurse-researchers with a career commitment to clinical research. Clinical nurse-investigators need mentors and role models, as well as satisfactory rewards, resources, and environmental or institutional support, to help them to develop and maintain research careers.

In academic and clinical institutions, there is often a lack of nurse-mentors and role models with a lifetime career commitment to research. Strong nurse-mentors who are productive in clinical research are important in facilitating research-intensive environments that foster the research development of predoctoral students and the career development of doctorate-prepared nurses who are beginning their clinical research programs. Nurse-researchers who work in low-intensity research environments without adequate mentors or role models often feel isolated and that they do not have the necessary collegial support to launch and maintain a career that is characterized by sustained clinical research productivity.

Most positions for clinical nurse-researchers are in academic settings, which have lower entry-level salaries and fewer rewards than positions in clinical institutions. Academic positions are not enticing to nurses who have made major financial investments in their doctoral education, while at the same time foregoing income they could have made if they had remained in their clinical positions. In addition, the work demands above and beyond the research responsibilities in academia are great, and they pose problems if the nurse-researcher is to achieve promotion and tenure. Doctorate-prepared nurses often find greater financial rewards and support in nonresearch roles, particularly in clinical settings. Therefore, a lifelong research career, which is most often based in a university, does not have great appeal for many nurses.

Heavy workloads are problematic for clinical nurse-researchers in both academic and clinical settings. In the academic setting this is especially true for undergraduate faculty with heavy responsibilities for student clinical supervision. Survey data from the NLN indicate that there is, on average, no time reported as being devoted to research by faculty teaching at the undergraduate level. Doctorate-prepared nurses employed in clinical settings often face a workload dilemma as well, because they have heavy administrative or managerial responsibilities that may not leave adequate time for clinical research.

Many nurses do not have adequate organizational and administrative support for a career in clinical research. Institutional support of research at all levels is necessary to facilitate research productivity and to foster research-intensive environments. This support is required in two forms: by the leadership at the university and school levels (or organizational and departmental levels) and through a valuing of research within the organizational culture. Researchers based in schools and departments of nursing require access to resources and rewards within their own divisions as well as in the broader institutional environment. Administrators often control the resources and rewards required to support the development of research careers and productivity. The policies of an institution often communicate institutional values that influence mores and norms and, thus, an organizational culture that can be supportive of research. Administrative behaviors and decisions at all levels are often important in helping to establish such a culture.

The careers of nurse-researchers could also be facilitated by bridging mechanisms between career steps in clinical research. In most cases, nurses reenter the practice arena between their educational degrees, which results in interruptions in research training. Although clinical experience is beneficial to the nurse-researcher because it helps to clarify research problems in need of investigation, such interruptions thwart progress in the research career and often keep nurse-investigators from proceeding with much-needed postdoctoral education. This problem can be addressed by making more flexible research awards available for clinical nurse-researchers. One approach that would help keep predoctoral trainees involved through postdoctoral education for up to five years would be to support three years of predoctoral training and to continue to support the trainee through two additional years of postdoctoral work. More flexible K series awards for nurses who require midcareer training or delayed postdoctoral experience would be useful.

Barriers

There are three major barriers to the training of clinical nurse-researchers. These include a lack of understanding of research training of nurses, lack of funds for research training and career development, and lack of awareness of the needs of new and established clinical nurse-investigators by administrators within the research environment.

Although research training of nurses begins early in their careers in the baccalaureate program, the public, other health care providers, and many nurses do not understand the nature, depth, or breadth of research training and opportunities that are received by clinical nurse-researchers. The nurse's role is still often perceived as totally delegated by the physician. There is not a clear understanding that nursing is a separate profession that defines the majority of its health care interventions independently and builds and seeks knowledge that will improve the quality and effectiveness of care through research. This lack of understanding of nursing and its role in health care research has not only limited the clinical nurse-researcher's access to necessary resources to conduct research programs but also to the funding necessary for research training.

Lack of funds for research training and development, particularly at the predoctoral and postdoctoral levels, has impeded the growth of an adequate pool of clinical nurse-researchers. Nurses who are interested in becoming clinical nurse-researchers are often older and have more financial responsibilities than trainees in other disciplines. In addition, research trainee support levels are very low compared with the salaries that can be earned by master's-prepared nurses who work in clinical settings. Hence, there is little financial incentive to pursue further training and a career in research.

Once clinical nurse-researchers receive their preparation, they often are employed in settings where administrators are unfamiliar with the needs and support required by young investigators to establish successful research programs and careers. As noted previously, it is not unusual for heavy workloads, isolation, lack of resources, and low-intensity research environments to mitigate against the productivity of new clinical nurse-researchers.

Recommendations

The task force recommends promotion of an institutional leadership that supports and values clinical nursing research and clinical nurse investigators, increased availability and levels of funding for research training and career development in clinical nursing research, and promotion of the education of the public and people in other health care disciplines regarding the research training of nurses.

References

American Nurses' Association, Commission on Nursing Research. 1981. Guidelines for the Investigative Functions of Nurses. Kansas City, Mo: American Nurses' Association.

Bednash, G., L.E. Berlin, and L. Chan. 1992. 1991–1992 Enrollment and Graduations in Baccalaureate and Graduate Programs in Nursing. Washington, D.C.: American Association of Colleges of Nursing.

National League for Nursing. 1989. National Data Review: 1988. Publication No. 19-2290. New York.

Polit, D., and B. Hungler. 1978. Nursing Research: Principles & Methods. Philadelphia: J.B. Lippincott.

U.S Department of Health and Human Services, Public Health Service, National Institutes of Health. 1989. Report of the 1989 National Institutes of Health Task Force on Nursing Research. National Institutes of Health Publication No. 89–487. Washington, D.C.

Wilson, H. 1985. Research in Nursing. Reading, Mass: Addison-Wesley.

Ziemer, M.M., J. Brown, M.L. Fitzpatrick, C. Manfredi, J. O'Leary, and T.M. Valiga. 1992. Doctoral programs in nursing: Philosophy, curricula, and program requirements. Professional Nursing 8(1):56–62.

CLINICAL RESEARCH IN PSYCHOLOGY

Psychologists who perform clinical research have commonalities and differences from other professional groups involved in the research endeavor. Scientific advances such as the proliferation of the knowledge base in the neurosciences have benefited many clinical researchers, including psychologists. Some professional barriers are also shared by psychologists and at least some other professional groups engaged in clinical research. Shared barriers include the erosion of federal support for graduate training and continuous financial disincentives to pursue research as opposed to clinical practice.

To provide a context for what follows, it may be helpful to describe some of psychology's relatively novel features as a profession and scientific discipline. One unusual characteristic is that training in the research enterprise begins at the undergraduate level and progresses continuously through the first several years of graduate school. It is not uncommon for promising young students to become involved in a laboratory under the tutelage of a research mentor, to author or coauthor one or more empirical publications before graduation, and to continue research, progressing toward a Ph.D. dissertation in the laboratory of a graduate school mentor. This progression reflects the strong emphasis that is placed on training in the scientific method at all phases in the educational process. The origins of this training philosophy reside in the beginning of academic psychology, which started with a tradition of experimentalism modeled after that in physics (Cronbach, 1957). The field's core scientific values have always included a commitment to empirical research and hypothesis testing. Only relatively recently has this orientation been brought to bear upon explicitly clinical research problems. Psychologists did not become extensively engaged in addressing clinical problems until World War II, when they were called to the task of developing personality tests to assess the fitness of potential recruits for military service. Clinical psychology only emerged as a subspecialty when, as the war effort continued, psychologists were recruited into psychiatric hospitals, initially to assist in the assessment and later in the treatment of combat veterans.

Once in the medical setting, their research expertise was enlisted to study a growing variety of health problems.

Clinical psychology's academic and scientific roots are preserved in its philosophy about the optimal balance between research and clinical training. Major professional accrediting groups have repeatedly endorsed the scientist-practitioner (or Boulder) model, which emphasizes a strong training base in science as a precondition for beginning to undertake thoughtful clinical practice. Unique among the professional groups drawn to clinical research, doctorates in clinical psychology complete at least three years of research-oriented training in the content and scientific methodology of the discipline before embarking upon the intensive clinical internship. The intent is to develop a conceptual framework that enables students to critically evaluate the scientific grounding of the current knowledge base rather than assimilating a static collection of facts (McGovern et al., 1991). An additional aim is to encourage students to adopt a scientific approach to clinical practice, generating hypotheses about the mechanisms that sustain maladaptive or unhealthy behaviors, consulting the relevant empirical literature, and subjecting their interventions to the test of clinical response. Because the modification of cognition and behavior is a core training area in most accredited programs (Sayette and Mayne, 1990), clinical psychologists are unusually well equipped to study and intervene in the behavioral factors that initiate and maintain a variety of psychological and physical disorders.

Throughout this appendix it will be important to note that other groups of psychologists are also well-trained to make important contributions to clinical research. Examples include Ph.D.s in the areas of developmental, personality, social, and experimental psychology. Although lacking specific training in techniques of clinical assessment and therapy, nonclinical psychologists also possess extremely strong grounding in research methodology. Nonclinical psychologists also possess intensive training in one or more of the areas of human learning, perception, cognition, motivation, physiology, emotion, and interpersonal behavior. This training background leaves both clinical and nonclinical psychologists well-equipped to make important discoveries about the mechanisms that give rise to mental and physical health problems.

Research Opportunities

Excellent scientific training has enabled Ph.D. psychologists to make important contributions to the understanding of many clinical problems. Substantial faculty expertise and research funding are already consolidated in certain domains (Sayette and Mayne, 1990), where the field is poised to fulfill its research promise.

Well-Established Areas of Investigation

Behavioral Medicine and Health Psychology Health psychology is a relatively new area of investigation that aims to understand the biopsychosocial factors that promote or prevent illness. Despite the field's youth, expertise and interest in behavioral medicine have grown rapidly, giving the area nearly twice the faculty and funding as any other domain of clinical psychology research (Sayette and Mayne, 1990). Two examples of psychologists' important contributions to clinical research in behavioral medicine concern cardiovascular risk factors and the influence of psychosocial factors on immune system function. Risk factors for cardiovascular disease have also been studied intensively, with much research focusing upon the type A personality, including its emergence during childhood. A significant new discovery concerns the heightened cardiovascular risk that is associated with repeated cycles of weight loss and gain. Although the underlying cause of the weight cycler's heightened risk remains unclear, the finding suggests a need to reevaluate potential health risks that may arise from the culturally ubiquitous practice of dieting.

Another area that holds enormous excitement and promise is psychoneuroimmunology, which examines the interdisciplinary interface among psychological, neural, and endocrine influences on the immune system. Understanding how psychosocial factors may mediate the initial susceptibility or the course of cancer or AIDS may one day enable clinicians to harness such influences in treatment.

Psychopathology Accredited clinical psychology programs possess resources in many areas of psychopathology. Expertise in schizophrenia and the affective disorders is well-established. During the past decade, new pools of talent and funding have emerged in the areas of anxiety disorders, eating disorders, and childhood psychopathology. Research in psychopathology is shedding light on genetic and psychosocial contributions to the etiology of mental disorders, their development across the life span, behavioral and pharmacologic treatments, and wider psychosocial problems, such as the homeless mentally ill.

Neuropsychology Embracing a broad knowledge base that reaches from molecular findings in the neurosciences to clinical rehabilitation efforts with brain-injured individuals, neuropsychology has become a well-established domain of inquiry. Neuropsychologists have profited from the emergence of new technologies in neuroimaging, which permit them to study the neural substrates for cognitive and affective processing of information. Findings are being applied to understand and remediate the behavioral and emotional effects of brain injury.

Children Psychologists have had a longstanding commitment to the study of children. Interest and expertise in assessing emerging cognitive capabilities have contributed to the development of programs like Head Start. Much current interest now focuses on the nature and origins of temperamental traits such as shyness and how these dovetail or clash with an individual's environmental niche. The socioemotional impacts of broader social influences including television, day care, and parental work roles have also been studied, as have a variety of societal problems. The latter include issues such as the short- and long-term effects of family conflict, abuse, criminality, and maternal psychopathology.

Aging Psychologists have also turned their attention to problems associated with aging, including determining the extent to which declining cognitive functions and deteriorating physical health are inevitable, as well as what can be done to delay or minimize their impacts. Studies are progressing on the development of family and community support systems, strategies for coping with chronic health problems, and the interaction between emotional and biological functioning.

Promising Newer Areas of Investigation

Clinical research into complex, entrenched sociobehavioral problems is less mature. Promising beginnings have been made, however, that put the field in a position to contribute significant advances to understanding and influencing some costly and demoralizing problems that plague U.S. society. Promising, high-need areas include the following.

Violence and Aggression At both individual and sociocultural levels, clinical psychology has begun to develop a knowledge base aimed at understanding the effects of such violent acts as homicide, rape, and child abuse on victims and survivors. Intervention methods are being developed to minimize that impact. In addition, a coherent pattern is starting to emerge from the multiple factors that cause an individual or group to commit violent acts, and deterrent interventions are beginning to show promise.

Substance Abuse At a time when intravenous drug abuse has become a major vehicle for the transmission of AIDS and drug-related crimes and violence plague many communities, the societal impact of substance abuse is only too apparent. Important progress has been made in unraveling the processes that lead to abuse and dependence upon a variety of psychoactive substances ranging from caffeine to tobacco, alcohol, opiates, and cocaine. One significant contribution to this area has been the discovery of conditioned physiological compensatory (drug-opposite) responses, whose activation thwarts the likelihood of death from drug overdose. A second area of progress concerns efforts to understand the nature and relapse relevance of the phenomenon of drug craving. A third concerns studies of nicotine's apparently increasing appeal to American females as a weight-suppressing agent, and the consequences of this phenomenon for initiating and sustaining cigarette smoking among females.

Prevention An overriding research opportunity that unites all of the areas previously mentioned involves psychological research on the prevention of clinical problems. Once established, the treatment refractoriness of chronic medical illness, psychopathology, violence, and substance abuse is impressive, arguing for the need for prevention before these disturbances become firmly entrenched. To be maximally successful, it is essential that preventive research and intervention be grounded upon a firm interdisciplinary base. For example, it is critical to muster the expertise of developmental psychologists who can tailor interventions to mesh with the capacities and interests of children. Similarly, population impact is maximized by interdisciplinary efforts that draw upon the skills of epidemiologists trained with a public health perspective. Clinical psychologists bring to the collaborative enterprise an extremely strong training background in research design and methods and an academic history of openness to interdisciplinary work. Their research expertise can be applied readily to almost any problem in which behavior potentially enhances or allays risk. This flexibility contributes to the broad diversity of clinical research opportunities in psychology.

Human Resources

There exists a large pool of psychologists who have been well-trained to conduct clinical research. The National Science Foundation's latest biennial survey registered 60,596 Ph.D. psychologists employed as scientists (Brush, 1991). More doctorates are awarded in the health service provider areas of psychology, of which the largest subdiscipline is clinical psychology, than in any other discipline of psychology. For example, of the 3,209 Ph.D.s awarded in 1989, approximately 1,840 doctorates were awarded in the subfields of clinical, counseling, and school psychology, with the remainder divided among six other subfields (National Research Council, 1990). Over half of full-time doctoral students (56 percent) and about two thirds of full-time master's students were enrolled in the health service provider subfields in 1989–1990 (Kohout et al., 1992).

The pool of students who want predoctoral training in clinical psychology remains deep; there are many more applicants for graduate school than there are slots available. This applicant pool is also quite intellectually talented. In

1989, the median Graduate Record Examination scores of students entering graduate training in psychology were: verbal, 601; quantitative, 620; total, 1,220. Separate figures could not be obtained for clinical psychology alone, but in the vast majority of psychology departments, the applicants' credentials are the most outstanding and the competition is keenest for admission into the clinical area.

It is difficult to ascertain that percentage of psychologists who engage in clinical research after completing the doctorate, but some estimates can be made. Considering clinical psychologists in particular, it can be inferred that those entering private practice are least likely to conduct research. Thus far, private practice has claimed only a minority of clinical psychologists. In 1983, for example, 30 percent of those clinical psychologists in the labor force were primarily self-employed. Of the remaining 70 percent, 24 percent were in academic positions, 22 percent were employed in hospitals and clinics, and the remainder were employed by government, industry, or the nonprofit sector, where there is at least the opportunity to engage in clinical research. Of nonclinical psychologists in the 1983 labor force, the vast majority (64 percent) were employed in academic positions (Institute of Medicine, 1985), where research is a primary activity. In total volume, the pool of psychologists who in 1991 identified themselves as scientists (n = 60,596) compares favorably with that of other groups of scientists who can potentially engage in clinical research (for example, medicine [n = 32,079]) (Brush, 1991). Also, at 36 percent, the representation of women in clinical psychology is the greatest of the scientific disciplines sampled by the National Science Foundation (Brush, 1991).

The number of women who receive training in psychology has increased dramatically. Women now constitute more than half of the applicant pool for graduate education in psychology, and they are in the majority as trainees in clinical psychology programs. In 1950 women received 37 percent of baccalaureate and 15 percent of doctoral degrees awarded in psychology. By 1988 women received 70 percent of baccalaureate and 55 percent of doctoral degrees, including 57 percent of the degrees in clinical psychology (National Science Foundation, 1990; Ostertag and McNamara, 1991). Women still hold only a minority of faculty positions, occupying slightly more than one fourth of the full-time faculty appointments in graduate departments of psychology (Kohout et al., 1992). More entry-level positions are opening to women, however. In 1989–1990, 48 percent of new appointments were made to women. Moreover, there are encouraging signs that the increasing "feminization" of the profession is not exacting a toll in loss of occupational prestige or salary (Ostertag and McNamara, 1991; Wicherski et al., 1992).

Asian, Hispanic, and African-American applicants remain very much in the minority, constituting 6 percent of full-time faculty members in graduate departments of psychology in 1989–1990 (Kohout et al., 1992). African-Americans constitute the largest single subgroup.

Intensive efforts to increase minority representation continue through fellowships and recruitment efforts at all levels of the academic ladder. In 1989–1990, 12 percent of new faculty appointments were made to members of minority groups (Kohout et al., 1992). Although the applicant pool remains small, the quality of minority student and faculty candidates is quite good. The diversity brought about by more women and minorities in clinical psychology has also broadened the field and enriched the knowledge base, especially in such areas as women's health, child and sexual abuse, and minority health.

The excellence of the pool of clinical psychology researchers is validated by their ability to compete successfully for federal research support. Even though the total dollar amount going to support behavioral research is relatively low (approximately 3.5 percent of the federal research support budget), psychologists (especially clinical psychologists) have a better than average "hit rate" for obtaining "approved and funded" grants. About 35 percent of the National Institute of Mental Health research dollars are awarded to psychologists, and 45 percent of the principal investigators supported are psychologists (Leshner, 1991).

Training

The education of psychologists traditionally has been characterized by the incorporation of strong training in research. Emphasis on the methods of science prior to professional training is uniquely associated with the training of psychologists. The scientific training begins early in the undergraduate curriculum and includes courses in experimental and laboratory methods as well as statistics. Experientially, psychology undergraduates participate in a variety of research activities, frequently serving as research assistants, which allows them to learn a variety of research skills. In many cases psychology undergraduates enter mentor relationships with faculty and become active members of ongoing research teams where they participate in the conceptualization, analysis of results, and preparation of manuscripts. As a result, many graduate with publications to their credit. Finally, but particularly important, is that the approach to understanding and interpreting the psychological literature is objective and critical. Hence, there is encouragement of the development of critical thinking skills. In general, through early socialization into the culture of science, the foundation for a scientific approach to the understanding of human behavior is laid.

Although there are diverse specialties within psychology, there are some common, unifying themes. These are found in the form of a shared undergraduate experience and a relatively common core background of knowledge in the areas of research design and experimental methodology, statistics, psychological measurement, individual differences, biological bases of behavior, social bases of behavior, and cognitive and affective bases of behavior. In short, psychology is the science of human behavior, and its trainees are uniquely qualified to study behavior from an integrative perspective, taking into account the biological, social, and individual factors associated with patterns of behavior.

The shared emphasis on the scientific method during all phases of training and the shared educational content concerning the mechanisms that govern learning, experience, and behavior equips those trained across all psychological specialties to conduct clinically related research. In addition to clinical psychologists, developmental, social, and experimental psychologists have made and continue to make important research contributions that affect the general health as well as the mental health of the nation.

The clinical psychologist is particularly well-suited to engage in clinical research because the model of training adhered to by most Ph.D. training programs is that of the scientist-practitioner, sometimes referred to as the Boulder model (for example, Belar and Perry, 1990; Raimy, 1949). This model calls for the integration of science and practice throughout the graduate training years. Thus, the clinical psychology trainee receives clinical and scientific training simultaneously. A particularly important aspect of this training is the reciprocal influence of each component on the other, resulting in continuous cross-fertilization (Kanfer, 1990). This model of training produces graduates who have a strong scientific approach to problem solving in the research laboratory as well as in clinical practice. These individuals are well-equipped to function in either the research or the practitioner role, or in both.

Following graduate course work, the clinical psychologist normally undertakes a one-year internship where there is additional intensive training in clinical assessment and intervention that continues in the scientist-practitioner tradition. Clinical psychologists are beginning to pursue postdoctoral training in increasing numbers. Some postdoctoral opportunities are to acquire further clinical training, some are to attain added research experience, and some are for both. The postdoctoral experience also allows for subspecialization in a domain of research or practice. Within the psychological research community, clinical psychologists are particularly well-suited to engage in research that pertains to understanding and modifying the basic mechanisms that govern maladaptive behavior patterns.

Barriers

Failure to Retain Clinical Psychologists as Researchers

Although it is difficult to ever know for certain how many psychologists are engaged in clinical research and whether this number is sufficient to meet the need for clinical researchers, there is consensus among the task force members that many well-trained, talented individuals who could engage in clinical research are no longer doing so. The bulk of these persons are clinical psychologists who never do a single study beyond their doctoral dissertation. The others gradually cease research activity and choose instead to concentrate on other activities, principally clinical work. The reasons for this "failure to retain" clinical researchers are many, but most reduce down to the simple fact that there are more disincentives to pursue or stay in a career that is research-intensive than there are positive incentives.

Economic disincentives deter many well-trained clinical psychologists from pursuing academic research careers. For example, in 1991–1992, the average academic year salary in a department of psychology for assistant professors who were between zero and five years beyond their Ph.D. was $35,000 (American Psychological Association, 1992). Postdoctoral positions pay still less, with many offering salaries in the low $20,000s. Many service agencies, in contrast, are willing and able to pay a new clinical Ph.D. a salary in excess of $60,000 to do full-time clinical practice. If, instead, the graduate chooses to go into independent practice, it is not uncommon for a clinical psychologist to gross over $100,000 once the practice has become established (a process that usually takes from two to five years).

It was formerly the case that clinical psychology Ph.D.s differed from their medical counterparts in lacking large debts that had to be repaid after graduation. This is no longer true, largely because of the erosion of federal funds for graduate training and the somewhat disproportionate loss of funds for graduate clinical training. In 1989 more than two-thirds of graduating psychologists had some level of debt to repay (Kohout et al., 1992). Of the enrolled full-time graduate students, almost half were relying primarily on self-support, and 95 percent had relied chiefly on personal financial resources at some point during their graduate education (Kohout et al., 1992). Graduates in clinical psychology had the highest levels of debt to repay and were less likely to have received federal fellowships or research and training grants than students in other nonclinical areas of psychology (Kohout et al., 1992). Graduate training funds in clinical psychology have eroded markedly during the past decade. For example, in 1977, 29 percent of clinical psychology graduates noted that federal fellowships and traineeships had provided the major support for their graduate training compared with 22 percent of psychology graduates in nonclinical areas. In 1986, by contrast, only six percent of new clinical psychology doctorates versus eight percent of nonclinical doctorates had relied primarily upon federal support for their graduate training. Although many major universities have been able to replace the lost federal training funds by using their own resources, it can no longer be assumed that the modal clinical psychology graduate contemplates professional options from a debt-free base. Research and academic settings need to take these market forces into account in setting salary levels for both incoming and continuing faculty, just as they do for other professional areas such as law, medicine, and business.

Clinical Ph.D.s who do enter academic positions, where research activity is desired and valued, soon encounter the frustration of competing for research funding in an environment of increasingly scarce funds to support even good-quality research. For example, although the National Institutes of Health budget has increased by more than 50 percent since 1980, the number of grants awarded annually has actually fallen by almost one third. At the National Science Foundation, only 30 percent of those who apply can hope to be funded (Holden, 1991). Although clinical psychologists have a relatively good "hit rate," their grant proposals are four times more likely to be unfunded than funded. If they turn to clinical practice to support their research and supplement their salaries, the time and energy requirements of clinical work soon swamp their ability to do research.

Powerful deterrents for clinical psychologists to remain in research can only be balanced by a concerted effort at all institutional levels to bolster the enticements to continue in research. One part of a solution will need to address the problem of noncompetitive salaries. As a beginning, there needs to be a mechanism whereby postdoctoral research positions in clinical psychology can be funded at more than minimal levels. A subsequent strategy, carrying on into the academic appointment, might be to allow clinical researchers who successfully compete for research awards to supplement their salaries from grants. In addition or as an alternative strategy, institutions might permit clinical faculty to supplement their salaries or their research resources by delivering some clinical services through a university clinic practice plan. This latter approach would have the added benefit of integrating clinical practice within the academic and research settings. University-based practice activities might also stimulate more clinical research, especially compared with the alternative, in which faculty divorce their clinical activities (and therefore their time and energy) from the university setting.

Greater institutional support is needed both to eliminate obstacles that plague the clinical research psychologist and to provide tangible resources to encourage research. An example of an obstacle is that in many clinical training programs course credit is no longer allocated for supervision of graduate students' clinical practicum work. Thus, in addition to the usual faculty course load involving lecture and seminar courses and research supervision, clinical faculty may shoulder, without credit, the extra burden of providing individual supervision for students engaged in clinical practice. Course credit needs to be awarded for clinical supervision. Another barrier has been the gradual erosion of the university's realization that preparation for engaging in research is an ongoing process. Researchers need to continually upgrade and refine their skills and knowledge by becoming immersed in the community of scholars in their particular area. Sabbaticals and release time from other academic duties to attend professional meetings are essential if clinical researchers are to remain competitive in the increasingly constricted funding arena. The ability to pursue these activities requires financial support that needs to be generated by university development offices. Although faculty sabbaticals offer an indispensable vehicle for rejuvenation, respecialization, or refinement and upgrading of skills, they are no longer available at many institutions. Task force members were in agreement that reestablishing paid sabbaticals for clinical researchers at five- to seven-year intervals throughout all levels of the career pathway offers one of the most effective incentives to retain researchers in clinical psychology.

Chilly Academic Climate for Women

The general difficulties of retaining clinical psychologists as researchers will now be influenced by the increasing proportion of women who are entering the profession. Great strides have been made in recruiting women into the early career stages as clinical psychology researchers. Women now constitute the majority of those entering graduate programs of clinical psychology, and almost half of new faculty appointments are being made to women. Continued initiatives, as well as the passage of time, will be required, however, before women achieve more than a toehold of representation in the academic community, and it will be still longer before balance is achieved at the upper levels of salary and academic rank. For example, despite new hiring initiatives, female graduate students still enter an academic environment in which women hold only a minority (about 25 percent) of faculty positions, and their representation at senior levels remains sparse. In 1989–1990, for example, women represented only 19 percent of tenured faculty (Kohout et al., 1992). The gains that have been made at the entry levels of academic rank are just beginning to be perceptible at higher levels. For example, in 1989–1990, women were more than twice as likely as men to be assistant professors, somewhat more likely to be associate professors, but almost a third less apt to be full professors (Kohout et al., 1992). Thus, although the situation is improving, female graduate students and faculty may still experience a sense of isolation in the academic environment and perceive a lack of support for their work. Until there is a critical mass of females within a department, networking needs to be done with women in other departments to provide support.

Retention of women at the upper rungs of the academic ladder will depend upon how successfully women are able to dovetail the demands of the tenure clock with those of the biological clock. Completing a Ph.D. and postdoctoral training places many women in their late twenties or early thirties by the time they obtain a first academic position. The tenure clock then allows five or six years to produce a sufficient volume of first-rate publications and grants to earn a permanent position. The demands of caring for young children during the tenure-probationary interval severely impede the pace of progress that is necessary to acquire tenure at many universities.

Alternatively, if a woman postpones childbearing, the tenure clock and the biological clock may seem to be running out in uncomfortably close proximity. A number of possible solutions have been proposed (Brush, 1991), including a longer tenure-probationary period, such as 9–10 years; one semester of paid "family care" leave; up to two years of unpaid leave for any reason; subsidized day care for preschool children; on a temporary non-tenure-track position for a qualified spouse when a nonuniversity position is unavailable. Such solutions are urgently needed if the intensive efforts that have successfully recruited women into the field are not to be wasted by having them drop out before they can contribute.

Chilly Academic Climate for Minorities

Much of what has been said about the retention of women can be reiterated for minorities, with the added comments that the problem is more acute and initial recruitment efforts have been less successful. In 1989–1990, minorities comprised 6 percent of full-time faculty members in U.S. departments of psychology, with African-Americans constituting the largest subgroup (Kohout et al., 1992). Minority representation also diminishes as academic rank increases: minorities comprise 13 percent of lecturer/instructors, 8 percent of assistant professors, 6 percent of associate professors, and 2 percent of full professors. Task force members felt that the most important corrective action is to remember that minority retention is a continuous process that begins rather than ends with successful recruitment of a minority student or faculty member. Efforts to combat isolation, to diversify the areas of study that are encouraged and rewarded for research and scholarship, and to enhance the flexibility of career timing all need to be encouraged.

Erosion of the Science Training Base by Professional Schools of Psychology

Until recent years, the bulk of clinical psychologists were trained as scientist-practitioners (the Boulder model) in university-based departments of psychology. This model builds practitioner training on top of a solid foundation in behavioral science. Today, however, approximately 50 percent of the doctorates in clinical psychology are awarded by "freestanding" professional schools of psychology, where scientific training clearly takes a back seat to preparing clinicians. Most professional schools lack the dissertation and the research requirements of Boulder model programs and greatly dilute the required training in scientific methods. The American Psychological Association has accredited

35 professional schools and estimates that from 33 to 59 percent of all doctoral students are currently enrolled in them (Craighead, 1991; Garfield, 1992).

Some professional school graduates are awarded the Psy.D. degree, but others are awarded the Ph.D. Thus, it now is difficult to determine by degree alone what the research training background has been for any given clinical psychologist. It would be difficult to overstate the degree to which the proliferation of professional schools has flooded the market with clinical psychologists. In the three-year period between 1978 and 1980, about 1,050 clinical psychologists a year received doctorates. In this three-year period alone, more clinical psychologists entered the field than were in the entire field 35 years earlier (Garfield, 1992). Unfortunately, it can no longer be assumed that a majority of these new clinical psychologists are well-equipped to engage in clinical research. Nor, certainly, can it be said that they are interested, since the vast majority of the clinical psychologists trained in professional schools enter non-research- or non-academic-related occupations. In contrast, students entering the university-based programs usually are seeking either research careers (a minority) or state an openness to combining research and clinical practice.

Since programs embracing a professional model are now producing about half of the new doctoral-level clinical psychologists, there can be no doubt that proliferation of the professional schools is serving to erode the base of scientific training of the profession as a whole. The solution to this problem will not be easy, but at least two paths can be recommended. First, the science training base should be strengthened in all clinical psychology programs, particularly in professional schools. Some movement in this direction is evident in the recommendations from the 1990 Report of the Joint Council on Professional Education in Psychology (Stigall et al., 1990), which reinforced the necessity for research training for all professional psychologists, including those being trained as practitioners. Accordingly, many professional schools have begun to strengthen their scientific training. Second, it is urged that the specific recommendations of the Utah Conference on Graduate Education and Training in Psychology (Beckman, 1987) be adopted. The Utah Conference advised that all nonuniversity-affiliated professional schools be required to have university affiliation by 1995 to receive continued accreditation by the American Psychological Association.

Increasingly Inflexible Licensing Requirements That Impede
Clinical Researchers' Eligibility for Licensure

A large proportion of clinical research in psychology involves evaluating the effectiveness of a modality of therapy or the mechanisms by which a treatment achieves its effects. The right to independently administer psychological treatment, even for primarily research purposes, is restricted to those who are licensed clinical psychologists, having met the licensing requirements of the state in which they reside. Eligibility for licensure depends partly upon passing a written national examination and partly upon performing a requisite number of hours of supervised psychological practice. Recent changes in the practice portion of the licensure requirements in most states have made it increasingly difficult for new clinical psychologists who engage in research or academic activities to achieve eligibility for licensure. Most states now require two years of postdoctoral experience to be eligible, and they will rarely credit instruction, research, or even the provision of clinical supervision as eligible practice activities. Many states specify that at least 10 or often 20 hours a week must be spent in direct client contact to meet the criteria for licensing. Moreover, it is often mandated that the practice requirements must be met during a consecutive two-year period. These time constraints make it very difficult if not impossible for a new Ph.D. who has chosen a research postdoctoral fellowship or an academic position to achieve eligibility for licensure while trying to meet research or tenure requirements. Increasingly, clinical researchers who wish to become licensed are needing to interrupt their research training or delay the start of an academic appointment to log in the necessary hours of supervised clinical practice. Nor can the individual with clinical research aspirations safely ignore or postpone the requirement for licensure, because potential employers fear that hiring an unlicensed psychologist will create insurance liabilities and jeopardize the site's professional accreditation.

The knowledge base that is the foundation for the practice of clinical psychology would clearly best be served by accommodating the professional needs of those who wish to integrate a career in clinical research and practice. Rigid licensure requirements that are increasingly unfriendly to the clinical researcher and academic do much to thwart this goal, adding to the list of factors that deter well-trained psychologists from embarking on clinical research careers. Solutions to this problem are badly needed and might take the form of expanding the definition of activities that are construed as psychological practice or increasing the flexibility of the temporal requirements for achieving licensure.

REFERENCES

American Psychological Association. 1992. 1991—1992 APA/COGDOP Survey of Graduate Departments of Psychology. Washington, D.C.: Education Directorate, American Psychological Association.
Belar, C., and N. Perry. 1990. Proceedings of the National Conference on Scientist-Practitioner Education and Training for the Professional Practice of Psychology. Sarasota, Fla.: Professional Resource Press.
Beckman, L., ed. 1987. Proceedings of the National Conference on Graduate Education in Psychology. American Psychologist 42(12).

Brush, S.G. 1991. Women in science and engineering. American Scientist 79:404–419.

Craighead, W.E. 1991. Division 12 meeting report. Clinical Science. APA Div. 12, Sec. 3, Spring Newsletter, pp. 2–3.

Cronbach, L.J. 1957. The two disciplines of scientific psychology. American Psychologist 12:671–684.

Garfield, S.L. 1992. Comments on "Retrospect: Psychology as a profession" by J. McKeen Cattell (1937). Journal of Consulting and Clinical Psychology 60:9–15.

Holden, C. 1991. Career trends for the 1990s. Science 252:1110–1120.

Institute of Medicine. 1985. Personnel needs and training for biomedical and behavioral research. The 1985 Report of the Committee on National Needs for Biomedical and Behavioral Research Personnel. Washington, D.C.: National Academy Press.

Kanfer, F.H. 1990. The scientist-practitioner connection: A bridge in need of consistent attention. Prof. Psychol. Res. Pract. 21:264–270.

Kohout, J., M. Wicherski, and B. Cooney. 1992. Characteristics of Graduate Departments of Psychology: 1989–90. Washington, D.C.: Education Directorate, American Psychological Association.

Leshner, A.I. 1991. Psychology research and NIMH: opportunities and challenges. Am. Psychol. 46:977–979.

McGovern, T.V., L. Furumoto, D.F. Halpern, G.A. Kimble, and W.J. McKeachie. 1991. Liberal education, study in depth, and the arts and sciences major—psychology. Am. Psychol. 46:598—605.

National Research Council. 1990. Survey of earned doctorates: 1980–89. National Research Council, Office of Scientific and Engineering Personnel. Washington, D.C.: National Academy Press.

Ostertag, P.A., and J.R. McNamara. 1991. "Feminization" of psychology: The changing sex ratio and its implications for the profession. Psychol. Women Q. 15:349–369.

Raimy, V.C. 1949. Training in Clinical Psychology. New York: Prentice-Hall.

Sayette, M.A., and T.J. Mayne. 1990. Survey of current clinical and research trends in clinical psychology. Am. Psychologist 45:1263–1266.

Stigall, T., et al. 1990. Report of the Joint Council on Professional Education in Psychology. Joint Council on Professional Education in Psychology.

Wicherski, M., J. Kohout, and B. Cooney. 1992. 1991–92 Faculty Salaries in Graduate Departments of Psychology. Washington, D.C.: Office of Demographic, Employment and Educational Research, American Psychological Association.

TASK FORCE MEMBERS

DOROTHY BROOTEN (Chair), Professor and Chair, Health Care of Women and Childbearing, Director, Low Birthweight Research Center, School of Nursing, University of Pennsylvania, Philadelphia, Pennsylvania

KAREN S. CALHOUN, Professor and Director of Clinical Training, Department of Psychology, University of Georgia, Athens, Georgia

ADA SUE HINSHAW, Director, National Center for Nursing Research,
National Institutes of Health, Bethesda, Maryland

ADA K. JACOX, Independence Foundation Chair in Health Policy, Johns
Hopkins University School of Nursing, Baltimore, Maryland

BONNIE J. SPRING, Professor, Department of Psychology, University of
Health Sciences, The Chicago Medical School and Health Scientist,
Veterans Administration Medical Center, North Chicago, Illinois

ORA L. STRICKLAND, Professor and Chair, Independence Foundation
Research, Emory University, Nell Hodgson Woodruff School of Nursing,
Atlanta, Georgia

SAMUEL M. TURNER, Professor of Psychiatry, Department of Psychiatry and
Behavioral Sciences, Medical University of South Carolina, Charleston,
South Carolina

KENNETH A. WALLSTON, Professor of Psychology, Vanderbilt University,
Nashville, Tennessee

Appendix C

Report of the Task Force on Clinical Research in Surgery

EXECUTIVE SUMMARY

Nearly all research performed by surgeons has a direct impact on or implications for patient care; therefore, the boundary between clinical and basic surgical research is almost nonexistent. In many areas of investigation, surgeons are uniquely positioned to bring the gains of fundamental advances in molecular biology and bioengineering to the patient's bedside.

Clinical research in surgery is currently inadequate in scope and, with some prominent exceptions, in quality. Greater and more meaningful collaboration between basic science and surgical departments needs to occur. The funding base in research is both inadequate and too narrow. One strategy is for surgeons and their professional associations to create a research foundation analogous to the Orthopaedics Research and Education Foundation (OREF). The OREF receives annual voluntary contributions from practicing orthopaedic surgeons and from industry. As an independent foundation with its own board of trustees, it undertakes peer review of both individual and institutional research proposals.

A second strategy for widening the base of surgical research is to develop collaboration between the military and civilian sectors. Military surgical training programs currently have inadequate experience for their residents in the management of major trauma, whereas civilian trauma centers, particularly those in central city areas, have inadequate personnel and funding. Training for military residents and continuing trauma and critical care experience for military surgeons can easily be provided in civilian trauma centers. All parties win in this arrangement: the military obtains the needed training in trauma, overworked surgical residents and faculty members in trauma centers would have time to train in or conduct research, and the care of the underserved patients in county hospitals would improve. The arrangement could also lead to collaborative research between universities and the military, allowing academic surgeons access to research funds in the U.S. Department of Defense.

The most important single reform necessary to promote clinical research by surgeons is for the National Institutes of Health (NIH) to implement true peer review. Of the more than 2,432 members of NIH study sections, only 21 are surgeons. There are only 5 surgeons among the 630 serving on institute review groups. Even in the surgery study sections, only a small minority are surgeons. Although surgeons have failed to take full advantage of NIH and U.S. Department of Veteran's Affairs (VA) career development awards, it should be noted that the guidelines for many of these grants appear to have been written with the express purpose of excluding surgeons. Career development awards must have the flexibility to allow surgeons the necessary time to enable them to maintain their operative surgical skills while developing academic careers.

The barriers to a career path in clinical research in surgery are similar to those in other disciplines, with some important differences. The length of training in surgery is very long, and the life of the academic surgeon is very busy, since one must maintain one's surgical skills to have credibility among one's peers. Research funding is also much more difficult for surgeons to obtain.

The task force makes the following recommendations:

• Increase meaningful collaboration between basic sciences and surgery by joint appointments of high-quality investigators.

• Propose to the American College of Surgeons the development of a research foundation, with contributions from surgeons and industry, to support research in surgery.

• Explore the development of collaboration between the military and civilian trauma centers; suggest that H. Mendez, Deputy Secretary of Defense for Health, be invited to testify before the full committee.

• NIH should undertake true peer review of proposals by surgeons by making the composition of surgical study sections at least 75 percent academic surgeons.

• Improve recruitment and retention of academic faculty in surgery through outreach programs to recruit students, minorities, and women; implementation of direct support of surgical research by the surgical community, and development of a formal program for the initial phase of faculty appointment of young academic surgeons.

• Special attention should be paid to the role of women in surgery; they should be recruited into Surgical Scientist Training Programs (SSTP) and given tenured positions, and special effort should be made to provide them mentors and role models.

• Similarly, minorities are underrepresented in surgery. The financial factor appears to be the *absolute* limiting factor for the career choices of minorities. Strategies are required to address this.

• Develop an NIH SST program and request that the Accreditation Committee for Graduate Medical Education (ACGME) facilitate development of accreditation of the SSTP track by the Residency Review Committee on Surgery.

• Shorten the length of clinical training in surgery and the surgical subspecialties.

DEFINING CLINICAL RESEARCH IN SURGERY

Nearly all research performed by surgeons can be regarded as clinical research. From the perspective of the task force, therefore, little is to be gained by trying to define the limits of clinical research in surgery. Examples of the kinds of research performed by surgeons are given below, and all are considered clinical research.

Examples of Human Studies

• prospective clinical trials in some aspect of surgical therapy or cancer treatment,
• research on human subjects that examines physiological alterations caused by surgery,
• studies of immunosuppression or prevention of rejection in transplant patients, and
• outcome studies of clinical therapy.

Examples of Animal Studies

• developing and testing of implantable devices, for example, artificial joints and prosthetic heart valves;
• developing new laparoscopic, endoscopic, and arthroscopic surgical instruments and procedures;
• organ, tissue, or cell transplantation with attendant studies in immunobiology and pathology;
• developing animal models of disease, for example, of acute pancreatitis or degenerative arthritis; and
• physiological studies of myocardial function, blood flow, gastrointestinal function, and so forth.

Studies at the Tissue, Cellular, and Molecular Level

- mechanisms of immunological tolerance,
- endothelial biology, and
- healing of wounds, bone, tendon, muscle, cartilage, nerve.

In all of the examples given above, the research is directly applicable to patient care. Nearly all surgical research is of this nature. As advances in molecular biology are made, surgeons must be ready to carry these advances to the bedside. Hence, a restrictive definition of clinical research that may have been appropriate 10 or 20 years ago is no longer acceptable.

IMPROVING CLINICAL RESEARCH IN SURGERY

The task force discussed the importance of having basic scientists as equal members in surgical departments. Having second-rate basic scientists that do research as "hired guns" is unacceptable. Indeed, especially in the era of unprecedented advances in biology, an opportune time exists for clinical departments to develop special collaboration with basic science departments. Outstanding basic scientists should be recruited jointly with basic science departments to have joint appointments in the basic science and clinical departments. The clinical departments would provide full-time employment, space, and research support. Individuals recruited in this fashion would be prized both by the basic scientists and clinicians, and they would be ideally situated to help bring the advances of modern science to the clinical arena.

RESOURCE BASE FOR CLINICAL RESEARCH IN SURGERY

Orthopedic Surgery

This surgical discipline has made impressive gains in providing a funding source and coordinating efforts to promote research, thanks to the vision of the leadership of the specialty. This effort is discussed as a potential model for other surgical disciplines.

OREF has established a fund to award grants for orthopaedic research. Contributions to this fund come from two sources. Voluntary contributions are supplied by the membership of the American Academy of Orthopaedic Surgery. A substantial proportion of orthopaedic surgeons in the country make an annual contribution of $1,000 to the fund, thus joining the "Order of Merit." OREF also receives unincumbered industrial contributions.

In 1991, OREF received $3.8 million in contributions and committed $3.7 million to 79 new grants. Although this funding amounts to only about 5 percent of all research expenditures in orthopaedics, it is being used in creative and effective ways including three career development awards, 23 individual investigator-initiated research grants, 9 resident research fellowships, 7 orthopaedic departmental progress grants, 19 state orthopaedic society grants, 4 clinical research lectureships, and 10 institutional grants. In addition, OREF will provide more than $55,000 to underwrite the American Orthopaedic Association Residents' Conference, the American Shoulder and Elbow Surgeons' Research Conference, and the 1992 Gordon Orthopaedic Conference on Orthopaedics. Recently, the OREF and the American Academy of Orthopaedic Surgeons have worked together to sponsor six two-year health services research fellowships that began in July 1993.

All OREF grants are awarded following rigorous peer review. Institutional grants usually involve site visits. In general, grants are given without providing for indirect costs, with some exceptions, in which individual grants may include approximately 15 percent overhead. The American Academy of Orthopaedic Surgeons has established and supports a Center for Research and a Council for Research. These units within the Academy help support the OREF and coordinate efforts to strengthen orthopaedic research at all levels.

The experience of OREF suggests a successful mechanism for distributing any unencumbered research support that may be obtained from industry. The task force believes that OREF, the American College of Surgeons, or similar organizations with proper peer review systems, rather than large organizations such as NIH, provide a better mechanism for allocating research endowment funds that may be developed with contributions from industry. Such a peripheral system of distribution is more likely to address the specific research needs of surgical disciplines. A brief description of the OREF is given at the end of this appendix.

NIH

A strong perception exists among surgeons that there is potential bias in the review process against proposals with surgeons as principal investigators. Fair critical review of surgical research proposals requires that review be conducted by individuals with appropriate surgical education and experience. In many instances the peer review process has not met this criteria and therefore is not true "peer review." Even when surgical study sections have been organized, the number of surgeons participating in these sections is frequently too small. For example, only three orthopaedic surgeons serve on the Orthopaedic and Musculoskeletal Study Section. While the total NIH funding for grants reviewed by the Orthopaedic and Musculoskeletal Study Section has increased, the number of grant awards with orthopaedic surgeons as principal investigators has declined over the past decade. Furthermore, of the 2,434 members of the NIH study sections, only 21 are surgeons, and only 5 of the 630 members of the institute review groups are surgeons. Even more critical, there are no surgeons on most of the NIH advisory councils that make final recommendations concerning funding.

The task force feels that the bias against surgery must be removed. This is best done by having true peer review and by having surgeons in the councils. A mechanism that may expand the pool of surgeons in study sections is to have a large panel of surgical experts who could be invited to serve as necessary.

A special problem was identified in trauma. Funding for research in trauma is shared by 3 federal agencies (NIH, the Centers for Disease Control and Prevention, and GMS). The arrangement is confusing to the investigator who wishes to apply for funding. Also, the responsibilities of each funding agency are unclear.

Department of Defense

Three compelling reasons were identified to support a proposal for cooperation between the U.S. Department of Defense and county hospitals. First, inadequate opportunities exist for the military to train in trauma during peacetime. Nationally, trauma care is concentrated largely in county hospitals. This vast experience could be made available for training of military residents and for providing continuing experience for surgeons in the military. Second, academic faculty members in county hospitals are overworked and have little opportunity to engage in research. The participation of military surgeons in trauma care in county hospitals would ameliorate this problem. Creative, collaborative research between the military and academic institutions could be developed in this way. The *quid pro quo* for resident training provided to the military might be direct provision of military funding for joint research efforts. Third, the large population of patients in county hospitals would be the beneficiary of such a collaboration. The problem of long delays experienced by patients who come to county hospitals could be alleviated.

It should be relatively easy to arrange for periods of training of the military surgical residents in civilian trauma centers. This arrangement would provide the needed training for the military while alleviating personnel shortages in trauma centers. Such arrangements have already been made in selected instances, such as the Martin Luther King Medical Center in Los Angeles and the Washington Hospital Center in Washington, D.C.

A second collaborative effort could be developed between the U.S. Department of Defense and VA hospitals. The task force suggests that VA hospitals are an ideal solution for the provision of care for the dependents of members of the military as the U.S. Department of Defense is closing down military bases and hospitals. This arrangement would reverse the declining census of many VA hospitals and would indirectly benefit clinical research.

BARRIERS TO CLINICAL RESEARCH
CAREERS IN SURGERY

Surgery, perhaps more than any other clinical discipline, requires an increase in its base in clinical research. Several reasons may be cited: (1) clinical research in surgery is currently inadequate in scope and, with some prominent exceptions, in quality; (2) clinical practice in surgery is lucrative and attracts increasing numbers of young surgeons away from academic careers; (3) even when surgeons have made a commitment to an academic career, the demands of patient care interfere with their ability to spend adequate time in research; (4) a perception abounds among surgeons that they are not given a fair chance in competition for NIH funding; and (5) the need to subject modes of surgical therapy to randomized clinical trials at their inception is great because operations become all too frequently accepted for general use prior to adequate proof of their efficacy.

Barriers

Barriers at Entry Level

General surgical residency is typically five years long. The programs that prepare residents for a career in academic surgery frequently require one or more additional years. If a resident wishes to specialize (for example, in cardio-thoracic, pediatric, vascular, plastic, or transplant surgery), a further two-year period of training is required. Young academic surgeon specialists usually start their careers between the ages of 34 and 36 years. The debt accumulated during medical school is significant, and the further indebtedness that must occur during specialty training is unappealing.

Barriers During Residency

Surgical residents have incurred debts of as much as $100,000 or more by the time they finish, and they frequently have spouses and children to support. The lure of a lucrative private practice is great. There are also few, well-established, productive clinician-scientists to serve as role models. Instead, residents see academic faculty members working very hard to fulfill their clinical and research commitments, and sometimes doing neither well.

Training in clinical research is not structured, and it is often inadequately supervised. The mentor or supervisor is frequently so preoccupied with clinical, teaching, and administrative duties that little time is available to teach and supervise the fellow. This phenomenon leads to disillusionment. No structured curriculum exists. The period of research training is frequently too short.

During their period of research training, surgical residents engage too frequently in "moonlighting." They can earn good sums of money staffing emergency rooms and intensive care units at night. This activity interferes with sound training in research and is detrimental to productivity in science.

The optimal timing of research training is not clear. If residents go into the laboratory at the end of the second year of clinical training, then they will have to do three clinical years after they complete their time in the laboratory. By the time they finish their residency, the data they accumulated in the laboratory may be too old for use as preliminary results for grant applications. If they go to the laboratory after the third year, they feel clinically uncomfortable when they return to the senior years of residency, when they are given significant responsibilities. On the other hand, if research training is not provided until after the completion of clinical training, two potential problems exist. First, the recruitment of bright residents into an academic career will have been missed by waiting so long. Second, if they train in research for two or more years after they complete their clinical training, they will feel clinically inadequate when they begin their careers.

Barriers After Residency

The barriers after residency are even more important and include the following.

• Academic departments are unable to nurture young faculty, which is evidenced by inadequate protected time for research because of pressure to produce clinical practice revenues; inadequate start-up funds; inadequate mentoring and guidance; and inadequate provision of good clinical experience. This problem creates a feeling of inadequacy and disappointment.
• There is difficulty in obtaining research funding.
• There is perceived instability of research funding. Even if they obtain their first grant, young academic faculty members are very uncertain whether they will receive continued funding.
• There is a threat of isolation and loss of clinical skills—the fear of the "rat surgeon" syndrome.

- The lure of clinical practice includes the interesting cases, the financial reward, and the ego satisfaction, with referrals of complex cases.

General Barriers to Surgical Research

General barriers in the way of a career in research include the following.

- a perception that surgeons are less able to perform serious research than other physicians and scientists,
- inadequacy of the peer review system for surgeons and the perception by surgeons that their proposals are reviewed unfairly,
- reluctance of third-party payers to pay the costs of care for patients participating in clinical research protocols,
- lack of adequate support from industry without strings attached, and
- need for the surgical department to value research as much as clinical practice.

Special Problems of Women in Surgery

For women, the years of training and of serving as junior faculty members in academic departments coincide with the childbearing period. In many instances, women are simultaneously subjected to the ticking of both the biological and the tenure time clocks. No provisions are made to alter the training program or the tenure time clock to accommodate the needs of women in surgery. Women in surgery have few role models, are frequently outside the information network, and choose to occupy the lower-echelon academic tracks. Their husbands are almost always either physicians or professionals in other fields, and frequently, the career needs of the husbands take priority. Such important requirements as day-care centers are rarely available. All of these problems add a different level of complexity to the choice of clinical research as a career path for women in surgery.

Minorities in Surgical Research Faculty Careers

The number of minorities in academic surgery is extremely low. Of the estimated 64,456 academic faculty members in medical schools, only 2,996 (or 4.6 percent) are underrepresented minorities. The recruitment of African-Americans and Hispanics into academic careers is especially difficult because the pool of qualified candidates is small and the financial difficulties of minorities are particularly severe because they frequently come from poor families who have been eagerly waiting for them to graduate and earn money in clinical practice. Even when minorities enter training in clinical research and are recruited into an academic track, they frequently are unable to sustain this position because of the financial needs of themselves and their family. In predominantly white medical schools, they have an uphill fight against prejudice. All too frequently the atmosphere is unwelcoming, even hostile, and is certainly not conducive to the enjoyable and productive pursuit of science. A critical lack of role models also exists. Of 5,293 surgical faculty 255 (4.8 percent) are non-Asian minorities; in othopaedic surgery, this number is 25 of 800 (3.1 percent).

HUMAN RESOURCES PROFILE AND TRAINING BACKGROUNDS OF THE PRESENT COHORT OF CLINICAL RESEARCHERS

No data are available to define the profiles of present cohorts of clinical researchers in surgery. A review of the top 10 NIH-funded surgical investigators shows that all are men, all but one are white, and all obtained their M.D.s at an early age and became full professors by age 40. They were all either Alpha Omega Alpha or Markle fellows. Few took formal research training. Unlike internal medicine, in which some 50 percent of the successful investigators had training links with NIH, only 2 of the 10 surgeons had similarly close links with NIH. Indeed, the single most important characteristic of these successful surgical investigators is that they are driven individuals. This cursory review seems to indicate that the quality of the individual, rather than his or her research training, was the key predictor to success.

The task force discussed the need for an NIH-sponsored surgical scientist development program. A key requirement of such a program would have to be flexibility: flexibility in the period of training, site of training, and program content.

EDUCATION AND TRAINING REQUIREMENTS FOR CLINICAL RESEARCH IN SURGERY

Three key requirements were considered essential in the training of surgeons in clinical research: motivated candidates, qualified and dedicated mentors, and flexibility. Unlike internists, surgeons need to maintain their technical skills. To do this, they must spend at least 50 percent of their time in clinical surgery. This requirement imposes the need for flexibility in designing training programs for surgeons.

The definition of clinical research done by surgeons should be very broad, because most research done in this discipline is prompted by clinical problems, even though it may utilize the most sophisticated techniques. Because this type of clinical research may vary from basic molecular biology to the development of new operative procedures or longitudinal study of patient disease outcome, the requirements for education and training cannot be rigid. Although the motivation of young surgeons and the provision of proper mentors and role models are crucial to capturing and retaining surgeons in the research field, it is also important that their initial research experience be accompanied by some kind of formal training. It is believed that too few surgeons are receiving such training at present, especially in the basic sciences. This seriously limits their ability to apply the new biology to the problems of surgical patients.

Mentors and role models can be identified in the backgrounds of most successful surgeon-scientists. This is perhaps the most important factor inspiring young surgeons to enter and succeed in research careers. The mentor and the role model may be the same or different people. For a young surgeon, role models within the field of surgery are indispensable, but they are suitable as mentors only if they are also scientists in the trainee's area of specific interest and are able to devote sufficient time to the task. In many departments of surgery they do not exist. In these instances mentors in other departments must be sought. They will often be Ph.D.s, and in any case they will usually be full-time, rather than part-time, scientists. Since being a mentor is a vital and time-consuming task, these individuals need to receive compensation, perhaps in the form of support of their own research programs.

The locus of the research training is important. Although it may take place in either a clinical or a basic science department, it is important that the parent department of surgery retain close ties with the trainee and the ultimate responsibility for overseeing the young surgeons training experience. In most instances this experience should last at least two years and should include rigorous course work in the discipline of interest. The curriculum, however, must be a flexible one, depending on the trainee's educational background and goals. Courses might vary from those in molecular biology to epidemiology and data collection. Some experience in writing manuscripts and grants would be valuable to all trainees. Individual work with mentors on hypothesis formulation and testing is also important.

Financial support for clinical research training in surgery is a major problem. Every advantage should be taken of existing sources of funding, such as Medical Scientist Training programs; National Research Service Award grants; NIH physician-scientist training programs; Howard Hughes medical student and postgraduate fellowships; Dana Foundation fellowships; VA grants; NIH research career development awards (RCDA), R29s, K04s, K08s, and K11s and various foundation- and industry-supported grants. Although surgeons have failed to take full advantage of these, it should be noted that many of them have guidelines that appear to have been written for the express purpose of excluding surgeons (on the basis of the fact that their clinical training is too long or that as junior faculty in surgical disciplines they now spend less than 75 percent of their time in research). It would be very helpful if some funding mechanisms that would be specifically intended to provide support for training in surgical research could be initiated. An NIH surgical scientist training program would be ideal. It is suggested that new grants be aimed at providing funding for technical help and supplies rather than stipends.

Although the research training of young surgeons is important, it is equally important to overcome this tendency to drift away from research as they mature (see the section on barriers). Because very few individuals will pursue clinical training programs in surgery unless they intend to practice actively, it is necessary to accept the concept that if surgeons are to be involved with investigation, they will pursue it on a less than full-time basis. Although this has certain disadvantages, the clinician- or surgeon-scientist has a unique perspective that is of special value in the pursuit of clinical research. Thus, in this discipline, at least the leaders need to be supported in their pursuit of dual goals. Since it is not intended that the research of these individuals be evaluated on a different scale than that of full-time scientists, it is especially important that they have sound training and that this training have adequate support.

It is unclear whether training should occur during or after residency. If research training does not occur during residency, the "entrapment" of bright individuals for academic careers might suffer. At the same time, the research training obtained and the data gathered during residency tend to lose currency by the time the clinical training is completed. Training ideally should occur during and immediately after the period of residency.

A major problem in the retention of academic surgeons in research was identified. All too frequently, an inadequate support system exists for the young surgeon taking a first academic appointment. Yet, this is the most crucial phase of the career of an academic surgeon. All of the resources and efforts expended in training such an individual are useless unless a system is provided for the smooth "reentry" into clinical surgery. Research time as well as good clinical experience must be provided and protected. Adequate laboratory space and start-up funds must be provided. The initial funding must be given for some three years to enable the individual to obtain an independent research grant. Initial funding support is currently provided haphazardly and inadequately by departments of surgery. With the changing medical economy, the ability of surgery departments to sustain this effort, even at an inadequate level, is questioned. Funding for the reentry phase ideally should be part and parcel of the training grant. Such an arrangement would ensure the highest possible retention of individuals trained in clinical research.

IMPLEMENTING CHANGES IN CLINICAL
RESEARCH TRAINING

Here, too, the unique needs of surgeons require flexibility. Important elements of the training program are as follows:

• Identification of a mentor: the individual must be well-qualified, dedicated, and able to provide the time needed for supervision.
• A minimum period of two years of supervised research is need. This period of time will need to be flexible to accommodate the needs of different surgical specialties.
• A didactic period of training appropriate for the unique needs of the specialty is needed. This aspect of the training should take place concurrently with the supervised research. Included here may be training in biostatistics, scientific instrumentation, scientific writing, computer science, and the auditing of graduate courses relevant to the individual's research needs.

The training program would be significantly enhanced if collaborations were created with established investigators, especially basic scientists. The training, however, should occur as much as possible in the surgical department, because this is an important method of enhancing the research that occurs in departments of surgery.

CHANGES IN SURGICAL RESIDENCY TRAINING

Basic residencies in all surgical specialties are a minimum of five years long. Specialization (thoracic, pediatric, vascular, critical care) requires additional residency times of one or two years. Adding adequate research training of 2 to 3 years extends residency training to 9 to 10 years for many surgeons.

Many surgical residents carry heavy indebtedness from undergraduate and medical school. Payback must begin at postgraduate year three (or sooner, if pending legislation is enacted). Research training is either omitted to facilitate earlier entry into practice to increase earnings and to pay back loans or it is chosen as a period of time to actively moonlight and earn money for debt repayment. If the research time is to be optimized, other mechanisms for payback should be initiated.

Residency programs can be restructured to permit shortening. General surgery programs can be shortened to four clinical years if one or two years of research are added; clinical exposure during the clinical residency must be intensified, however, so that the research-track residents are at least as well prepared as others and are fully able to meet board requirements.

RECOMMENDATIONS

Collaboration Between Basic Sciences and Department of Surgery

The quality of clinical research and training in surgery is significantly enhanced when basic scientists are full members of departments of surgery. The recruitment of such individuals should be made jointly with the basic science departments, and the recruits should have joint appointments in surgery and the basic science department. In this way, quality investigators can be recruited to surgery, which should provide full-time equivalents, space, and resources. These individuals will have credibility in the basic sciences and will be equal members in the department of surgery. They will serve as the vehicle for developing collaborative research between clinicians and basic scientists. The will also play an important role in the training of surgeons in clinical research. In the era of swift and explosive developments in biomedical science, collaboration between basic science and clinical departments is crucial to rapidly bringing advances in molecular biology to the bedside.

Proposal to American College of Surgeons Board of Regents to Undertake Direct Support of Research by Surgeons

The American College of Surgeons has demonstrated success in raising contributions from its members. The OREF has been highly successful in raising funds, improving the general funding of orthopaedic research, in greatly improving the amount of quality research, and in giving contributors a direct sense of pride and accomplishment in their contributions.

The task force recommends that the American College of Surgeons should undertake direct support of research by surgeons. This can best be implemented through its Surgical Research and Education Committee (SREC).

1. Funds should be raised directly and earmarked to be spent directly (not invested) on research.
2. Allocation of funds should:
   a. be made to different disciplines (cardiothoracic surgery, general surgery, ophthalmology, and obstetrics and gynecology, for example) in proportion to the amounts donated by members to these different disciplines;

    b. be limited (initially at least) to two years of support for the purpose of initiating research plans to secure preliminary data that would allow for application for NIH or other funding. These funds may also serve as bridging grants. (Initial amounts: $50,000–$70,000).

    3. Distribution of funds by independently appointed study sections with a small nucleus of experts and a large network of approved ad hoc reviewers. Plans would be to have a simple application form prepared for quick (within six months) review.

    4. Yearly research progress reports will go to the American College of Surgeons for distribution to SREC contributors. The reports should include lists of publications, reprints, and evidence of progress in securing further research support and in academic progress (promotion, new appointments, appearances at national meetings, and election to learned societies, for example).

    5. Contributors should receive highly visible recognition:

        a. letter of commendation,

        b. lapel pins (nine years or $1,000/yr, for example),

        c. banners with donor names ($5,000/yr),

        d. publication of the contributor's name in the *College Bulletin*.

    6. To raise funds, consider turning the project over to:

        a. new independent committee or department, or

        b. a committee of fellows (or fellowship contributors) with or without help from fundraising consultants already in place.

NIH—Peer Review

The single most important reform necessary to promote clinical research by surgeons is to implement what is already a salient principle of grant evaluation–peer review. This means not only that grant proposals from academic surgeons should go to surgical study sections but that the proposals should be evaluated by academic surgeons, even if the proposal deals with basic science, such as molecular biology, signal-transduction mechanisms, or ligand-receptor interactions in cellular or humoral immunology. The current composition of surgery study sections shows the following: in Surgery and Bioengineering Study Section, 8 surgeons of 18 members; in Surgery, Anesthesiology and Trauma Study Section, 7 surgeons of 18 members; in the Orthopaedic and Musculoskeletal Study Section, 4 surgeons of 18 members. Surgery study sections should be made up of at least 75 percent surgeons. The task force believes that it is no exaggeration to say that all progress in clinical research is contingent upon the basic premise of peer review, a premise on which all levels of NIH evaluation are posited. The executive secretary could obtain a list of qualified experts from the American College of Surgeons' Surgery Research and Education Committee. The explanation for failure of peer review classically given by executive secretaries is that the membership of surgical study sections is limited to only a few areas of basic science expertise. The answer, of course, is to get outside help. The executive secretary could identify a large group of experts on whom they could call.

Collaboration Between Military and Civilian Sectors

Discussion should be initiated among appropriate personnel in the U.S. Department of Defense, such as H. Mendez, Deputy Secretary of Defense for Health, and the Institute of Medicine Committee on Career Paths for Clinical Research to explore options for increased military-civilian coordination. An opportunity appears to exist to enhance the training as well as the research opportunities by using civilian trauma centers for the training of military surgical residents.

Recruitment and Retention of Academic Faculty in Surgery

1. Outreach programs should be developed to recruit medical students. Recruitment of underrepresented minorities is especially important and may require financial support during medical school, and every attempt should be made to secure role models and dedicated mentors.

2. Instill flexibility into mechanisms of NIH support of clinical research:
   • Develop a surgical scientist track (analogous to the pediatric track) at NIH.
   • Institute a program for direct support of surgical research by the American College of Surgeons. (The Fellowship Committee could conduct a fundraising campaign to raise money to be spent directly— not invested—for support of research. Provide no funds for salary, and aim at $50,000–$70,000 for two years to allow start-up funds to be used to gather preliminary data, thus answering the most critical need of young investigators.) Funds will be allocated in proportion to discipline of origin. Funds should be distributed by independent reviewers, and money raised by private practitioners should be coordinated on a regional basis.
   • Simplify and decentralize mechanisms for review of training proposals. Introduce flexibility in the duration of research and sites of training, and require an absolute divorce from clinical duties.

3. Identify the mentor and, after proper vetting, reward the mentor with the money for research costs of the applicant. The importance of the mentor or role model (who are often not the same) is underappreciated.

4. Mechanisms for the evaluation of success or failure must be structured into the program. This should go on for at least 10 years and should provide specific data on the scholarly contributions of trainees.

5. To initiate formal programs for reentry, consider provision of a portion of grant funds for a three- to five-year period after the formal research years to support the continuation of studies. These funds might be crucial in locking the trainee into a lifetime of investigation. Provision of the salary will give the department a chance to demonstrate its commitment. There should be protection of time and effort in the years coming out of training.

Women in Surgical Research Faculty Careers

1. Recruitment of women into surgical scientist training programs (SSTPs) should be encouraged. Promising female students should be identified and actively recruited and supported in surgical residencies.

2. Retention of female faculty in tenure-track positions should be facilitated through extensions of time to tenure by academic institutions and recognition of childbearing time demands.

3. Mentors and sponsors for women in SSTPs should be actively sought. Female surgeons in tenure-track positions should be identified and sponsored in academic surgery by senior academic surgeons within and outside their institutions. Special seminars and training sessions for women surgical scientists should be regularly conducted by NIH and by surgical societies such as the Association of Academic Surgeons and Society of University Surgeons. These societies should develop a mechanism to assist in grant preparation and to conduct prereviews.

4. Academic medical centers with women in tenure-track positions in surgery should be strongly encouraged to develop and provide readily accessible day-care facilities.

5. A national system of identification of professional couples in which the wife is a surgical scientist should be developed to assist in spouse placement. Academic institutions should be encouraged to facilitate two-career appointments.

Under-represented Minorities in Academic Surgery

Targeted funds from government and the private sector should be established to enable poor but talented young men and women to enter training in clinical research in surgery. The financial factor is often the *absolute* limiting factor in the career choices of minorities. The need for mentors and role models is even greater for minority students and residents than for others. Robert Wood

Johnson Foundation scholarships are a successful model for this purpose, but these scholarships may need to start early, perhaps in the last year of medical school.

Development of NIH Surgical Scientist Training Program

Current medical scientist training programs offered by NIH do not meet the needs for training physician-scientists in the surgical disciplines. Few surgeons have participated in these programs because the program time commitments required in each year make it difficult for awardees to develop and maintain surgical clinical skills and may extend the total length of training beyond medical school to as much as 10 years or more, leaving many individuals with substantial debt.

Completion of surgical clinical education frequently requires seven years or more following medical school. Development and maintenance of the high level of technical skills and knowledge necessary for the practice of surgery requires commitment of 20 or more hours a week to clinical practice. The available NIH-sponsored research training programs specify that the awardees must dedicate substantially more than 50 percent of their time to research and therefore make it difficult for surgeons to develop and maintain their skills. Limitations on the levels of compensation awardees may receive make these programs substantially less attractive than full-time clinical practice.

Recommendation

NIH should develop SSTPs with the intent of increasing the number of independent clinical investigators in the surgical disciplines. To be effective these programs should include the following features:

- Integration into surgical education: SST programs should allow the awardees to continue to maintain and develop their clinical skills.
- Minimize increased length of training: SST programs should be organized so that the effect on the total length of training is minimized. This may be accomplished by developing combined clinical specialty and research training programs.
- Emphasis on research related to surgical treatment: SST programs should emphasize surgical treatment of clinical problems such as traumatic injuries, cancer, and congenital deformities.
- Require close supervision by experienced scientists: SST awardees should work initially under the close supervision of an experienced scientist.

• Flexible time requirements: SST programs should allow awardees to begin the training program at different times during training, return to clinical training, and then return to research. During research training, awardees should be allowed sufficient time to maintain their clinical skills.

• Flexible levels of financial support: SST programs should allow awardees to receive levels of compensation that correspond to their level of education and experience. This may be accomplished through joint sponsorship of surgical scientist training programs by NIH and academic programs or surgical professional societies or foundations.

Institution of Changes in Surgical Residency Training

Institutions intending to implement an SST program in a residency program should define the structure of their program in their application to the Residency Review Committee (RRC). The RRC for surgery should define special requirements for such programs and include evaluation of this component of the program in its accreditation process. These requirements should include:

• criteria for the recruitment and selection of SSTP candidates, including identification of candidates in medical school;
• identification and description of research resources available to the SSTP, including the track record of the research program(s);
• identification of faculty mentors including established surgeon-scientists;
• description of the structure of the training program, including the proposed training in research methodology, techniques, and statistics;
• a plan whereby the clinical training, including the chief residency, will be accomplished in four clinical years; equivalency in surgical experience must be demonstrated, and requirements of the American Board of Surgery must be fully met; and
• a plan for retention of the SSTP appointee in academic surgery following completion of residency.

ACGME should facilitate the development of accreditation of the SSTP track by the RRC for surgery. The research program itself will not be subject to accreditation; rather, the accreditation process should address (1) the plan for research training and resources, (2) the fulfillment of all RRC and American Board of Surgery requirements in a four-year clinical program, and (3) monitoring of the success of SSTP appointees in certification by the American Board of Surgery. Debt repayment, deferral, or forgiveness should be a foremost consideration in any SSTP.

ORTHOPAEDIC RESEARCH AND
EDUCATION FOUNDATION

The Orthopaedic Research and Education Foundation (OREF) began as an effort by orthopaedic surgeons to increase support for orthopaedic research. It initially depended on voluntary contributions by practicing orthopaedic surgeons. Although it has been encouraged and supported by the American Academy of Orthopaedic Surgeons (AAOS) and the Orthopaedic Research Society (ORS), OREF is an independent foundation with its own board of trustees.

OREF consists of a board of trustees, a paid executive director and several administrative support personnel. Volunteers serve on peer review panels for individual and institutional grants.

The trustees are the governing body of OREF. They are independent of any other organization, and OREF is administratively and legally an independent foundation. OREF does accept recommendations for areas of research emphasis and types of programs from other orthopaedic organizations.

OREF provides several different types of grants including: investigator-initiated grants, resident research grants, institutional grants to orthopaedic departments, and career development grants. All grants are reviewed by a peer review panel. These panels are independent of other orthopaedic organizations. In 1991, OREF received $3.8 million in contributions and committed $3.7 million to 79 new grants.

AAOS supports the efforts of OREF by recognizing donors at the AAOS annual meeting and by supporting the efforts to increase contributions to OREF by orthopaedic surgeons and industry. AAOS may initiate a more direct effort to solicit contributions from AAOS fellows. AAOS has established and supports a Center for Research and a Council for Research. These units within the AAOS help to support OREF and coordinate efforts to strengthen orthopaedic research at all levels. ORS frequently supplies reviewers for OREF grants and supports the efforts of OREF to increase contributions to orthopaedic research.

TASK FORCE MEMBERS

HAILE T. DEBAS (Chair), Professor and Chairman, Department of Surgery, University of California at San Francisco, San Francisco, California

CLYDE F. BARKER, Professor and Chairman, Department of Surgery, University of Pennsylvania Medical Center, Philadelphia, Pennsylvania

JOSEPH BUCKWALTER, Professor, Department of Orthopaedics, University of Iowa Hospital, Iowa City, Iowa

OLGA JONASSON, Professor and Chairman, Department of Surgery, Ohio State University, Columbus, Ohio

FRANK R. LEWIS, Jr., Professor of Surgery, Chief of Surgery, San Francisco General Hospital, University of California at San Francisco, San Francisco, California

JAMES C. THOMPSON, John Woods Harris Professor and Chairman, Department of Surgery, The University of Texas Medical Branch, Galveston, Texas

SAMUEL A. WELLS, Jr., Bixby Professor of Surgery and Chairman, Department of Surgery, School of Medicine, Washington University, St. Louis, Missouri

Appendix D

Agenda for the Workshop on Clinical Research and Training: Spotlight on Funding

June 12–13, 1992
Cecil and Ida Green Building
Room 104
2001 Wisconsin Avenue, NW
Washington, D.C.

Friday, June 12

8:00   Registration and Coffee

8:30   Welcome and Introductions
- Robert Collins, Workshop Chair

8:35   Committee Overview
- William Kelley, Committee Chair

8:45   Keynote Address
- James Wyngaarden, Duke University and National Academy of Sciences

9:15   ***FEDERAL SUPPORT FOR PATIENT-ORIENTED CLINICAL RESEARCH***

Discussion Leader: Mary Charlson

9:20   Overview of Federal Sponsorship of Patient-oriented Clinical Research
- William Raub, White House Office of Science and Technology Policy

9:45   Reactions from Federal Agencies
         -   Darrell Regier, Director, Division of Clinical Research, NIMH
         -   Dennis Smith, Associate Director for Medical Research,
             Department Veterans Affairs
         -   Ira Raskin, Agency for Health Care Policy and Research

10:15   Panel/Committee Discussion

11:00   **BREAK**

11:15   *PRIVATE SECTOR FUNDING*

         Discussion Leader: Irving Fox

11:20   Funding by the Pharmaceutical/Biotechnology Industry
         -   Louis Lasagna, Tufts University

11:30   University/Industry Cooperative Funding Ventures
         -   Virginia Weldon, Monsanto Corporation

11:40   Nonprofit Sponsors
         -   Thomas Langfitt, Pew Charitable Trusts

11:50   Panel/Committee Discussion

12:40   **LUNCH**

1:30   *SHARING THE COSTS OF CLINICAL RESEARCH:
         I.   THIRD-PARTY PAYERS*

         Discussion Leader: Karen Antman

1:40   Role of Third-Party Payment Decisions on Clinical Research
         -   Michael Friedman, National Cancer Institute

1:50   Blue Cross/Blue Shield
         -   Ralph Schafferzick, Formerly with Blue Cross/Blue Shield of
             California

2:00   Private Insurers
         -   James Mulvihill, Travelers Insurance Company

2:10 ·   Health Maintenance Organizations
         -   Robert Goodman, US HealthCare, Inc.

2:20   Panel/Committee Discussion

3:15   **BREAK**

3:30   *SHARING THE COSTS OF CLINICAL RESEARCH:*
        II. HOSPITALS AND ACADEMIC HEALTH CENTERS

        Discussion Leader: William Kelley

3:35   NIH Intramural and Extramural Funding
        - John Diggs, Deputy Director for Extramural Research, NIH

3:45   Teaching Hospitals
        - Jerome Grossman, New England Medical Center

3:55   Academic Health Centers
        - David Challoner, University of Florida

4:05   Hospital-Based Clinical Research
        - Ruth Hanft, The Geroge Washington University

4:15   A Clinical Investigator's Perspective
        - John Glick, University of Pennsylvania

4:25   Panel/Committee Discussion

5:15   Concluding Remarks by Rapporteur
        - Eli Ginzberg, Columbia University

5:30   Adjourn

5:30   **RECEPTION AND DINNER**

Saturday, June 13

8:00   Continental Breakfast

8:30   *FOCUS ON HUMAN RESOURCES*

        Discussion Leader: John Stobo

8:30   Overview of Barriers to Careers in Clinical Research
        - John Stobo, Johns Hopkins University

8:45   Organizational Barriers (Medical Schools)
        - Alfred Fishmam, University of Pennsylvania

9:00   Indebtedness - Congressional Perspective
        -   Van Dunn, Senate Labor and Human Resources Committee

9:15   Indebtedness - Medical School's Perspective
        -   Julie Disa, Johns Hopkins University

9:30   Panel/Committee Discussion

10:00   **BREAK**

10:15   *FINANCING CLINICAL RESEARCH TRAINING*

        Discussion Leader: Albert Mulley

10:15   NRSA Training
        -   Charlotte Kuh, Educational Testing Service

10:30   American Cancer Society Program
        -   Virgil Loeb, Washington University

10:45   Nonprofit Organizations
        -   Richard Reynolds, Robert Wood Johnson Foundation

11:00   Medical Scientist Training Program
        -   Harold Swartz, Dartmouth Medical School

11:15   Panel/Committee Discussion

11:45   Concluding Remarks by Rapporteur
        -   E.H. Ahrens, Rockefeller University

Appendix E

Contributors

This Appendix recognizes a number of individuals who contributed in various ways to this study who are not recognized in other sections of the report or appendixes. Many served on planning committees in the early stages of the project; whereas others contributed written materials, data, or provided testimony to the committee during the study. The committee wishes to extend their appreciation to all investigators and administrators who have contributed. The committee extends a special note of gratitude to Dr. Judith Vaitukaitis, now the Director of the National Center for Research Resources, without whose assistance this study could not have been performed. The provided herein reflects the contributor's position at the time of interaction with the committee.

WILLIAM B. ABRAMS, Executive Director, Scientific Development, Merck Sharp & Dohme Research, Laboratories, West Point, Pennsylvania

STEPHEN A. BARKANIC, Program Officer, Undergraduate Science Education Program, Howard Hughes Medical Institute, Bethesda, Maryland

J. CLAUDE BENNETT, Professor and Chairman, Department of Medicine, University of Alabama School of Medicine, Birmingham, Alabama

ROBERT BERLINER, Yale University School of Medicine, New Haven, Connecticut

BRUCE BRUNDAGE, Professor of Medicine and Chief of Cardiology, Department of Medicine, University of Illinois at Chicago, Chicago, Illinois

LOUIS CANTILENA, Program Director, Division of Clinical Pharmacology, Uniformed Services University of Health Sciences, Bethesda, Maryland

SAM C. CARRIER, Provost, Oberlin College, Oberlin, Ohio

SEU LAIN CHEN, Division of Research Grants , National Institutes of Health, Bethesda, Maryland

DARYL CHUBIN, Senior Associate, U.S. Congress Office of Technology Assessment, Washington, D.C.

BARBARA FILNER, Program Officer, Graduate Science Education Program, Howard Hughes Medical Institute, Bethesda, Maryland

MARC S. GOLDSTEIN, Director, Research Services, American Physical Therapy Association, Alexandria, Virginia

RICHARD GREENE, Director, Center for Medical Effectiveness Research, Agency for Health Care Policy and Research, Rockville, Maryland

M. CAROLYN HARDEGREE, Director, Office of Biologics Research, Food and Drug Administration, Bethesda, Maryland

BERNADINE P. HEALY, Director, National Institutes of Health, Bethesda, Maryland

MARC HOROWITZ, Director, Loan Repayment Program, Office of AIDS Research, National Institutes of Health, Bethesda, Maryland

PAUL JOLLY, Associate Vice President, Section for Operational Studies, Association of American Medical Schools, Washington, D.C.

SHERRY KERAMIDAS, Associate Executive Vice President for Research and Education, American Physical Therapy Association, Alexandria, Virginia

CARL KUPFER, Director, National Eye Institute, National Institutes of Health, Bethesda, Maryland

JOHN LASZLO, American Cancer Society, Atlanta, Georgia

CLAUDE LENFANT, Director, National Heart, Lung, and Blood Institute, National Institutes of Health, Bethesda, Maryland

ROBERT MOORE, Division of Research Grants, National Institutes of Health, Bethesda, Maryland

ROBERT C. NELSON, Director, Office of Professional Development and Staff College, Center for Drug Evaluation and Research, Food and Drug Administration, Rockville, Maryland

EDWARD H. O'NEIL, Director, Pew Health Professions Program, Duke University, Durham, North Carolina

CARL C. PECK, Director, Center for Drug Evaluation and Research, Food and Drug Administration, Rockville, Maryland

JOHN T. POTTS, Jr., Professor and Chairman, Department of Medicine, Massachusetts General Hospital, Harvard Medical School, Boston Massachusetts.

THOMAS C. PURCELL, Director, Division of Training and Manpower Development, Centers for Disease Control, National Institute for Occupational Safety and Health, Cincinnati, Ohio

PAULA RANDOLPH, Elementary Teacher, Redmond School District, Redmond, Washington

MICHAEL ROSENBLATT, Senior Vice President for Research, Merck, Sharp & Dohme Laboratories, West Point, Pennsylvania

WALTER T. SCHAFFER, Research Training and Research Resources Officer, Office of Extramural Programs, National Institutes of Health, Bethesda, Maryland

ELAINE SEYMOUR, Bureau of Sociological Research, Department of Sociology, University of Colorado at Boulder, Boulder, Colorado

CHARLES SHERMAN, Office of Medical Applications of Research, National Institutes of Health, Bethesda, Maryland

LOUIS M. SHERWOOD, Executive Vice President, World Wide Development, Merck Sharp & Dohme Research Laboratories, Rahway, New Jersey

SAMUEL O. THIER, Former President, Institute of Medicine, National Academy of Sciences, Washington, D.C.

PHILIP TOSKES, University of Florida School of Medicine, Gainsville, Florida

JUDITH VAITUKAITIS, Deputy Director for Extramural Research Resources, National Center for Research Resources, National Institutes of Health, Bethesda, Maryland

DAVID DAVIS-VAN ATTA, Program Officer, Howard Hughes Medical Institute, Bethesda, Maryland

STEVEN WEISS, E. Gifford and Love Barnett Upjohn Professor of Internal Medicine and Oncology, University of Michigan Medical Center, Department of Internal Medicine, Division of Hematology/Oncology, Ann Arbor, Michigan

KERN WILDENTHAL, University of Texas Southwestern Medical Center, Dallas, Texas

ROGER L. WILLIAMS, Director, Office of Generic Drugs, Food and Drug Administration, Rockville, Maryland

JANET WOODCOCK, Deputy Director, CBER, Food and Drug Administration, Bethesda, Maryland

ROBERT YOUNG, President, Fox Chase Cancer Center, Philadelphia, Pennsylvania

KATHRYN ZOON, Director, CBER, Food and Drug Administration, Bethesda, Maryland

Appendix F

Biographies of Committee Members

WILLIAM N. KELLEY, M.D., is the Executive Vice President of the University of Pennsylvania, with responsibilities as Chief Executive Officer for the Medical Center, Dean of the School of Medicine, and Robert G. Dunlop Professor of Medicine and Biochemistry and Biophysics. He has held this position since October 1, 1989. Over the years, Dr. Kelley has played an important personal role in research, patient care, and teaching. At the time of his move to the University of Pennsylvania, he had served continuously as a principal investigator on investigator-initiated grants from the National Institutes of Health, principal investigator at the NIH-funded Michigan Multipurpose Arthritis Center, and principal investigator on the program project proposal entitled "Experimental Models of Gene Therapy," which was the first program project in the field of gene therapy funded by NIH. In his own research, he was the first to directly administer a human gene in vivo and obtain expression in an experimental animal. He was honored to serve as the keynote speaker at the First International Congress of Human Gene Therapy in Beijing, China, in October 1992. Dr. Kelley has had an opportunity to serve as president or chairman of six national professional organizations. He also currently serves as Chairman of the Membership Committee of the Institute of Medicine of the National Academy of Sciences. His honors include the John Phillips Memorial Award and medal of the American College of Physicians for his contributions to American medicine. Prior to his position at the University of Pennsylvania, Dr. Kelley was the John G. Searle Professor and Chairman of the Department of Internal Medicine and Professor of Biological Chemistry at the University of Michigan. He was Chief of Rheumatic and Genetic Diseases at the Duke University Medical Center prior to moving to Michigan. Dr. Kelley received his undergraduate and medical degrees from Emory University in Atlanta and training in internal medicine, rheumatology and genetics at the University of Texas Southwestern Medical School and Parkland Memorial Hospital in Dallas, the Massachusetts General Hospital and Harvard Medical School in Boston, and the National Institutes of Health in Bethesda, where he received the John D. Lane Award of the U.S. Public Health Service for his research contributions. Dr. Kelley's bibliography lists in excess of 240 publications and 12 books, and he has participated as a member of the editorial boards of 12 medical journals. He is the founder and senior editor of *The Textbook of Rheumatology*, which is now in its 4th edition, and is the founder and editor-in-chief of *The Textbook of Internal Medicine*.

KAREN H. ANTMAN, M.D., is Professor of Medicine and Chief of the Division of Medical Oncology at Columbia-Presbyterian Medical Center. Dr. Antman received her M.D. from the College of Physicians & Surgeons of Columbia University and joined the Harvard Medical School faculty in 1979. She previously was Associate Professor at the Harvard Medical School, where she was Clinical Director of the Dana Farber Cancer Institute and Beth Israel Hospital Solid Tumor Autologous Marrow Program and coordinated the sarcoma and mesothelioma clinical research and treatment programs at the Dana Farber Cancer Institute. Dr. Antman moved to Columbia-Presbyterian Medical Center in 1993. She has published extensively on bone marrow transplantation, hematopoietic cytokines, and sarcomas and mesotheliomas, and is coeditor of two textbooks, *Asbestos Related Malignancy* and *High Dose Cancer Therapy*. The latter examines the state of the art of bone marrow transplantation, hematopoietic stem cells and hematopoietic cytokines. The solid tumor marrow transplant program under her direction initially began pilot trials of new regimens in incurable breast cancer and other solid tumors on the basis of laboratory-based observations and has expanded to randomized trials with significantly less toxic regimens with curative intent. She has consulted for the U.S. Department of Justice on asbestos-related malignancies and served on the Health and Human Services Advisory Board Study of Coverage of Investigational Therapy, on the Physicians Payment Review Commission/American Medical Association Consensus Panel for Evaluation and Management of Services, and on the Harvard Resource Based Relative Value Scale Technical Consulting Panel. She is currently an associate editor of *Cancer Research*, is on the editorial board of *Annals of Internal Medicine* and the *New England Journal of Medicine*, and is president of the American Society for Clinical Oncology.

DOROTHY BROOTEN, Ph.D., R.N., is the Director of the Center for Low Birthweight: Prevention and Care, Professor in the Health Care of Women and Childbearing Dvision at the University of Pennsylvania School of Nursing, and the Overseers Term Chair in Perinatal Research. She is a member of the

Institute of Medicine. She is a former member of the governing council of the American Academy of Nursing and was cochair of the expert panel on Prevention and Care of Low Birthweight Infants for the National Center for Nursing Research at the National Institutes of Health. She is also a member of the Nursing Research Study section of NIH. Dr. Brooten was awarded the first Baxter Foundation Episteme Award from Sigma Theta Tau International, which acknowledges a major breakthrough in nursing knowledge development. She received the award for her randomized clinical trial on "Early Discharge of Very Low Birthweight Infants." The title Episteme Luareate was conferred upon her. Her study was published in the *New England Journal of Medicine* and received national and international coverage in the print media and on the Cable News Network as well as on local television newscasts across the country. The study represented a milestone for nursing research.

MARY E. CHARLSON, M.D., is an Associate Professor of Medicine and Chief of the Division of Internal Medicine at Cornell University Medical College. After completing her residency at Johns Hopkins Hospital, she graduated from the Robert Wood Johnson Clinical Scholar Program at Yale University. After joining the faculty at Cornell, she founded the Clinical Epidemiology Unit and a multidisciplinary research methodology group. She has published extensively on research methodology for clinical research and on strategies for measuring and improving prognoses and outcomes. She is the author of over 60 publications and serves on the editorial board of the *Journal of Clinical Epidemiology*. She is actively involved in the conduct of patient-oriented clinical investigation.

ROBERT C. COLLINS, M.D., is Frances Stark Professor and Chairman, Department of Neurology, University of California, Los Angeles (UCLA). Dr. Collins was recruited to the Chairmanship at UCLA in 1987 from Washington University, where he was Professor of Neurology and of Anatomy and Neurobiology. At UCLA, Dr. Collins is Director of the Read Neurological Research Center, which in the past five years has expanded programs in molecular and cellular neurosciences as well as in human brain mapping targeted on human neurological diseases. The Center is known for its work on multiple sclerosis, epilepsy, Parkinson's disease, Alzheimer's disease, neurootology, and neuroimaging. Prior to his appointment, Dr. Collin's research explored basic mechanisms of cerebellar metabolism and blood flow in experimental animals. A graduate of Cornell University Medical School, he completed an internship at Massachusetts General Hospital, research training at the National Institutes of Health, and neurology training at Cornell-New York Hospital before moving to Washington University. Dr. Collins is a coeditor of *Neurobiology of Disease*, a textbook for medical students. He serves on the editorial board of *Annals of Neurology*, and is co-founding editor of *Clinical Neuroscience*. He serves on committees for the American Neurological Association, National Institute of Neurological Diseases and Stroke, and the Institute of Medicine.

HAILE T. DEBAS, M.D., is Professor and Chairman of the Department of Surgery at the University of California, San Francisco (UCSF). He was born in Eritrea. He obtained his medical degree from McGill University in 1963 and completed his surgical residency at the University of British Columbia, where he later joined the faculty. In 1980, Dr. Debas was appointed Professor of Surgery at the University of California, Los Angeles, Chief of Gastrointestinal Surgery at Wadsworth Veterans Administration Medical Center, and Key Investigator at the Center for Ulcer and Research and Education (CURE). In 1985, he moved to the University of Washington in Seattle as Professor and Chief of Gastrointestinal Surgery. He was named Chair of the Department of Surgery at UCSF in 1987. In addition to being a member of the Institute of Medicine, Dr. Debas is involved in the following organizations: Director, American Board of Surgery; American College of Surgeons; American Surgical Association; Internatinal Hepato-Biliary Pancreatic Association; Society for Surgery of the Alimentary Tract; American Gastroenterological Association; Association of Academic Minority Physicians; and Pacific Coast Surgical Society. His university service includes: Chair of the UCSF Academic Senate and cochair, UCSF Planning Committee for the 21st Century. He also serves on the editorial boards of the following publications: *Gastroenterology, American Journal of Surgery, Western Journal of Medicine*, and *Regulatory Peptide Letter*. Dr. Debas's major research interests are peptic ulcer, gastrointestinal endocrinology, and gastrointestinal physiology.

WILLIAM L. DEWEY, Ph.D., is Vice President for Research and Graduate Studies and Professor of Pharmacology, Virginia Commonwealth University (VCU). Dr. Dewey joined VCU in 1972 as an Associate Professor after serving as Assistant Professor of Pharmacology at the University of North Carolina for three years. He was promoted to the rank of Full Professor in 1976. In 1981, he was named Assistant Dean in the School of Graduate Studies, and in 1982 he became the Associate Dean of the VCU School of Basic Health Sciences. He was named Associate Provost for Research and Graduate Studies in 1987, a post he held until promoted to his current position in 1992. Dr. Dewey has authored or coauthored approximately 250 papers, book chapters, or review articles as well as over 250 abstracts on the pharmacology of drug abuse. He has served as the primary adviser for 15 doctoral students and one master's degree recipient. Twenty-nine postdoctoral fellows or foreign scientists have studied in his laboratory. He served as President of the American Society for Pharmacology and Experimental Therapeutics, the Federation of American Societies for Experimental Biology, and the College on Problems of Drug Dependence as well as serving as Chairman of Study Sections for the National

Institute on Drug Abuse. He has served as field editor for the *Journal of Pharmacology and Experimental Therapeutics* and currently serves on the National Advisory Council for the National Institute on Drug Abuse.

JANICE ELECTA GREEN DOUGLAS, M.D., is a graduate of Fisk University and Meharry Medical College. She began her formal training in biomedical research supported by National Institutes of Health Endocrinology Training Fellowship at Vanderbilt University School of Medicine, where she also served as an Instructor in the Department of Medicine. She continued her research training in Bethesda, Maryland, as a Senior Staff Fellow at the National Institutes of Health, National Institute of Child Health and Human Development, Section on Hormonal Regulation. She is currently a Professor of Medicine and Professor of Physiology and Biophysics at Case Western Reserve University School of Medicine. She is also the Director of the Endocrinology and Hypertension Division. In addition, she was appointed Vice Chairperson for Academic Affairs for the Department of Medicine in 1991. Dr. Douglas is internationally renowned as a physician-scientist and conducts studies on cellular and molecular mechanisms of blood pressure regulation with a focus on the renin angiotensin system and racial/ethnic diversity in the pathophysiology of essential hypertension. She is author or coauthor of many medical publications and is (or has been) a member of editorial boards and publication committees, and has been associate editor (or guest editor) for a number of prestigious medical journals, including the *Journal of Clinical Investigation, American Journal of Physiology, Journal of Laboratory and Clinical Medicine, Circulation, Ethnicity and Disease,* and the *Endocrine Society,* to name a few. She has been elected to membership in a number of prestigious organizations for physician scientists, including the American Society for Clinical Investigation and the Association for American Physicians, and she is a fellow of the High Blood Pressure Council of the American Heart Association, the Association for Academic Minority Physicians, and the Central Society for Clinical Research. Dr. Douglas has served on numerous National Institutes of Health review and advisory committees, U.S. Department of Veterans Affairs Merit Review Board for Cardiovascular Studies, and the Council for the National Heart, Lung, and Blood Institute (NHLBI). This Council is the principal advisory body to the NHLBI, makes decisions about research and training support, and advises on programmatic issues. She is currently serving on an advisory group for President Clinton's White House Task Force on Health Reform.

IRVING H. FOX, M.D., is Vice President of Medical Affairs, Biogen, Inc. Dr. Fox joined Biogen in 1991 following a 17-year career in academic medicine. During 13 years at the University of Michigan, Dr. Fox held positions that included Program Director of the Clinical Research Center at the University of Michigan Hospital (1978–1990) and Interim Division Chief in

Rheumatology. His academic appointments include full professorships in internal medicine (1978–1990) and biological chemistry (1984–1990) at the University of Michigan. He is currently Clinical Professor of Medicine at Harvard Medical School and Clinical Associate at the Massachusetts General Hospital. A well-known medical scientist, Dr. Fox has consulted on many task forces and committees including the National Institute of Arthritis and Musculoskeletal and Skin Diseases Task Force for the National Institutes of Health (1991 to present). Among his many memberships in professional societies are the American Society for Clinical Investigation, American Society for Biological Chemistry and Molecular Biology, American College of Physicians, American Federation for Clinical Research, and American College of Rheumatology. Dr. Fox has published more than 110 peer-reviewed articles in scientific journals and over 75 review articles and chapters in medical textbooks.

ROBERT J. GENCO, D.D.S., Ph.D., is the Distinguished Professor of Oral Biology and Periodontology; Chair, Department of Oral Biology; and Associate Dean for Graduate Studies and Research, State University of New York (SUNY) at Buffalo School of Dental Medicine. Professor Genco joined SUNY Buffalo in 1967 after completing his Ph.D. degree and clinical training in Periodontology at the University of Pennsylvania. His work since then has involved laboratory and clinical studies of the causes, prevention, and treatment of oral diseases including dental caries and periodontal disease. He established a periodontal clinical training program in 1968, which combined a Ph.D. in oral biology with clinical specialty training, that has resulted in the training of a number of successful clinician-scientists who are presently active in research and academics throughout the country. In 1977, he founded the Periodontal Disease Research Center at SUNY Buffalo, which is one of five national centers dedicated to evaluation of clinical advances in periodontology. He edited *Contemporary Periodontics* with Drs. Henry Goldman and Walter Cohen, a popular text among dental students and residents in the United States and other countries. He has been active in many professional organizations and was chairman of the Dental Section of the American Association for the Advancement of Science. In 1985 he was President of the American Association for Dental Research, and in 1991 he served as President of the International Association for Dental Research, which has over 9,000 members. Since 1988 Dr. Genco has been the editor of the *Journal of Periodontology* and was recently awarded the Gold Medal for Excellence in Research by the American Dental Association. Dr. Genco has also been a member of the Institute of Medicine since 1988.

DAVID J. KUPFER, M.D., is Professor and Chairman of the Department of Psychiatry and Professor of Behavioral Neuroscience at the University of Pittsburgh School of Medicine. He received his bachelor (magna cum laude) and M.D. degrees from Yale University. Following completion of an internship, Dr. Kupfer continued his postgraduate clinical and research training at the Yale-New Haven Hospital and at the National Institute of Mental Health. In 1969, he was appointed an Assistant Professor of Psychiatry at Yale University School of Medicine. Dr. Kupfer joined the faculty at the University of Pittsburgh in 1973 as an Associate Professor of Psychiatry and Director of Research and Research Training at Western Psychiatric Institute and Clinic. In 1975, he became Professor of Psychiatry and Chairman of the Department in 1983. For more than 20 years, Dr. Kupfer's research has focused primarily on the conceptualization, diagnosis, and treatment of mood disorders. He has written more than 500 articles, books, and book chapters examining the use of medication in recurrent depression, the causes of depression, and the relationship between biological rhythms, sleep, and depression. In recognition of his contribution to the field, Dr. Kupfer has been the recipient of numerous awards and honors, including the A.E. Bennett Research Award in Clinical Science, the Anna-Monika Foundation Prize, the Daniel E. Efron Award, the Twenty-Sixth Annual Award of the Institute of Pennsylvania Hospital in Memory of Edward A. Strecker, M.D., and the William R. McAlpin, Jr., Research Achievement Award. He was elected to the Institute of Medicine in 1990.

NICHOLAS F. LARUSSO, M.D., is Professor of Medicine and Professor of Biochemistry and Molecular Biology, Mayo Medical School, Clinic and Foundation, Rochester, Minnesota. Dr. LaRusso received his undergraduate degree in biology (magna cum laude) from Boston College and his M.D. degree from New York Medical College. The majority of his clinical training in internal medicine and gastroenterology, in which he is board certified, was received at the Mayo Graduate School. His initial research training was as a National Institutes of Health postdoctoral research fellow at the Mayo Clinic and subsequently as a Mayo Foundation scholar and guest investigator in the Department of Biochemical Cytology at the Rockefeller University, where he worked with the Nobel Laureate Christian de Duve. He joined the faculty of the Mayo Medical School in 1977, and in 1990 became Chairman of the Division of Gastroenterology, a position he currently holds. Dr. LaRusso is involved in both basic and patient-oriented clinical research. His basic research focuses on digestion and transport in hepatic epithelia and has been supported by NIH since 1978; he currently holds a MERIT award from NIH for this research. In addition, he is currently involved in industry- and federally funded research on the pathophysiology and therapy of hepatobiliary diseases. In 1991, he became Editor of *Gastroenterology*, the premier subspecialty journal in the field.

ALBERT G. MULLEY, Jr., M.D., is Associate Professor of Medicine and Associate Professor of Health Policy at Harvard Medical School, Chief of the General Internal Medicine Division and Director of the Medical Practices Evaluation Center at Massachusetts General Hospital. After receiving degrees in medicine and public policy from Harvard, he completed his residency training in internal medicine at Massachusetts General Hospital. He is author and editor of the text *Primary Care Medicine*, and of many articles in the medical and health services research literature. Dr. Mulley's recent research has focused on the use of decision analysis, outcomes research, and preference assessment methods to distinguish between warranted and unwarranted variations in clinical practice. This work has led to development of research instruments and approaches, including shared decision-making programs utilizing interactive videodisc technology to inform patients about treatment options and to catalyze large-scale prospective clinical trials.

JOHN D. STOBO, M.D., is the William Osler Professor of Medicine and Director of the Department of Medicine at the Johns Hopkins University School of Medicine and Physician-in-Chief for the Johns Hopkins Hospital. He received his B.A. from Dartmouth College and his M.D. from the State University of New York at Buffalo. Dr. Stobo was an intern and assistant resident and served as chief medical resident on the Osler Medical Service of the Johns Hopkins Hospital. He is a member of the Institute of Medicine and currently serves on the Board of Governors of the American Board of Internal Medicine and serves as Secretary/Treasurer of the Association of Professors of Medicine.

MYRON L. WEISFELDT, M.D., is the Chair of the Department of Medicine, the Samuel Bard Professor of Medicine, and Director of the Medical Service and Head of the Cardiovascular Center at Columbia-Presbyterian Medical Center in New York. Following two years of college at Northwestern University he entered a five-year medical school program at the Johns Hopkins University School of Medicine. During medical school he spent a pivotal year in research training at the National Institutes of Health (NIH) studying cardiovascular physiology. After graduating from medical school, Dr. Weisfeldt performed an internship and one year of residency in internal medicine at Columbia-Presbyterian Medical Center. Dr. Weisfeldt then spent two years at NIH performing research on cardiovascular aging and then completed his residency and fellowship training at the Massachusetts General Hospital in Boston. He became a faculty member at Johns Hopkins in 1972. Dr. Weisfeldt's research interests have included reperfusion injury following a period of ischemia or reduced blood flow, the relaxation phase of cardiac contraction and the relationship of relaxation properties to heart failure, and the mechanisms of blood movement during cardiopulmonary resuscitation. In 1975, Dr. Weisfeldt was appointed Director of the Cardiology Division at Johns Hopkins University School of Medicine. Three years later he was promoted to full professor and appointed the Robert L. Levy Professor of Cardiology. Dr. Weisfeldt moved to Columbia-Presbyterian Medical Center in 1991. He currently serves on the editorial boards of the journals *Circulation, Circulation Research,* and the *Journal of the American College of Cardiology.* Dr. Weisfeldt served as President of the American Heart Association in 1990. From 1987 to 1990 he was Chairman of the Cardiology Advisory Committee to the National Heart, Lung, and Blood Institute of NIH.

CATHERINE M. WILFERT, M.D., received her B.A. with distinction from Stanford University in 1958 and her M.D., cum laude, from Harvard Medical School in 1962. After completing one year of internal medicine residency on the Harvard Service at the Boston City Hospital, she entered pediatric residency at the Bowman-Gray School of Medicine in Winston-Salem, North Carolina, and Children's Hospital Medical Center of Boston. Two years of fellowship in infectious diseases under the direction of Dr. John F. Enders and Dr. Samuel Katz were completed in 1967, at which time she became a faculty member in pediatrics at Harvard. In 1969 Dr. Wilfert was appointed Assistant Professor of Pediatrics at Duke University School of Medicine and was promoted to Professor in 1980, and she remains Chief of the Division of Infectious Diseases in the Department of Pediatrics at the present time. Her career in infectious diseases has included clinical investigations of a variety of immunogens in children and service on the Microbiology and Infectious Diseases Advisory Committee of the National Institute of Allergy and Infectious Diseases, as well as being Chair of the Advisory Committee on Immunization Practices for the Centers for Disease Control and Prevention. Recently she has been the principal investigator of the Pediatric AIDS Clinical Trial Unit and in that capacity has formed a statewide consortium of Pediatric Centers caring for children with human immunodeficiency virus infection to provide access to the clinical trials as well as to regionalize care. Dr. Wilfert has also been a member of the Advisory Committee to the Center for Biologics Evaluation and Research and has been the Chair of the Pediatric Committee of the AIDS Clinical Trials Group.

Glossary

AAMC	Association of American Medical Colleges
AAP	American Association of Physicians
ABIM	American Board of Internal Medicine
ADAMHA	Alcohol, Drug Abuse, and Mental Health Administration
AFOSR	Air Force Office of Scientific Research
AHCPR	Agency for Health Care Policy and Research
AMA	American Medical Association
BRASS	Biomedical Research Assistant Saturday Scholars
CAP	Clinical Associates Program
CDCP	Centers for Disease Control and Prevention
CDER	Center for Drug Evaluation and Research
CIA	Clinical Investigator Award
CIP	Clinical Investigator Pathway
CRADA	Cooperative Research and Economic Development Agreements
CRCM	Comprehensive Regional Center for Minorities
CRISP	Computerized Retrieval of Information on Research Projects
CSP	Clinical Scholars Program
DHHS	Department of Health and Human Services
DOD	Department of Defense
DRG	Division of Research Grants
DRR	Division of Research Resources
DVA	Department of Veterans Affairs
EIS	Epidemic Intelligence Service

FDA	Food and Drug Administration
FCCSET	Federal Coordinating Committee on Science, Engineering, and Technology
GAO	General Accounting Office
GCRC	General Clinical Research Centers
GME	Graduate Medical Education
GPEP	General Professional Education of the Physician
GUIRR	Government-University-Industry Research Roundtable
HCFA	Health Care Financing Administration
HFRA	Health Research Facilities Act
HIV	Human Immunodeficiency Virus
HHMI	Howard Hughes Medical Institute
HPSP	Health Professional Scholarship Programs
HRA	Health Resources Administration
HSA	Health Services Administration
IOM	Institute of Medicine
IRB	Institutional Review Boards
IRG	initial review groups
LCME	Liaison Committee for Medical Education
MARC	Minority Access to Research Careers
MBRS	Minority Biomedical Research Support
MEDTEP	Medical Treatment Effectiveness Program
MRO	Medical research organizations
MSTP	Medical Scientist Training Program
NHSC	National Health Service Corps
NIMH	National Institute of Mental Health
NIDRR	National Institute on Disability and Rehabilitation Research
NIDA	National Institute of Drug Abuse
NIAAA	National Institute of Alcohol and Alcohol Abuse
NCI	National Cancer Institute
NCHS	National Center for Health Services Research
NCHSR	National Center for Health Statistics
NCNR	National Center for Nursing Research
NCRR	National Center for Research Resources
NEI	National Eye Institute
NHLBI	National Heart, Lung, and Blood Institute
NIA	National Institute of Aging
NIAID	National Institute of Allergy and Infectious Diseases
NIAMS	National Institute of Arthritis, Musculoskeletal and Skin Diseases

NIDCD	National Institute of Deafness and Communicative Disorders
NICHD	National Institute of Child and Human Development
NIDDK	National Institute of Diabetes, Digestive and Kidney Diseases
NIDR	National Institute for Dental Research
NIGMS	National Institute of General Medical Sciences
NINDS	National Institute of Neurological Diseases and Stroke
NIOSH	National Institute of Occupational Safety and Health
NOAA	National Oceanic and Atmospheric Administration
NRC	National Research Council
NRSA	National Research Service Awards
NSB	National Science Board
NSF	National Science Foundation
OASH	Office of the Assistant Secretary for Health
OHRST	Office of Health Research, Statistics, and Technology
OMAR	Office of Medical Applications of Research
OMB	Office of Management and Budget
ONR	Office of Naval Research
OREF	Orthopedic Research and Education Foundation
OTA	Office of Technology Assessment
P01	Program Project Grant
PCAST	President's Council on Science and Technology
PHS	Public Health Service
PORT	Patient Outcomes Research Teams
PSA	Physician-Scientist Award
R01	Traditional Research Project Grant
RCDA	Research Career Development Award
RCT	Randomized clinical trial
REU	Research Experiences for Undergraduates
R&D	Research and development
RPG	Research project grants
RRC	Residency Review Committees
SEPA	Science Education Partnership
SSTP	Surgical Scientist Training Program
SURF	Summer Undergraduate Research Fellowships
URAP	Undergraduate Research Associates Program
USAMRDC	U.S. Army Medical Research and Development Command
VHA	Voluntary health agencies
WHSC	White House Science Council

Index

A

Academic health centers
  career path of researchers in, 5, 13–14
  clinical care component in, 21, 28, 53
  in clinical research oversight, 6
  cost of graduate medical education, 21, 28
  definition, 13
  disincentives for clinical research in, 53–55
  faculty demographics, 45–50
  faculty growth in, 43–44
  faculty tracks in, 55–57
  funding for research in, 20–21
  growth of, 28
  in health care plan benefit design, 21
  health care reform and, 5, 8
  health research spending by, 63
  historical development, 43–44
  number of, 43, 44
  patient access, 21
  recognition for researchers in, 13–14, 28–29, 50–55, 60
  recommendations, 13–16, 20–21
  research infrastructure, 14–15, 60–61
  research involvement of faculty, 50
  role of, 2, 21
  technology assessment in, 21
  See also Medical school(s)
Academic-industry linkages, 110
  benefits for academic institutions, 209
  commercialization of research findings, 205–206
  concerns about, 210, 216, 217
  conflict of commitment in, 214–215
  conflict of interest in, 20, 213–214
  current context, 199–200, 216–217
  exclusivity of research findings, 212–213
  history of, 197–199
  industry benefits, 207–209
  management of, 215
  objections to, 200
  objectives of, 20, 200
  prevalence, 206–207
  proprietary rights issues in, 210–212
  recommendations, 20
  research culture in, 201–202
  research goals and, 211
  types of, 202–205
Accreditation/certification
  agencies, 16
  in clinical psychology, 277–278

as disincentive to research, 18, 57,
    166–167
of medical schools, 167
problems in, 4
recommendations, 16–18
residency review committees, 17, 164–
    165
specialty board certification, 18, 166–
    167
Accreditation Committee for Graduate
    Medical Education, 16, 17
Agency for Health Care Policy and
    Research, 27
    budget, 101, 188
    outcomes research, 100–101
    role of, 99
AIDS, 67, 97, 99
AIDS Research Debt Relief Program, 12,
    190
Alcohol, Drug Abuse and Mental Health
    Administration (ADAMHA), 64,
    69, 73–76, 136
Alliance for Aging Research, 19, 119
American Academy of Orthopaedic
    Surgeons, 284–285, 300
American Association for the
    Advancement of Science, 137
American Association of Physicians, 56
American Board of Internal Medicine, 166
American Board of Medical Specialties,
    16, 18, 166
American Cancer Society, 107, 189
American College of Surgeons, 294–295
American Federation of Clinical Research,
    56
American Heart Association, 107, 189
American Lung Association, 107
American Society for Clinical
    Investigation, 24, 56
Anesthesiology, 166
Armed Services Health Professional
    Scholarship, 157–159
Association of American Medical
    Colleges, 147, 214
Atherogenesis, 26
Autologous bone marrow transplantation,
    114

B

Basic science research
    clinical research and, 27, 28–29, 35,
        55–57
    disease-related, 34
    in medical schools, 28–29, 55–57
    medical student interest in, 147
    NIH grants, 93–94
    surgical research, 284, 294
*Biomedical and Behavioral Research
    Scientists: Their Training and
    Supply,* 30
Biomedical Research and Development
    Price Index, 76
Biotechnology research, 110–111, 199
Breast cancer, 26
    autologous bone marrow
        transplantation for, 114

C

California Institute of Technology, 133
Carnegie Mellon University, 133
Centers for Disease Control and
    Prevention, 12, 67
    research spending, 98–99
    research training in, 187–188
    role of, 98
Clinical Associate Physician program, 12,
    186
Clinical research
    background papers for evaluation of,
        38
    classification of activities in, 7, 32–34,
        88
    contribution of, 1, 24, 41–42
    cost of, 79
    data collection/analysis for evaluation
        of, 7, 29, 44
    definition, 3, 30–31, 32, 34–35, 87–88,
        92–93
    evaluation strategy, 29–31, 36–40
    future challenges to, 4–6, 41–42
    future needs in, 3–4, 6, 25–27, 35, 41,
        216–217
    historical development, 24–29

institutional obstacles to, 5
oversight, 5, 6, 7, 18–20
researcher demographics, 44–50
role of, 27, 193–194
scope of, 24–29, 34, 36
supply of researchers, 2, 4, 6, 27, 29
See also Human research; Training for
    research
Clinical Scholars Program, 190
Clinical trials, 5
consortia for conduct of, 204
historical development, 25
third-party payers and, 115–116
Compensation for researchers, 12
in academic-industry collaboration,
    203, 204, 213
in academic settings, 13–14
as career path disincentive, 59–60
in clinical psychology, 272–273
in Department of Veterans Affairs, 103
educational debt burden and, 160, 190
Conflict of interest issues, 20, 213–214
Consulting, 203
Cost of training
in academic health centers, 21–22
as disincentive to research career, 4,
    42, 60, 156, 159–160
recommendations, 12–13
tuition debt relief program, 12–13, 189
See also Funding/funding issues
Cystic fibrosis, 26

D

Dentistry, 3, 142
clinical research in, 239–251
curriculum, 124
human research training, 11
recommendations, 240, 243–244, 245–
    247, 249–250
schools, 248–250
Department of Agriculture, 12, 67
Department of Defense, 12, 67, 105, 131,
    286–287, 296
Department of Education, 12, 67, 105
Department of Energy, 12, 67

Department of Health and Human
    Services, 12, 73
health research spending, 67
Department of Veterans Affairs, 12, 67,
    282
budget, 102, 103–104
organizational structure, 101
research activities, 101–103
research training in, 188
Dermatology, 166
Disabilities, students with, 137
Disincentives for research career, 42–43
career compensation as, 12, 59–60
clinical care responsibilities as, 170
in clinical psychology, 272–278
duration of training as, 4, 12, 42, 55,
    150, 162
educational costs as, 4, 12, 42, 60, 156,
    159–160, 190
evaluation of, 29–31
lack of exposure to research practice
    as, 167–168
lack of role models or mentors as, 4,
    29, 58–59
lifestyle factors, 29, 42, 59–60
in medical education, 53–55, 144–145,
    167–170
for newly independent investigators, 8,
    53
professional status of research as, 4,
    12, 28–29, 42, 55, 194
recertification requirements, 18, 57,
    166–167
timing of training and, 169
Doctor–patient relationship, 113, 203
Duke University, 151

E

Ethics, 155, 192, 203

F

F32 awards, 170, 171, 173–175, 178
Federal Coordinating Council on Science,
    Engineering and Technology,
    128, 130, 131

Federal government
   in clinical research oversight, 6, 18–19
   commercial use of research funded by,
      212–213
   departmental support for human
      research, 12, 67, 101–105
   in development of academic medical
      centers, 44
   health research support, 9–10, 63, 65,
      67, 120, 197, 198–199, 202
   in improvement of research training,
      194–195
   legislative encouragement of research,
      198–199
   medical school scholarships, 158
   postdoctoral training funded by, 170
   in precollege science preparation, 131
   training program outcomes, 188–189
   undergraduate science programs, 134–
      136
   See also specific agency or department
First Investigator Research Support and
      Transition, 8
Food and Drug Administration, 115, 188,
      200
Foundations, 106–107, 189, 190
Four Schools Physician Scientist Program
      in Internal Medicine, 151
Funding/funding issues
   academic health centers, 20–21
   academic-industry collaborations, 203,
      204, 205
   average cost of research grant, 102
   basic research, clinical research vs.,
      28–29
   in Centers for Disease Control and
      Prevention, 98–99
   central management of, 19
   clinical psychology, 270–271
   comparative cost of human research,
      79
   in cooperative model of research
      management, 118–121
   cost of medical education, 156–160
   data for evaluation of, 5, 64
   Department of Defense research
      spending, 105

Department of Education research
      spending, 105
   in Department of Veterans Affairs,
      102, 103–104
   faculty, support for, 193–194
   in General Clinical Research Centers,
      97
   government support, 9–10, 64–67, 197,
      198–199
   grant size, 76
   grant writing skills, 10
   health research spending, 63
   historical development, 27–28, 64–65,
      197
   human research programs, 58
   industry-sponsored research, 109–111,
      197, 198
   Medical Scientist Training Program,
      11, 12, 152
   minority access to science careers,
      134–136
   NIH extramural research, 72–77
   NIH human research, 81–95
   NIH research centers, 95–96
   nonprofit organizations, research
      spending in, 106, 107, 108
   postdoctoral research training, 171–178
   precollege science preparation, 130–131
   privately supported research training,
      189
   research career development awards,
      184–185
   research training programs, 11, 151, 192
   social context, 202
   support of newly independent
      investigators, 8, 53
   in surgical career, 291–292
   third-party payers in clinical research,
      112–118
   training in, 192
   training related to subsequent grant
      success, 178, 182–184, 186
   tuition debt relief, 12–13, 189
   undergraduate science preparation,
      134–136
*Funding Health Sciences Research: A
   Strategy to Restore Balance,* 31

G

General Clinical Research Centers
  evaluation of, 194
  funding, 97
  future of, 97
  historical development, 96, 97
  number of, 9
  organizational structure, 96
  recommendations, 9, 12
  research activities in, 97
  role of, 96
  training of researchers in, 97, 186
Genetic engineering, 1–2, 26
Genome mapping, 1, 23, 26
Government-University-Industry Research
    Roundtable, 119
Grant preparation, 10
  as distraction from research, 74–76
  training in, 192

H

Harvard Clinical Effectiveness Program,
    189, 191
Health care reform, 23–24
  clinical research and, 2, 5, 8, 18, 41–42
  medical innovation and, 110
  support for clinical research and, 118
Howard Hughes Medical Center, 108–
    109, 151
Human immunodeficiency virus, 2, 24,
    97, 98, 99
Human research
  activities in, 36, 93
  cost of, 79
  data needs, 7
  definition, 3, 93
  diversity of, 3
  in F32 awards, 173–175
  in K awards, 185
  in NIH, 81–95
  R01 grants for, 5, 39, 185
  recommendations for NIH in, 6–7, 8,
    9–11, 12–13
  resources assessment, 29–30
  See also Clinical research

I

Imaging technology, 23
Incentives for research career
  in development of research
    infrastructure, 14–15, 28
  mentor role, 58–59, 168–169
  need for, 6
  professional recognition, 13–14
  recommendations, 12–13
  tuition debt relief, 12–13, 190
  See also Disincentives for research
    career
Intellectual property rights, 199, 204,
    207
  in academic-industry linkages, 210–
    212
  corporations owned by academic
    institutions, 206
Internal medicine, 166

J

J. David Gladstone Foundation
    Laboratories for Cardiovascular
    Disease, 108
Johns Hopkins University, 56, 151, 192
Joint Commission for Accreditation of
    Health Care Organizations, 16

K

K awards, 10, 170, 184–185

L

Legal issues
  in academic-industry linkages, 212
  antitrust law and cooperative research,
    119
  intellectual property rights, 199, 204,
    207, 210–212
  reimbursement issues, 113–114
Liaison Committee for Medical
    Education, 16, 17, 167

M

Managed care, 110
Managed competition, 5
March of Dimes-Birth Defects
    Foundation, 107
Mayo Clinic, 191
McMaster University, 192
M.D.s
    dual-degree program, 151–152
    laboratory-research training, 150
    medical school faculty, 44–46, 50
    in Medical Scientist Training Program,
        154
    as NIH grant recipients, 28, 77–79, 85,
        172, 173, 175–176, 178
    in NIH peer review groups, 82
    number of, 44–45
    postdoctoral training, 182–184
    research training after medical school,
        163
    See also Postgraduate medical
        education
Medicaid, 112
Medical research organizations, 108–109
Medical school(s)
    accreditation, 167
    costs, 21, 156–160
    curriculum, 15, 17, 145–147
    dual-degree programs, 151–152
    faculty, clinical or preclinical
        distribution of, 45–46
    faculty degrees, 45
    faculty demographics, 46–48
    faculty growth, 28, 43–44
    faculty research activity, 50
    historical development, 42–43, 142–
        143
    laboratory training in, 146
    Medical Scientist Training Program in,
        152–155
    model training programs, 189–192
    postgraduate research training, 160–
        170
    in promoting research careers, 144–
        145
    research training programs in, 151

student demographics, 143–144
student exposure to research, 15, 148–
    150
student interest in research, 145, 147–
    148
time demands in, and research, 150
tuition debt relief, 12–13, 189
See also Academic health centers
Medical Scientist Training Program, 11,
    12, 152–155
Medicare, 21, 64, 110, 112
Minorities
    in clinical psychology, 270, 276
    in medical school, 143–144
    on medical school faculty, 49–50
    in medicine, 127
    in surgical science, 289–290, 297–298
    in undergraduate science, 134, 136,
        137
Molecular biology, 1–2, 25
Multidisciplinary research, 8, 61
Muscular Dystrophy Association, 107

N

National Center for Health Statistics, 99
National Center for Nursing Research, 3
National Easter Seal Society, 107
National Health Service Corps, 157–159
National Institute of Mental Health, 271
National Institute of Occupational Safety
    and Health, 98–99
National Institute on Disability and
    Rehabilitation Research, 104
National Institutes of Health (NIH), 131
    appropriations to, 9–10
    biotechnology research, 111
    budget history, 67, 76–77
    Computerized Retrieval of Information
        on Research Projects, 88–90
    data collection, 7, 82–84
    degrees of grant recipients, 77–79, 85
    in evaluation of training programs, 10,
        11
    extramural research, 67–69, 72–77

General Clinical Research Centers, 96–97

grant applications received by, 78, 84–85

human research funding, 81–95

intramural research, 67, 69–72

Medical Scientist Training Program, 152–155

Minority Access to Research Careers program, 134

Minority Biomedical Research Support, 136

multidisciplinary research in, 8

Office of Medical Applications of Research data, 87–88

oversight role, 7

peer review process, 77, 79–82, 282, 285–286, 295–296

postdoctoral research training in, 170, 171–176, 180–184

recommendations for, 6–7, 8, 9–11, 12–13

research career development awards, 10, 184–185

research settings, 8, 95–98

Research Supplements for Underrepresented Minorities, 136

study sections, 7, 81–82, 282, 285–286, 295–296

surgical research in, 285–286, 290, 298–299

in training of researchers, 71, 178–180

National Oceanic and Atmospheric Administration, 131

National Research Service Awards, 30, 170

National Science Foundation, 12, 67, 131, 136, 137

Research Experiences for Undergraduates, 134–136

New investigators, 8, 53

Nonprofit organizations, 106–109

Nursing

clinical research in, 3, 253–264

doctoral programs, 124

training, 142

O

Outcomes research

in Agency for Health Care Policy and Research, 100–101

in dentistry, 250

General Clinical Research Centers for, 9

in human research, 81

role of, 2, 27

status of, 41

third-party payers in, 116

Oversight

of academic-industry linkages, 20, 215

current problems in, 5, 18–19

interorganizational interdisciplinary group for, 117

model of, 118–121

of NIH study sections, 7

recommendations, 6, 19–20

P

Patent & Trademarks Act, 199

Patient-oriented clinical research. *See* Human research

Peer Evaluation of Extramural Research, 7

Peer review, NIH, 7, 77, 79–82, 282, 285–286, 295–296

Pharmaceutical industry

corporations owned by academic institutions, 206

new drug development, 109, 110

reimbursement concerns, 115

research spending, 109, 110, 197, 209

Ph.D.s

dual-degree programs, 151

educational debt, 189

on medical school faculty, 45–46, 50, 55

as NIH grant recipients, 28, 77–79, 85, 172–176, 178, 182

in nursing, 257–259

training, 150, 161–162, 182–184

Positional cloning, 1

Postgraduate medical education
    design of research programs in, 161–163
    mentoring in, 168–169
    quality of research training in, 167–168
    recommendations, 16
    residency review committees in, 164–165
    role of research training in, 160–161
    specialty certification, 166–167
    timing of research training in, 169–170
Primary and secondary school science, 125, 126
    classroom experience, 127–129
    evaluation of, 132
    federal programs, 131
    role of, 127
    science fairs, 129
    special initiatives, 129–130
    teacher preparation, 128
    trends, 130–131
Private sector
    in clinical research oversight, 6, 18–19
    clinical researchers in, 42, 208–209
    corporations owned by academic institutions, 206
    in funding of evaluative science centers, 11
    in funding of research training, 11
    health research spending, 63, 65
    industry-sponsored research, 63, 109–111, 197–198
    medical research organizations, 108–109
    medical school research programs funded by, 151
    nonprofit organizations, 106–109
    research culture in, 201–202
    research training in, 170–171, 189–190
    voluntary health agencies, 107
    See also Academic-industry linkages
Prostate hypertrophy, 27
Psychology
    clinical research in, 265–278
    training, 142

R

R01 grants, 72
    award size, 76
    distribution of, 84–95
    duration of, 74–76
    evaluation of, 39
    human research in, 5, 39, 185
Research design
    historical development, 25
    human studies, unique features of, 79–81
    obstacles in clinical studies, 55, 57
    resource demands, 5
    subject enrollment, 42
    third-party payers in, 116
    training in, 162–163, 167, 191–192
Research infrastructure
    in academic settings, 14–15, 60–61
    as career path incentive, 60
Residency review committees, 17, 164–165
Resources for Clinical Investigation, 30
Review of the National Institutes of Health Biomedical Research Training Programs, 176–177
Robert Wood Johnson Clinical Scholars Program, 189, 190
Role model or mentoring relationships, 4
    faculty responsibility and, 193
    good qualities in, 59
    institutional recognition of, 14
    postgraduate medical education, 168–169
    role of, 58–59
    in surgical careers, 291, 296
Rush Medical College, 146

S

Science fairs and competitions, 129
SEMATECH, 119–120, 205
Stanford University, 191
Surgical research
    barriers to, 287–290
    current status of, 281

Medical Scientist Training Program
and, 154
resource base, 284–287
strategies for improving, 281–283,
293–299
types of, 283–284

T

T32 awards, 10, 170, 171, 178
T35 grants, 151
Technology assessment, 21, 114–115
Technology development, 1–2, 23, 123
academic health centers in, 21
in academic research culture, 201
clinical research and, 2
in commercial research culture, 201–
202
commercialization of academic
research, 205–206
health care reform and, 110
intellectual property rights, 199
outcomes research and, 2, 21
regionalization of, 21
Technology transfer, 20
academic-industry collaboration, 20,
205
biotechnology, 199
federal initiatives, 198
training for, 28, 216
Third-party payers
clinical research and, 64, 112–114,
117–118, 121
concerns of, 114–116
data collection by, 116–117
in research design and data analysis,
116–117
support for academic health centers,
20–21
Training for research
in clinical psychology, 265–266, 269–
278
in dentistry, 124, 244–247
in Department of Veterans Affairs, 103
in dual-degree programs, 151–152

duration of, 4, 12, 42, 150, 161–163,
169–170, 183
effecting change in, 194–195
faculty needs, 193–194
federally supported non-NIH, 188–189
in General Clinical Research Centers,
97
goals of, 124–125
historical development, 43–44
importance of, 193–194
laboratory-based model, 57–58
laboratory experience, 150
in medical school, 123–124, 145–147,
151, 191–192
in Medical Scientist Training Program,
152–155
medical student interest in, 145, 147–
148
model programs, 10–11, 188, 190–192
NIH intramural programs in, 71
in nursing, 257–264
obstacles to, 125–126, 168–170
postdoctoral, 161–163, 170–176, 180–
184
postgraduate, 16, 160–170
primary and secondary school
preparation, 125, 126, 127–132
in private sector, 170–171
privately funded, 189–190
program evaluation, 10–11, 12, 17, 18,
176–180, 194
recommendations, 10–11
recruitment for, 176–177
research methodology, 162–163, 191–
192
residency review committee
requirements, 264–265
scientific ethics as element of, 155,
192
social demographic context, 125, 126–
127
specialty board certification and, 166–
167
status of, 4, 5
subsequent grant success and, 178,
182–184, 186
in surgery, 287–292, 298–299

technology transfer as element of, 216
trends, 28–29
undergraduate student preparation,
132–142
Tufts University, 56

U

Undergraduate science preparation
criticisms of, 136–137
design of, 138–140
effectiveness of, 137–138
federal programs, 134–136
improvements in, 141–142
institutional efforts, 133
role of, 140–141
science majors, 132
University of California, 191
University of Kentucky, 133, 140

University of Michigan, 55, 190–191
University of Pennsylvania, 151
University of Puerto Rico, 140

V

Voluntary health agencies, 107

W

Washington University, 151
Women
in clinical psychology, 270, 275–276
in clinical research, 48–49
on medical school faculty, 46–48, 49–
50
physicians, 44–45, 48–49, 127, 143
in surgical science, 282–283, 289, 297
in undergraduate science, 136–137